# Clinical Assessment
## *of* Neuromusculoskeletal
## Disorders

# Clinical Assessment
## *of* Neuromusculoskeletal Disorders

### Gary M. Greenstein, D.C.

Assistant Professor of Clinical Sciences
University of Bridgeport College of Chiropractic
Bridgeport, Connecticut;
Postgraduate Faculty
Los Angeles College of Chiropractic
Whittier, California

with 26 clinical cases
and 164 illustrations

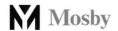 Mosby

St. Louis  Baltimore  Boston
Carlsbad  Chicago  Naples  New York  Philadelphia  Portland
London  Madrid  Mexico City  Singapore  Sydney  Tokyo  Toronto  Wiesbaden

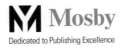

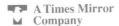

**Publisher:**  Don Ladig
**Executive Editor:**  Martha Sasser
**Developmental Editor:**  Kellie F. White
**Project Manager:**  Dana Peick
**Project Specialist:**  Catherine Albright
**Manufacturing Manager:**  Betty Richmond
**Designer:**  Amy Buxton

Printed in the United States of America
Composition by TCSystems, Inc.
Printing and binding by Maple-Vail, Binghampton

Mosby–Year Book, Inc.
11830 Westline Industrial Drive
St. Louis, Missouri 63146

**Library of Congress Cataloging-in-Publication Data**

Clinical assessment of neuromusculoskeletal disorders : with 26
   clinical cases / [edited by] Gary M. Greenstein.
        p.     cm.
     Includes bibliographical references and index.
     ISBN 0-8151-3948-9 (alk. paper)
     1. Musculoskeletal system—Diseases—Case studies.
   2. Neuromuscular diseases—Case studies.   I. Greenstein, Gary M.
     [DNLM:   1. Neuromuscular Diseases—problems.   2. Neuromuscular
   Diseases—case studies.   3. Chiropractic—problems.
   4. Chiropractic—case studies.     WE 18.2 C641 1997]
   RC925.5.C565     1997
   616.7—dc20
   DNLM/DLC
   for Library of Congress                                          96–19078
                                                                         CIP

96 97 98 99 00 / 9 8 7 6 5 4 3 2 1

# Contributors

**Cynthia Baum, D.C., D.A.C.B.R.**
Postgraduate Faculty,
Los Angeles College of
  Chiropractic,
Whittier, California;
Private Practice,
Canoga Park, California

**Raymond Brodeur, D.C., Ph.D.**
Assistant Professor,
Department of Biomechanics,
Michigan State University,
East Lansing, Michigan

**Bruce Carr, D.C., Ph.D.**
Associate Professor of Basic Science,
Department of Anatomy,
Los Angeles College of
  Chiropractic,
Whittier, California

**Jeffrey Cooley, D.C., D.A.C.B.R.**
Associate Professor of Clinical
  Science,
Department of Radiology,
Los Angeles College of
  Chiropractic,
Whittier, California

**Gregory Cramer, D.C., Ph.D.**
Associate Professor and
  Chairperson,
Department of Anatomy,
The National College of
  Chiropractic,
Lumbard, Illinois

**Darryl Curl, D.C., D.D.S.**
Associate Professor,
Department of Clinical Sciences,
Los Angeles College of
  Chiropractic,
Whittier, California

**J. Paul Ellis, M.S.(R.), Ph.D.
(candidate)**
Assistant Professor in Basic Science
  and Research Divisions;

Assistant Professor,
Department of Anatomy,
Logan Chiropractic College,
Chesterfield, Missouri

**Emile Goubran, M.D., Ph.D.**
Professor and Division Chairperson,
Department of Anatomy,
Los Angeles College of
  Chiropractic,
Whittier, California

**Gary M. Greenstein, D.C.**
Assistant Professor of Clinical
  Sciences,
University of Bridgeport College of
  Chiropractic,
Bridgeport, Connecticut

**Warren Hammer, D.C., M.S.,
D.A.B.C.O.**
Private Practice,
Norwalk, Connecticut

**Charles N.R. Henderson, D.C.,
Ph.D.**
Assistant Professor of Anatomy,
Palmer Chiropractic University,
Research Fellow,
Palmer Center for Chiropractic
  Research,
Davenport, Iowa

**Gary Lindquist, D.C., D.A.C.B.R.,
L.A.C.C.**
Postgraduate Faculty,
Los Angeles College of
  Chiropractic,
Whittier, California;
Private Practice,
Canoga Park, California

**Timothy Mick, D.C., D.A.C.B.R.**
Associate Professor and
  Chairperson of Radiology,
Northwestern College of
  Chiropractic,
Bloomington, Minnesota

**Jeddeo Paul, Ph.D.**
Professor of Basic Science,
University of Bridgeport College of
  Chiropractic,
Bridgeport, Connecticut

**Chae-Song Ro, M.D., Ph.D.**
Associate Professor,
Department of Anatomy,
The National College of
  Chiropractic,
Lombard, Illinois

**Edward Rothman, D.C.,
D.A.B.C.O.**
Private Practice,
Portland, Oregon

**Gary Schultz, D.C., D.A.C.B.R.**
Associate Professor and
  Chairperson of Radiology,
Los Angeles College of
  Chiropractic,
Whittier, California

**Dorrie Talmage, D.C., D.A.B.C.O.**
Assistant Professor,
Department of Clinical Sciences,
Los Angeles College of
  Chiropractic,
Whittier, California

**Gene Tobias, Ph.D.**
Professor,
Department of Anatomy,
Los Angeles College of
  Chiropractic,
Whittier, California

**Tuan Tran, D.C., Ph.D.**
Professor and Chairperson of
  Anatomy,
Los Angeles College of
  Chiropractic,
Whittier, California

v

# Foreword

The past three decades have seen major changes sweep across professional education. Although no specific individual or institution is credited with initiating dramatic educational reforms, McMaster University Medical School in Hamilton, Ontario is considered the birthplace for many reactive instructional strategies and curricular innovations. Also notable are the efforts at Harvard Medical School to develop a problem-based curriculum that has been highly acclaimed. Many authorities in the field of professional education also point to the 1984 General Professional Education of the Physician (GPEP) report "Physicians for the Twenty-First Century," which outlined important considerations for medical school curricula in preparation for education of clinicians into the next century. Before publication of this report, many leading educators had been experimenting and perfecting innovative instructional strategies that were directed toward active learning. This approach was in contrast to the normal passive learning mode that focused upon the instructor as the "wellspring of all knowledge" and forced students to sit passively through endless lectures.

Notable among these innovative teachers is Howard Barrows, a medical educator from Southern Illinois University. He and his team of educators refined the process of what is now known as problem-based learning. Although this term is used for a variety of instructional strategies today, its main theme is the use of problems as the central teaching strategy. Thus, in the context of professional education, clinical problems form the core of the instructional strategy. There is particular value in this approach because it integrates basic science facts with clinical decision making.

This activity may take many forms depending upon the instructional strategy selected. Should self-directed learning be an objective of the exercise, a small-group tutorial has been recommended as the desired setting.

In the small-group tutorial the focus of learning is on the student, with the clinical case being the instrument to guide the learning and the faculty member the facilitator of learning. Several hundreds of articles have been written about problem-based learning and the variations that are being developed. This book is a representation of the refinement and further innovative approaches to problem-based learning.

Active learning strategies have been used not only within individual courses to modify or enhance the learning process, but they have also altered the course of entire curricula within various professions and have thus dramatically influenced students, faculty, and institutions. In all cases, specific outcomes should be established that will guide the development and implementation of the instructional strategy. Several key outcomes have been noted for problem-based instructional modules, which have been developed and implemented in many professional institutions. These outcomes may be utilized as guideposts for further instructional strategies designed to enhance the education of professionals in a variety of settings.

## DEVELOP STUDENTS AS SELF-DIRECTED LEARNERS

This rather obvious outcome often does not receive adequate attention when problem-based instructional programs are designed in self-directed learning, the instructional emphasis shifts from the regular classroom activities of case-based learning to the library or learning resource center. Students who utilize the library as a repository of informational resources must be able to easily access information beyond the books and periodicals on the shelves. Attention must be paid to the acquisition of informational databases and CD-ROM discs and these resources should be made easily accessible to large groups of students.

Developing self-directed learners also requires a retooling of faculty and their approaches to teaching. With the lecture diminishing in importance and the addition of small-group discussions, faculty are experiencing a dramatic shift in their jobs. This requires institutions to invest in the development of resources that will provide faculty with the necessary information and assistance to tackle new tasks.

## ENHANCE COMMUNICATION SKILLS OF STUDENTS

Students enrolled in professional programs will be caring for and interactive with the public. The appalling fact is that the current professional educational system provides little direction or assistance in communication. The small-group tutorial places students in an environment in which communication skills must be utilized effectively. A major role of the faculty facilitator is to encourage the participation of all students in the discussion. During the second group session each student must make a formal presentation of a specific assignment to the rest of the members; thus, each student assumes a teaching role. This skill is also enhanced through a variety of other instructional strategies, most notably the clinical case presentation utilized in both pre-clinical and clinical settings. These instructional strategies thus provide opportunities to develop and enhance the communication skills that today's professionals must have to interact with the public, the profession, and associated health-care professionals.

## LOWER THE BARRIERS BETWEEN FACULTY AND STUDENTS

For centuries faculty have hidden behind the podium in the lecture hall. This effective barrier kept students "at bay" and provided the faculty member with a sense of revered isolation. Problem-based learning strategies greatly cut down this isolationist approach to teaching. Small-group tutorials normally have a faculty/student ratio of 1 : 10, which considerably increases the contact with students. Because the tutorial is also less formal than a lecture, there is considerably more interaction, which is often missing in the mainstream of higher education. Student and faculty satisfaction ratings of this outcome have been extremely high. The setting of the tutorial actually leads to greater communication, not only during the activity, but also throughout the program and student opinon surveys report faculty as being more accessible. Thus professional education (a stressful experience to say the least) is infused with some humaneness and caring, both qualities that are highly desirable in the health-care arena.

## DEVELOP PROBLEM-SOLVING SKILLS

Professional educators generally agree that improving student's problem-solving skills will enhance their clinical decision-making ability. Problem-solving skills are best honed where the students are dealing with a real or simulated clinical case. A variety of instructional strategies utilize the problem-solving approach. The paper case that is patterned within this book attempts to simulate the doctor-patient interaction through the use of information directly related to patient outcomes. This places the student in a learning environment that simulates the clinical workplace. Through the logical sequence of following a case from the initial presentation through the treatment regimen, the student begins to recognize the process of gathering data, interpreting that data, considering hypotheses, testing those hypotheses, and ultimately, arriving at a working diagnosis. These are all steps that mimic the thought process of any health-care provider. By emphasizing this approach on numerous occasions, the student begins to develop clinical judgement. Thus, the critical thinking process used in problem solving can become an integral aspect of learning during the earliest stages of a student's professional education.

## ENHANCE APPLICATION OF BASIC SCIENCE KNOWLEDGE

Perhaps the complaints heard most frequently by any dean at a professional school are those related to the lack of clinical application of basic science information. Many faculty are comfortable within the confines of their disciplines and for reasons both personal and academic, have been reluctant to allow clinical application into their classrooms. The fact, however, is, and this has been confirmed by educators, that the basic science knowledge within a discipline is actually better understood when it is applied to a clinical setting.

In a problem-based curriculum, students continually comment on how real and applicable the basic science information becomes once it is taught within the context of a clinical case. The many cases represented within this book emphasize this concept. However, many other disciplines within the curriculum such as biochemistry, neuroscience, and human physiology also utilize this method to enhance learning, and all have created clinical cases such as these as a primary instructional method to apply basic facts and concepts. Student satisfaction with this approach is high and faculty have broadened their scope of instructional design and added to their own clinical knowledge.

## RETAIN COGNITIVE KNOWLEDGE

Faculty may initially be concerned that students will not be able to learn pertinent facts and concepts outside the context of a lecture. Some administrators have also voiced concern that students will not be able to pass nationally standardized tests that emphasize cognitive recall if the learning process has focused on problem solving. These concerns have been dispelled by the experience of the many who have embraced the problem-centered approach to professional education. Several noted medical schools and at least one chiropractic college have observed that student scores on these nationally standardized tests have either improved or remained about the same. In several instances student testimony indicates that they were better prepared to answer some questions because they recalled the clinical case in which the information was presented. If scores are the same or better, student satisfaction higher, and faculty growth and development blooming, there should be no reason for an institution to turn its back on problem-based instructional strategies. Perhaps entropy has truly taken over the educational enterprise!

## CONCLUSION

This book represents more than a compilation of selected cases. It proposes an integration of facts and concepts that transcend the barriers of academic and clinical disciplines. The chapters are arranged by anatomic region with appropriate cases representative of associated problems. However, the information contained within each case broadens the reader's perception beyond simple anatomic and physiologic concepts. The authors provide a complete review of the structure and function of the region, as well as an exhaustive description of the diagnostic regimens that should be considered. A few patient management issues are addressed that are directly relevant to the case. Thus, the text leads the reader beyond the simple sleuthing of a diagnostician and through a thorough discussion of the key scientific issues that should be comprehended.

The many authors who have given so much of themselves to produce this book should not only be applauded for their efforts but hailed as pioneers within the professional educational community. They have trodden a difficult path that has often led to increased work and frustration. Yet they have been dedicated to the task of enhancing the learning process beyond their specific disciplines. These faculty have learned much about the educational process through teamwork, which emphasizes the importance of both process and product. They are educators in the truest sense, having exceeded the boundaries of their own education to provide students with learning opportunities that will benefit them in all aspects of their clinical practice. Many have devoted themselves to excellence, a quality that is often heralded, yet seldom observed. Even the casual observer of this text will note the educational benefit that is offered to both faculty and students. This is not just a fad. Utilizing problem-based instructional strategies will enrich the lives of all those who participate, faculty and student alike. My highest regards go to all who enter this gateway to learning and tread the paths of educational excellence.

*The wise man must remember that while he is a descendent of the past, he is a parent of the future.*

Herbert Spencer

*Gary A. Miller, Ph.D.*
Dean of Academic Affairs
Los Angeles College of Chiropractic,
Vice Provost
Biola University

# Preface

The educational process of the health professional who treats and educates patients with neuromusculoskeletal (NMS) problems is undergoing a revolution. Education has switched from daily 8-hour lectures to a more thought-provoking atmosphere in which students are allowed to explore the literature and to come up with their own answers. This text is designed to help the educator achieve this goal of problem case–based education. To the practitioner who treats NMS patients this text provides challenges to explore alternative treatments and to develop treatment and management protocols.

The purpose of this text is to

- bring to the forefront basic science explanations of the NMS system, its function, and treatment and management application to the patient
- facilitate discussion on treatment and management protocols for the patient with NMS problems
- encourage new avenues of investigation by the reader and researcher in the field of conservative care of the NMS system
- assist the educator, either undergraduate or postgraduate, to develop a new way of teaching by thought-provoking case-based presentations.

The text achieves the first goal by applying up-to-date information on the basic science of the NMS system and its relevance to diagnosis. The first section of this text presents 26 cases that come from clinicians' offices. Each case presentation has case objectives that provoke readers to increase their understanding of the patient's problem. Each case asks readers to develop and justify patient protocols.

The remaining chapters answer the case objectives. There is a suggested reading list of selected articles and texts that will help the reader investigate the case objectives at the end of each chapter. The treatment and management chapter (Chapter 7) ties basic science with a general treatment protocol of the patient with an NMS problem. A Glossary of terms assists the reader in understanding medical and scientific terminology. The glossary attempts to increase communication and understanding amongst the different professions that treat NMS problems.

The second goal is achieved by the case objectives. The reader is asked to develop a treatment and management protocol and to discuss cotreatment and referral of the patient. In many of the cases, referral pain occurs from other anatomic structures (for example, the liver) and the patient must be referred to another clinician. This text will facilitate discussion between the student and clinician regarding what is best for the patient.

The third goal is to encourage the reader to investigate new and innovative treatments in the conservative care of patients with NMS problems. In Chapter 7 a treatment and management protocol is developed that, hopefully, will provoke the reader to further investigate the function of the musculoskeletal system and how to assist it in proper healing.

The text is arranged to assist the educator to teach students with a new flavor and appreciation for the NMS system. By presenting cases that are from field practitioners, there is a new sharing of information that helps the "dry" material of basic science come alive and become intriguing to the student.

The combination of basic science theory and clinical case presentations will hopefully lead to better treatment and management protocols. The development of more comprehensive treatment and management protocols leads to a better understanding and cooperation among the different disciplines that treat NMS problems because the ultimate goal is to do what is best for the patient.

*Gary M. Greenstein*

# Introduction

Welcome to the world of problem case–based learning. In the first chapter, 26 clinical cases are presented that are from clinician's offices. These cases are presented in narrative form with provocative questions (case objectives) that "tickle the reader's inquisitiveness." Following each narrative are case objectives and questions that are case problems that help the reader tie together basic science principles and clinical case presentations. The goal of this text is to help the reader learn basic science material needed to answer clinical presentations that lead to more accurate diagnoses and treatment and management protocols of neuromusculoskeletal disease. The text is arranged so that in the first chapter the reader is exposed to the cases and the case objectives and questions. The following chapters present material that will help the reader answer the case objectives and questions. In a subject of this magnitude not all the answers can be given in one text. At the end of each chapter there is a reference and suggested reading list that will help the reader answer the case objectives in more detail. There are six chapters that follow the cases. Chapter 2 deals with the neuroscience of the neuromusculoskeletal system; the three chapters that follow are regionally divided—head and neck, spine, and extremities. Chapter 6 discusses gait, and Chapter 7 focuses on treatment and management protocols. The text ends with a glossary of terms to assist the reader with common scientific and medical terminology used in neuromusculoskeletal science. The authors hope that the experience of problem case–based learning is enjoyed by all readers, regardless of whether they are in the first year of education or are practicing clinicians.

# Acknowledgments

Special thanks is offered to the people who guided me through the roads of my education and who taught me the value of seeking knowledge: Dr. Manohar Panjabi, Joanne Duranceau, and Donald Summers. They inspired and guided me during my education at Yale University. Without them this text would have been only a dream.

Special thanks also goes to President Reed Phillips, Vice-President Alan Adams, and Academic Dean Gary Miller at the Los Angeles College of Chiropractic. Their determination to promote higher education and initiate problem-based learning at the college was a rewarding and fulfilling experience that led to the writing of this text. Gratitude is also due to Nehmat Sabb and Shoreh Saljooghi for their librarian expertise.

Without the assistance and support of the following instructors and students at the University of Bridgeport College of Chiropractic and at the Los Angeles College of Chiropractic, this text would not have come to fruition. The editor would like to thank Dr. Debra Burns, Dr. Rose Galiger, Dr. Stephen Perle, Dr. Terence Perrault, Dr. John Hsieh, Dr. Jeffery Berube, Dr. Phillip Merker, and Mr. Clark Danielson for their constructive comments on the manuscript as it was being written. Sincere gratitude is expressed to the clinicians who contributed cases used in this text: Drs. Bruce Carr, Darryl Curl, Emile Goubran, Warren Hammer, Nicholas Palmieri, Michael Reife, John Scaringe, Gene Tobias, Alfred Traina, and Michael Yoel.

Further gratitude is expressed to the people at Mosby: Martha Sasser for her guidance, Amy Dubin for her assistance, and especially Kellie White for her perseverance and confidence in this project. A special thanks is also offered to Sarah Crenshaw McQueen for her exceptional abilities as medical illustrator.

Dr. Tim Mick wishes to thank Arne Krogsveen and Corneil Blatz for their assistance in preparing the radiographs appearing in his section on the radiology of the upper extremity.

# Contents

# CHAPTER 1

# The cases

Hector M. is a 29-year-old man who complains of muscle weakness in both arms and blurred vision. He states that the blurred vision began 2 days previously and that he is currently experiencing weakness in both arms, which seems to be worsening. He is not in pain and does not recall any injury that preceded these problems. He states that 3 days previously he had used an organophosphate insecticide on the crops of his family farm. Hector has not had any previous health problems and describes himself as a hearty eater and a hard worker. He claims that he usually has the strength to keep working on the farm from dawn to dusk, 6 days a week. He is accustomed to having three well-balanced meals a day. He does not smoke but occasionally drinks beer on hot days or after a soccer match. He plays club soccer in a local men's league on weekends with his brothers and friends.

An examination of Hector's medical history does not reveal any previous illnesses, vaccinations, or injections that would cause the symptoms. He takes no medications other than aspirin occasionally for minor aches and pains.

Hector M.'s family history reveals that his parents and grandparents are living and are in good health. His brothers are healthy and do not have complaints similar to Hector's.

• What could be happening to Hector?

### *Examination*
Vital signs.
    Blood pressure: 126/86 mm Hg
    Pulse rate: 74 beats/min
    Repiration rate: 13 breaths/min
    Temperature: 98.4° F
    Height: 5'8''
    Weight: 155 lbs
The patient looks tan and athletic, but when seated, his posture is slumped. The patient has muscle weakness in both arms and shoulders. The passive range of motion of the joints of the upper extremity is normal. Both eyes exhibit ptosis. His breathing appears to be labored, and he has difficulty speaking.

The upper extremity muscle strength scores are +4 (on a 5-point scale) and are bilaterally symmetric. There is no sensory loss and the deep tendon reflexes (DTRs) have a score of +2 and are bilaterally symmetric. Tromner's reflex is absent, Adson's, Allen's and Tinel's tests are normal, the pupils are dilated and unresponsive to light, and there are no significant findings on static or motion palpation.

Laboratory blood analysis reveals a normal complete blood count and normal levels of (CBC), serum albumin, $K^+$, $Ca^{+2}$, creatine kinase, and thyroid hormone. The Tensilon test is positive. Nerve conduction velocity (NCV) is within normal limits, but the electromyogram (EMG) is abnormal, revealing a decrease in muscle electric activity with eventual disappearance of activity on the EMG during continuous voluntary muscle contraction. Muscle-evoked response reveals repetitive nerve stimulation to show a gradual reduction in the muscle response.

• How does this information add to the determination of what is happening to Hector?

### Case OBJECTIVES
1. Explain the neuroanatomy of the peripheral nerve and the physiologic events that occur in the transmission of a nerve impulse.
2. Describe the neuroanatomy of the synaptic junction.
3. Describe the biochemical reaction for the synthesis and degradation of the neurotransmitter at the neuromuscular junction.
4. Describe and explain the events that occur during synaptic transmission at the neuromuscular junction. What is a Tensilon test? How does it relate to the neuromuscular junction?
5. Describe the facilitative and inhibitory neurotransmitters of the central nervous system (CNS) and peripheral nervous system (PNS).
6. Describe muscle histology and physiology of striated muscle. How does this information relate to the case?
7. Explain the effects of myasthenia gravis (MG) on synaptic transmission at the neuromuscular junction.
8. Describe and discuss the findings in the history, physical examination, and special studies that are unique to myasthenia gravis.
9. Differentiate myasthenia gravis (mg) from Lambert-Eaton syndrome. What are the similarities and differences in the history and physical examination findings?
10. List the differential diagnoses. Compare and contrast these diseases.
11. Describe a treatment and management protocol for the working diagnosis. Educate the patient about his or her disease. To which medical specialist would this patient be referred? What are the immediate, intermediate, and long-term goals for this patient?

**CASE 2**

Patricia P., a 34-year-old housewife, reports to your office complaining of lower back pain, weakness in both legs, and overall fatigue. Pat reports that her lower back pain began about 2 weeks previously and describes the pain as a constant, dull ache that is limited to her lower back. She recalls no trauma preceding the onset of pain. Pain is constant. She is annoyed with the pain and feels as though she is growing prematurely old. Nothing alleviates the pain: she has tried changing posture, hot baths, and sleeping with more or fewer pillows. Her weakness and fatigue have been "coming on" for the previous 6 months or more. Her right leg, especially, feels weak and "funny" if she walks or stands for prolonged periods. The weakness in her left leg comes and goes. She also states that her right hand feels weak. Overall, she doesn't seem to have the energy she used to have. She is sleeping 10 hours almost every night, however she is still feeling tired. By early evening she just wants to go to bed; sometimes she feels dizzy and has trouble reading in the afternoon or evening. She says, "I saw my eye doctor last week and told her I am having trouble focussing and that I am seeing double sometimes; she gave me new contacts and said my prescription has actually improved."

A review of Pat's systems does not reveal any changes in bowel habits or urination. She does not complain of any sudden weight loss or gain and her health has been generally good until the onset of the problems described. She has not had any recent vaccinations or illnesses. She does not smoke, drinks socially, eats a "well-balanced" diet, exercises little, and takes no other medications. She works part-time in a business with her uncle.

Pat is married and has two children (a 6-year-old boy and a 2-year-old girl). There is no family history of cancer, diabetes, or high blood pressure; her father is deceased (he died of a heart attack). Her mother is 73 years old and in good health. She has no siblings.

• What could be happening to Pat?

### Examination
Vital signs.

  Blood pressure: 125/84 mm Hg
  Pulse rate: 70 beats/min
  Respiration rate: 15 breaths/min
  Temperature: 98.6° F
  Height: 5'5''
  Weight: 122 lb

General inspection reveals a healthy-looking, moderately overweight, middle-aged, adult female. Examination of the eyes, ears, nose, and throat is unremarkable. The lymph nodes are not palpable and the abdomen is supple with no indication of pathology. Inspection of the spine reveals no redness, swellings, or discolorations of the skin or surrounding tissues. It is noted that as Pat walks, her right lower extremity is slightly ataxic.

Palpation of the spine reveals bilateral paraspinal musculature tightness.

### Range of motion
Range of motion (ROM) of the spine is within normal limits; however, on active and passive flexion in the lumbar spine, there is mild aching pain at the end of the range. Active range of motion of the lower extremities, especially on the right side, is very difficult to evaluate because the patient is not able to control her movements sufficiently.

### Orthopedic examination
The straight leg raise is negative, Lhermittes sign is positive, and passive motion is not easy because the patient has diffi-

culty relaxing the musculature to allow motion. Left leg motion is easier.

### Muscle testing
The patient has difficulty controlling muscle action. The hand grasp is within normal limits, but thumb opposition is not easily accomplished in the right hand. Mild muscle spasticity is noted in the right knee, ankle, and foot.

### Neurologic examination

| Deep tendon reflex level | left | right |
|---|---|---|
| C5 | +2 | +2 |
| C6 | +2 | +2 |
| C7 | +2 | +3 |
| L4 | +3 | +3 |
| S1 | +3 | +4 |

*Scale 0 to +4*

There is some loss of sensation (pinwheel, sharp and dull) over the right leg and foot, whereas all other limbs have normal sensation; stereognosis and graphesthesia are within normal limits. Dysdiadochokinesia, point-to-hand test, and finger-to-nose test can be performed, but ataxic motions are noted with the eyes open or closed. Romberg's test shows that the patient has trouble keeping her balance, both with eyes open and with eyes closed. The heel-to-shin test is difficult for the patient to perform and Babinski's reflex is not present. Tests for cranial nerve functions are all within normal limits.

### Radiologic examination
An x-ray examination is deferred at this time.

### Laboratory examination
The CBC and urinalysis (UA) are normal, with no indication of anemia or infection. The erythrocyte sedimentation rate (ESR) and thyroid panel values are within normal limits.

### Special tests
Spinal tap: increased cerebrospinal fluid (CSF) protein is detected.

Magnetic resonance imaging (MRI): several sites of increased signal density in the brain white matter are located in the area of the precentral gyrus and frontal lobe bilaterally. Somatosensory evoked potentials (SSEP) and visual and auditory evoked potentials are both abnormal.

• How does this information contribute to the understanding of Pat's symptoms?

### Case OBJECTIVES

1. Describe the neuroanatomy of the brain and spinal cord that is relevant to this case.
2. Describe the neuroanatomy of the tracts needed for sensation and motor activity in the brain and spinal cord and discuss the relevance of this information to the case.
3. Explain the anatomic and physiologic bases of hyper-reflexic myotactic reflexes and pathologic reflexes.
4. Explain the neuroscience for the clinical tests used to evaluate the function of the CNS.
5. Differentiate the clinical findings in an upper motor neu-

ron lesion (UMNL) and a lower motor neuron lesion (LMNL). Define the common terminology used to describe a UMNL and a LMNL.

6. Discuss the pathologic changes that occur to the neurologic system in a patient with multiple sclerosis (MS).

7. Differentiate the objective findings in MS and amyotrophic lateral sclerosis (ALS). Educate the patient about MS.

8. List the differential diagnoses. Compare and contrast these diseases.

9. Educate the patient about the working diagnosis. Explain the role of the physiatrist and the physical therapist in treating this patient's illness. What are the immediate, intermediate, and long-term goals for this patient?

10. Explain the difference between reactivation and rehabilitation. Which therapy does this patient need? What is proprioceptive neuromuscular facilitation (PNF) and how will it benefit this patient?

## CASE 3

George E., a 26-year-old paramedic, comes to your office complaining of paralysis of the right side of his face. He had been to the emergency room the previous evening and was told he has Bell's palsy. He was given prednisone (40 mg daily) and advised that the condition would likely resolve within 5 to 7 days.

His problem began the previous day after he awoke from a nap. He initially attributed it to a lack of sleep but became concerned when he noted difficulty with speech. He reports being unable to close his right eye, frown, or move his forehead and is drooling when he tries to talk, but he is in no pain. He denies any recent infections, tick bites, dental work, or trauma. No other complaints or problems are present.

His family history and medical history are unremarkable. He completed the vaccination series for hepatitis B about 4 months earlier. He denies taking any prescribed medications.

• What could be happening to George?
• What physical examination procedures would you deem necessary to diagnose George's condition?

### Examination
Vital signs.
    Blood pressure: 126/78 mm Hg
    Pulse rate: 72 beats/min
    Repiration rate: 14 breaths/min
    Temperature: 98.6° F
    Height: 5'8''
    Weight: 170 lb
On inspection, George's face reveals flaccidity on the right side. There are no masses, hematomas, or ulcerations. His skin is supple, and no dermatologic abnormalities are noted. Lymphadenopathy is not present. The eyes, ears, nose, and throat are normal. Palpation does not reveal any muscle splinting or unusual masses. His thyroid, parotid, and mandibular glands are supple. The thyroid gland moves appropriately when George is asked to swallow, and there are no lymph node enlargements. Examination of his facial expressions reveals complete paralysis of the right side of the face, with inability to close his eye, lift his eyelid, smile, or pucker his lips.

### Range of motion
The range of motion of the cervical spine is within normal limits. Motion restrictions are noted on the right occiput—cervical vertebral 1 (C1), right rotation at C1 to C2, and left lateral bending at C4 to C5. Muscle activity on the right side of the face does not change as active and passive motion of the cervical spine is tested.

### Orthopedic and neurologic examinations
All orthopedic and muscle tests of the cervical spine are within normal limits. George's test is unremarkable. The examination of the cranial nerves (CNs) is within normal limits except for CN VII. The score for muscles of facial expression is 0 on the right side (a score of +5 is considered normal). The patient cannot pucker, blow, furrow his forehead, or blink his right eye. A nonresponsive Chovstek's test is obtained over the right temporomandibular joint. George has lost the sense of taste on the anterior two thirds of his tongue. The DTRs of the upper extremities have a score of +2 and are bilaterally symmetric.

### Radiologic and laboratory examinations
X-ray films of the skull and neck do not reveal any masses, fractures, or other pathology. A CBC, UA, and ESR are within normal limits.

• How does this information help in the determination of what is wrong with George?
• How does the anatomy of the cranial nerves help explain George's facial movement?

### Case OBJECTIVES

1. Describe the neuroanatomy of the sensory and motor systems related to this case. Include upper motor and lower motor neuron innervation.

2. Describe the neuroanatomy of CN V and CN VII and their innervations. Describe Chovstek's test and its relationship to CN VII.

3. Describe the correlation between a nerve impulse and a striated muscle contraction.

5. Relate the objective clinical findings to neuroanatomy of CN VII.

6. Describe the objective neurologic tests used by the clinician to determine the location of the lesion.

7. List the differential diagnoses. Differentiate the objective facial findings in Bell's palsy from that of a cerebral vascular accident (CVA) and transient ischemic attack (TIA).

8. Describe the treatment and management protocol for this patient. Is this patient a candidate for adjustment or manipulation? If so, why? What is the protocol for further evaluation if the patient's condition does not improve in a given period of time? Would you refer this patient? If so, to whom?

9. Describe the immediate, intermediate, and long-term goals for this patient.

## CASE 4

Lou M., a 72-year-old man, is seen at your office with a complaint of left sided lower back pain. He had a cerebral vascular accident (CVA) 3 years previously and now has trouble communicating. The stroke has affected the right side of

Lou's upper and lower extremities and face. His right upper extremity displays a flexion pattern, and there is an extensor thrust of the right lower extremity.

His wife states that the lower back pain began 2 weeks previously "for no apparent reason." She states that his back pain is a dull ache that is relieved after a back rub at night. She mentions that although he is unable to sit for a long period of time, he has not complained of pain going down either leg. Lou seems to have an increase in pain toward the end of the day and sometimes needs to lie down and rest. His only medication is a daily aspirin. He has not had bowel or bladder problems.

Lou's medical history reveals that his CVA was caused by an embolus. During his 2-month hospitalization, he received physical therapy for 4 weeks. His condition has not improved over the years. Before the CVA he was in apparent good health. His family history reveals that his father died of a stroke at the age of 88, and his mother died of hypertension at the age of 80. His wife is 70 years old and healthy. His two sons (aged 37 and 34) are both in good health.

- What could be happening to Lou?

### Examination

Vital signs.
    Blood pressure: 130/84 mm Hg
    Pulse rate: 73 beats/min
    Respiration rate: 13 breaths/min
    Temperature: 98.4° F
    Height: 5'3"
    Weight: 160 lb

Inspection of the patient reveals paralysis of the right side of the face. Flaccid paralysis below his right eye involves the cheek and mouth. He cannot smile or frown but can wrinkle his forehead and blink his eye. He can protrude his tongue without deviation. His right upper extremity is adducted at the shoulder, but flexed and supinated at the elbow. His wrist is flexed and his hand is in a fist. The muscles of the upper extremity are spastic and display the clasp-knife phenomenon when stretched. In the seated position, Lou has trouble bending his right knee, and his right foot is inverted and plantar-flexed. Point tenderness and spasm are noted in the erector muscle of the spine in the left lumbar spine area.

Analysis of Lou's gait reveals an extensor thrust of the right lower extremity. While standing stationary, he adjusts most of his weight on the left side. Plumb-line evaluation reveals an increase in lumbar lordosis and a left lateral sway. A spinal curvature with the apex at T10 on the right is noted. The pelvis is level, the right shoulder is higher than the left, and the head is laterally bent to the right.

### Range of motion

The patient attempts range of motion of the lumbar spine but is unable to accomplish it because he has difficulty maintaining balance. In the seated position the patient is able to touch his toes, bend laterally, and rotate at the waist. The pain is reproduced on flexion of the lumbar spine at the end of the range and on extension.

### Orthopedic examination

Provocative tests are negative for straight leg raise (SLR), Becterew's test, and Valsalva's maneuver.

### Neurologic examination

Sensory evaluation reveals no paresthesias or dysesthesias in the lower extremities. Reflexes are +4 on the right and +2 on the left in the upper and lower extremities. Babinski's reflex is present on the right side but not on the left. Muscle testing cannot be performed on the involved side. Muscle strength on the left side is normal; however, the patient has difficulty following instructions.

### Radiologic examination:

An x-ray examination of this patient's lower back is deferred at this time.

- How does this information help determine what is wrong with Lou?

### Case OBJECTIVES

1. Describe the neuroanatomy of the brain and spinal cord that explains the patient's symptoms.
2. Describe the vasculature of the brain and spinal cord and how it relates to this case.
3. Describe the neuroanatomy of speech and present the relevance to this case.
4. Describe the differences between an UMNL and a LMNL.
5. Define ataxia, athetosis, spasticity, and rigidity. What neuroanatomic structures cause these findings?
6. Describe the neuroanatomic structures that exist in the precentral gyrus, the basal ganglia, and the cerebellum of the brain.
7. Describe the relationship between the precentral gyrus, the basal ganglia, and the cerebellum during human motion.
8. Describe and rationalize a treatment and management program for this patient. Would you adjust or manipulate this patient? If so, how? What are the goals for electric stimulation and moist heat packs? What are proprioceptive neuromuscular facilitation (PNF) exercises?

### CASE 5

John F., a 66-year-old man, comes to your office with the complaint of right-hand weakness and difficulty in movement. He states that this problem began 1 year previously for no apparent reason. The hand symptoms have progressively worsened, a hand tremor (4 to 5 tremors per second) is now noted at rest, and John is having problems with his other extremities also. Although he has no pain, he states that his muscles feel hard, and that, at times, it is difficult to flex and extend his knees and elbows. Movement of the extremities is stiff and it is hard for John to walk. He appears to have a shuffling (festinating) type of gait. The tremor in the right hand is present only when the hand is at rest, not when it is in motion. No position seems to relieve his symptoms. The stiffness and difficulty with movement are increasing with time. He does not have problems with bowel or bladder functions, nor with hearing, speaking, or seeing.

John's medical history is unremarkable, with the usual vaccinations and childhood diseases but there is nothing that can account for the present symptoms.

His family history reveals that he is an only child and that both parents died in their 90s of unknown illnesses. His wife is healthy and they have four children who are all in good health.

- What could be happening to John?

### Examination

Vital signs.
    Blood pressure: 134/88 mm Hg
    Pulse rate: 78 beats/min
    Respiration rate: 15 breaths/min
    Temperature: 98.6° F
    Height: 6'2"
    Weight: 163 lb

Mr. F is a healthy looking man who appears to be alert and well-oriented. He performs appropriately on knowledge and memory function tests, being able to recite the names of the last five presidents and count backward by threes. His knowledge of world events is substantial, and there does not appear to be any memory deficit. He is lacking in facial expressions.

Examination of the eyes, ears, nose, and throat is unremarkable. The cranial nerve examination is within normal limits and corneal, Chvostek's, direct, and consensual light reflexes are intact.

### Range of motion

A range-of-motion test of the extremities reveals muscle spasticity of the right wrist and elbow flexors and extensors. John has trouble moving his right wrist and elbow throughout their ranges. Mild bilateral spasticity and rigidity of the quadriceps and gastrocnemus muscles are also noted. Motion does not cause pain.

### Orthopedic examination

Orthopedic tests are deferred at this time.

### Neurologic examination

Neurologic examinations reveals that responses to light touch, pain, and vibration are within normal limits and that the pathologic reflexes are not present. Superficial reflexes are present with no deviations. Muscle strength tests reveal weakness of the flexors and extensors of the right wrist, and the right hand grasp is significantly weaker than the left hand grasp. Graphesthesia, stereognosis, and two-point discrimination are within normal limits. Romberg's test reveals mild swaying, and the patient seems to lean forward more than is usual. The finger-to-finger and finger-to-nose tests are within normal limits.

### Radiologic examination

An x-ray examination is deferred at this time.

### Laboratory examination

A CBC, UA, and creatine phosphokinase (CPK) are all within normal limits.

- From the information provided above what could be happening to John?

### Case OBJECTIVES

1. Identify the structures of the CNS associated with motor activity.
2. Describe the neuroanatomy of the basal ganglia.
3. Describe the interrelationships of the cerebral cortex, basal ganglia, and cerebellum during human motion.
4. Define spasticity, tremor, athetosis, ataxia, chorea, and ballism.
5. Describe the different tremors and how they relate to this case.
6. Explain the anatomic and physiologic basis of hyperreflexia, myotactic reflexes, and pathologic reflexes.
7. Classify the different types of nerve and muscle abnormalities.
8. Describe the differences between the history and physical examination in myasthenia gravis (Case 1), multiple sclerosis (Case 2), cerebral vascular accident (Case 3), and Parkinson's disease (Case 4).
9. Develop a list of differential diagnoses. Compare and contrast these diseases.
10. Describe the treatment and management of Parkinson's disease. What are the immediate, intermediate, and long-term goals for this patient? Educate the patient about his condition. What part of the basal ganglia is involved in this disease? What are the different signs and symptoms a patient would have if different parts of the basal ganglia have lesions?

### CASE 6

Dorothy M., a 23-year-old woman, is seen in your office with the complaint of a severe headache. She walks into your office with a protected type of posture. She is supporting her head with her right hand, appears pale, and is wearing sunglasses. Her gait has a resemblance to "walking on egg shells." She describes the headache as a severe throbbing type of pain that has been present for the past 2 hours. She states that her headaches occur twice monthly.

Her first symptom was a stiff neck that has progressed to a deep, throbbing pain located in the right temporal region of her head. She can recognize the onset of a headache because her eyes become very sensitive to bright lights, and she sees halos around objects. Her stomach is always upset when these headaches develop and, on occasion, vomiting occurs. These headaches have been present since she was 17 years old but Dorothy does not recall how they started. Migraine was diagnosed by her family clinician and she was treated with an ergotamine (Cafergot), which gives her relief but makes her very drowsy. She rates the headache pain as an 8 on a 0 to 10 scale (10 being the pain score for a miscarriage).

Dorothy gets relief from sleep or by lying in a comfortable position without moving her neck. Psychologic stress seems to play a minor role in her headache presentation. If she does not rest, the headache intensifies, and she "loses control" of her pain.

Dorothy's medical history is unremarkable. She has had the usual childhood diseases and has never been hospitalized. She does not take any other medications or vitamins.

She has two older brothers. Both are in good health and do not suffer from headaches. Both her parents (her mother is 64 years old and her father is 67 years old) are alive and in good health. Dorothy recalls her mother having headaches when she was younger but not after she reached menopause. Dorothy's husband is 26 years old and has no health complaints.

- What anatomic structures could be contributing to Dorothy's headache?
- What additional tests would you perform during the physical examination of this patient?

### Examination
Vital signs.
Blood pressure: 123/82 mm Hg
Pulse rate: 71 beats/min
Respiration rate: 13 breaths/min
Temperature: 97.3° F
Height 5'4"
Weight 128 lb

The patient is in acute distress. An observation of her face and neck reveals no obvious swellings or deviations. She appears pale and feels cool and clammy to touch. Examination of her eyes, ears, nose, and throat reveals normal findings. The lymph nodes and thyroid are normal on palpation. Point tenderness is located throughout the cervical spine. Trigger points are located bilaterally at the level of C2 to C4 in the posterior cervical musculature and refer pain to the right temporal area. Her posterior cervical musculature is very tight and feels boardlike. During palpation of the scalp the patient states that she is hypersensitive to touch. The patient also has cold hands at the time of examination.

### Range of motion
An evaluation of the active and passive ranges of motion of the cervical spine reveals a decrease in range on extension, right lateral bending, and left rotation with the exacerbation of the patient's complaints.

### Orthopedic examination
Orthopedic provocative tests do not indicate radiculopathy; however, the patient's complaints are exacerbated on cervical distraction.

### Muscle testing
The patient is unable to tolerate muscle testing of the head and neck because of the increase in pain and a feeling of nauseousness.

End-feel motion palpation evaluation reveals joint restrictions at C1 to C2 on right rotation (at 20 degrees) and restrictions at C3 to C7 on left lateral bending. George's test for vertebral artery compromise is negative.

### Neurologic examination
Sensory evaluation of light touch indicates slight hypersensitivity of the right upper extremity when compared to the left. Cranial-nerve function is within normal limits. Deep tendon reflexes for the upper extremity have a score of +2 and are symmetric. Pathologic reflexes are not present. Strength tests of the upper extremity are within normal limits.

### Radiologic examination
A three-view cervical spine radiographic series shows no indication of fracture or tumor. Bone density is normal and there is no indication of spondylolisthesis or spondylolysis. George's line is curvilinear with no noticeable defects.

- How does this information add to the determination of what is going on with Dorothy?

### Case OBJECTIVES
1. Define a cervicogenic headache.
2. Describe the neuroanatomy of the trigeminocervical nucleus.
3. Describe the neuroanatomy of the trigeminal nerve (CN V) and its role in this case.
4. Describe the embryology and neuroanatomy of referral pain. What referral patterns can appear in a patient with cervicogenic headache?
5. Describe the anatomy of the upper cervical spine and its role in this case.
6. Describe the anatomic structures that are tested by the provocative tests. What do these test results reveal about the cause of this patient's problem?
7. Describe the radiologic views for the cervical spine. What is George's line? What anatomic structures are being viewed on each x-ray film?
8. Describe the differences in the history and physical examination between a patient with a cervicogenic headache and a patient with a common or classical migraine headache.
9. Develop a list of differential diagnoses. Compare and contrast these diseases.
10. Describe the treatment and management protocols for this patient. What would be the immediate, intermediate, and long-term goals? Would you adjust this patient? Why and where?
11. Describe the physiologic therapeutic techniques that might be used in this case. What are the therapeutic goals of these techniques?

## CASE 7

Steven D., a 36-year-old construction worker, is seen at your office with the complaint of a right-sided headache and ear pain. He states that the pain is located in the right temporal and frontal areas of the head and along the anterior border of the ear. He adds that the pain has been present for the past 3 months and is getting worse. Steven describes the headache as a dull ache in the right temporal and frontal area and the ear pain, as a deep and diffuse ache. He rates his head and ear pain as a 7 on a 1 to 10 scale (10 being the score for the pain he felt when he fractured his femur about 5 years previously at work). The headaches are related to inadequate sleep or rest. He further adds that if he gets less than the 8 hours he requires in order to feel rested, he tends to feel fatigued, and this precipitates his headache and ear pain.

Steven describes other situations that can trigger or worsen his symptoms, in particular, stress on his job. He also adds that if he eats quickly or opens his mouth wide, the headache will occur. Additionally, he indicates that he is unable to chew hard food; and, chewing gum or hard food for prolonged periods of time causes his headache and ear pain to recur and worsen.

He does not recall any traumatic event that may have initiated his headache and ear pain, but he does remember being hit in the left jaw many years previously. And he states that since that time, he has had difficulty opening his mouth in a normal fashion. He mentions that he grinds his teeth but is unaware of how long he has been doing it.

Steve reports that he wore braces on his teeth between 13 and 17 years of age. He has noticed that his teeth are not as straight as they were when the braces were removed.

The patient states that he is otherwise healthy. His ears were recently examined and did not display any ear pathology. His family history is unremarkable.

- What could be happening to Steve?
- Which physical examination tests are dictated from Steven's history?

### *Examination*

Vital signs.

Blood pressure: 126/82 mm Hg
Pulse rate: 74 beats/min
Respiration rate: 14 breaths/min
Temperature: 98.4° F
Height: 5'8"
Weight: 225 lb

Inspection of the head and ear do not reveal any visual abnormalities. Palpation of the head and neck area reveals normal lymph nodes and a supple thyroid gland. Palpation of the area surrounding the right temporomandibular joint (TMJ) reveals some muscle tightness of the masseter muscle. Upon further palpation a trigger point in the masseter muscle is detected that causes pain in the temporofrontal region of the right side of the head as well as in the ear. Direct palpation of the left TMJ reveals an irregularity in the joint motion when the patient attempts to open his mouth. The right TMJ palpates normally and no irregular motions are detected. Palpation of the ear structure does not reveal pain or point tenderness.

Range of motion of the TMJ reveals that Steve cannot open his mouth to a normal full dimension. He can open his mouth only to about 43 mm (versus a normal dimension of 50 mm). When he does open his jaw a deviation to the left is noticed. Muscle testing of the masseter and pterygoid muscles gives a score of +5. The jaw jerk is scored +2.

An oral examination reveals that Steve's posterior teeth, especially the molars, have flattened surfaces. On further questioning he states that he is aware of clenching his jaw a great deal during the day, particularly when upset.

### *Range of motion*

Active and passive ranges of motion of the cervical spine are unremarkable.

### *Orthopedic and neurologic examinations*

Orthopedic and neurologic examinations of the cervical spine are unremarkable and within normal limits.

### *Radiologic examination*

Radiographs of the TMJ reveal that the joints are normal in appearance, with the heads of the mandible appearing to be symmetric, cylindrical, smooth, and properly positioned when the mouth is closed.

- How does this information contribute to the understanding of Steve's problem?

### Case OBJECTIVES

1. Define myofascial pain syndrome.
2. Describe the anatomy and biomechanics of the TMJ. Incorporate the nociceptive neuroanatomy of the TMJ.
3. Define a trigger point. What are the similarities and differences between a trigger point and a tender point? What is bruxism?
4. Describe the recent neuroanatomic theories of referral pain. What are the possible pain referral patterns that can be precipitated from a lesion of the TMJ?
5. Describe the similarities and differences between myofas-

cial pain syndrome, fibromyalgia, polymyalgia rheumatica, and polymyositis.

6. Describe the provocative tests used to evaluate the TMJ. What anatomic structures are these tests evaluating and what does a positive finding indicate?
7. Describe the radiologic views taken to evaluate the TMJ. What anatomic structures are observed on each view?
8. Develop a list of differential diagnoses. Compare and contrast these diseases.
9. Describe and perform a treatment and management protocol for this patient. Would you adjust or manipulate the TMJ? If so, how? What are your immediate, intermediate, and long-term goals?
10. Discuss cotreatment protocols for a patient with a TMJ problem.

## CASE 8

Aaron R., a 23-year-old artist, visits your office with the complaint of headache and pain in the neck and shoulders. Aaron had been involved in an automobile accident the previous day. He states that he was stopped at a stop sign when his vehicle was hit in the rear by a car traveling at approximately 25 miles/hour. The other driver claimed not to have seen the stop sign or Aaron's car because he was preoccupied. Aaron can recall the entire accident and he did not hit his head. The police were called and a report was filed. The paramedics came to the scene, but Aaron refused to go to the hospital.

Aaron did not have any neck pain until this morning, at which time he claims his pain was severe with a rating of 6 (10 being the score for the pain after he hit his thumb with a hammer). Both his shoulders feel very stiff, and he has an occipital headache. He has no trouble seeing, speaking, or hearing and has not felt nauseous. He localizes the pain to the suboccipital area, the posterior cervical spine, and the midtrapezius area of both shoulders. The neck and shoulder pain increased as the day progressed and he has a bad occipital headache. Aaron describes his pain as a dull ache and admits he cannot rotate his head without having pain in the cervical spine. He has no difficulty sleeping, swallowing, or eating, his appetite has not changed, and he does not hear any ringing in his ears.

His medical history is unrevealing. He has had the usual vaccinations with no sequelae. His father died of a heart attack and his mother is in a convalescent home.

- What could be happening to Aaron?
- What are the cervical spine biomechanics in a rear-end collision?
- What procedures would you perform during the physical examination?

### *Examination*

Vital signs.

Blood pressure: 120/76 mm Hg
Pulse rate: 62 beats/min
Respiration rate: 14 breaths/min
Temperature: 98.4° F
Height: 5'6"
Weight 155 lb

A limited mental exam does not reveal any memory abnormalities.

Inspection of the head and neck and examination of the eyes, ears, nose, and throat are unrevealing. There is no bruising, nor are any hematomas present. Palpation of the head and neck does not reveal any unusual swellings, bumps, or bruises. Muscle spasm is noted in the cervical musculature, namely the scalene and the sternocleidomastoid (SCM) muscles of the lateral and anterior aspects of the cervical spine, respectively. All internal organs of the cervical spine (the thyroid gland and arteries) are unremarkable. George's test for vertebral artery compromise is negative. Point tenderness is located at the middle and upper trapezius muscles and at the mid-SCM muscles bilaterally.

### Range of motion and orthopedic examination
Active and passive ranges of motion are limited in all directions with pain at the end of the range. Provocative tests reveal an increase in cervical spine pain during distraction and a relief from pain during compression. The headache increases with cervical distraction. Shoulder depression leads to pain in the ipsilateral trapezius and scalene muscles.

Shoulder range of motion is within normal limits except for stiffness in the midtrapezius muscle at the end of abduction.

Orthopedic tests for injury to the shoulder joints are negative.

### Neurologic examination
Tests for vision, speech, hearing, cranial nerve function, the vestibular system, and all sensations are unremarkable and within normal limits. Sensory tests for light touch, pain, and temperature are within normal limits and are bilaterally symmetric. All myotactic reflexes are scored a +2 and are bilaterally symmetric.

### Radiologic examination
A Davis series of the cervical spine reveals normal bony architecture. Soft tissues are normal in appearance, George's line is unbroken, and the retrotrachial and retropharangeal spaces are within normal limits. The cervical lordotic curve is straightened. A flexion and extension series reveals limited motion from C4 to C7.

### Laboratory examination
Laboratory studies are deferred at this time.

- How does this information assist you in determining what is wrong with Aaron?

### Case OBJECTIVES

1. Describe the anatomy and biomechanics of the cervical spine.
2. Describe the pathomechanics of a cervical spine whiplash injury caused by a rear-end collision.
3. Describe the anatomy of a suboccipital headache. What anatomic structures could be causing this pain distribution?
4. Differentiate the pain presentations from C1, C2, and C3. How do these pain presentations differ from a suboccipital headache? What provocative tests would help differentiate these anatomic structures?
5. Describe the inflammatory response to soft tissue injury. Of what importance is the inflammatory response to soft tissue healing?
6. Describe the steps needed for soft tissue healing.
7. Describe the history and physical examination findings in a patient who has sustained a whiplash injury.
8. Describe the x-ray examinations needed to evaluate a cervical spine whiplash injury.
9. Develop a list of differential diagnoses. Compare and contrast these diseases.
10. Develop a treatment and management protocol for this patient. What are the immediate, intermediate, and long-term goals of this diagnosis? What type of manipulation or adjustment procedures would be used on this patient?
11. Define Melzak and Wall's pain-gait theory. Of what significance is this theory in the treatment of Aaron's whiplash?

### CASE 9

Jim F., a 47-year-old housepainter, comes to your office with the complaint of right-sided neck pain, headaches, and pain extending into the right forearm and hand. Mr. F. states that the pain in the neck and the right lateral forearm has been present for 7 months and is progressively getting worse. The headaches have been present for the past 4 weeks and are increasing in frequency. The headache occurs more commonly toward the end of the work day, is diffusely present over the entire head, and gives him the feeling of wearing a tight headband. He describes the neck pain as a continuous, dull ache. When he extends, rotates, and laterally bends his head to the right his pain becomes sharp and intensifies in the lateral forearm and thumb. The pain feels as though a red-hot poker is extending into his hand and thumb. Tucking his chin to his chest or stretching his neck to the left provides temporary relief in the neck and forearm. Jim states that the headaches subside, and the neck and forearm pain decrease when he takes Motrin. He had also noticed a decrease in the frequency and severity of the headaches when he was on a short 4-day vacation with his wife.

Jim's medical history reveals that he drinks a six-pack of beer daily and works 50 hours a week. He smokes approximately one pack of cigarettes daily. He does not take any recreational or prescribed drugs.

The patient further reveals that his daughter and her three young children have moved into his home after her separation from her husband. Jim's family history reveals that his father died of a heart attack 6 years previously and that his mother and his two younger brothers, who are successful carpenters, have no medical problems.

- What anatomic structures could be causing Jim's problems?
- What procedures would you perform in your physical examination of this patient?

### Examination
Vital signs.
Blood pressure: 165/98 mm Hg
Pulse rate: 76 beats/min
Respiration rate: 14 breaths/min
Temperature: 98.7° F
Height: 5'9''
Weight: 175 lb

A physical examination of the chest, abdomen, eyes, ears, nose, and throat is within normal limits. Static palpation reveals a normal posture with a slightly exaggerated lumbar curve and an enlarged abdomen. Motion palpation reveals tight posterior neck muscles with restrictions in the lower cervical spine (C4 to T1) in extension and right lateral bending. Trigger points are found on the right side at the spinal levels of C2, C5, and T1.

### Range of motion

Active and passive extension, right rotation, and right lateral bending of the neck cause the neck and forearm pain to increase.

Active and passive neck flexion and left lateral bending provides slight relief of pain. The patient's headaches do not change with motion. George's test is negative for vertebral artery compromise.

### Orthopedic provocative examination

The cervical compression test reproduces the patient's pain and arm symptoms. Cervical distraction relieves the pain. The patient's pain is reproduced by Valsalva's maneuver and Dejerine's triad. The extension of the right wrist is not as strong as is left wrist extension.

### Neurologic examination

Examination of the 12 cranial nerves reveals normal findings. The right brachioradialis reflex is decreased. Light touch reveals a decrease in sensation over the palmar aspect of the right thumb and thenar eminence.

### Radiologic examination

A radiologic evaluation reveals that cervical lordosis is 28 degrees. Anterior osteophytes with spondylosis are present at C5 to C7 and there is uncinate process hypertrophy of C4 to C7. Encroachment of the intervertebral foramen (IVF) occurs between C5 and C6 and between C6 and C7. The discs between C4 and C5, between C5 and C6, and between C6 and C7 are narrowed. George's line is uninterrupted.

### Laboratory examination

The serum triglyceride level is 180 mg/dl (normal 35 to 160 mg/dL) and the total serum cholesterol level is 230 mg/dl (normal 150 to 240 mg/dl). The low density lipoprotein (LDL) level is 205 mg/dl (normal <170 mg/dl), whereas the high density lipoprotein (HDL) level is 25 mg/dl (normal 29 to 72 mg/dl).

- How does this information add to the determination of what is wrong with Jim?

### Case OBJECTIVES

1. Describe the anatomic boundaries of the cervical intervertebral foramen (IVF). How do these boundaries differ in the thoracic and the lumbar spine?
2. Describe the anatomic structures located in the cervical IVF. What other anatomic structures are in proximity to the cervical IVF?
3. Define and describe George's test. What are Maigne's and DeKleijn's maneuvers?
4. Describe the biomechanics (osteokinetic and arthrokinetic) of the cervical IVF. How does this information explain the pain presentations during certain cervical spine motions in this case?
5. Describe the radiographic views needed to observe the cervical IVF. What anatomic structures does each view present?
6. Describe the laboratory results. What do they indicate about this patient's condition and overall health?
7. Describe organic diseases that could mimic this case presentation.
8. Develop a list of differential diagnoses. Compare and contrast these diseases.
9. Explain the pain-spasm-pain reflex.
10. Describe the treatment and management protocol for this patient. What are the immediate, intermediate, and long-term goals? Is cotreatment necessary?

## CASE 10

James Q., a 31-year-old male accountant, complains of left-sided neck pain and numbness and tingling in the left-arm. His neck symptoms began approximately 3 years previously after an automobile accident. His vehicle was hit from behind by another automobile. His neck injury was diagnosed as a whiplash injury from which he never fully recovered. He describes the neck pain as a continual dull ache that does not refer to any other spinal location. The numbness and tingling in his left arm have been gradually increasing over the previous 6 months. His neck and upper extremity symptoms greatly increase when he bends his head laterally toward the right or when he abducts and externally rotates his left shoulder. The arm paresthesias start at the posterior aspect of his shoulder, proceed down the triceps into the medial aspect of his forearm to the fourth and fifth digits of his hand. His left hand feels "cooler" in the area of numbness and tingling. However, if he avoids placing his arm or neck in these positions, the pain in the neck is mild and the arm paresthesias do not occur. He is left-handed and his problems are bothersome, because they cause him to take frequent work breaks. Jim has no trouble holding objects, nor does he have problems with hearing, speaking, or seeing.

Jim has not had any other medical problems and his family history is unremarkable. He considers himself healthy except for this complaint, but admits that he is overweight and does not get enough exercise.

- What could be happening to Jim?

### Examination

Vital signs.
   Blood pressure: 126/82 mm Hg
   Pulse rate: 78 beats/min
   Respiration rate: 14 breaths/min
   Temperature: 98.8° F
   Height: 5'10"
   Weight: 160 lb

Inspection of the cervical spine and left upper extremity is unrevealing. There are no bruises or swellings in any area. Palpation of the cervical spine reveals point tenderness and muscle spasm located at the left scalenes, the SCM, and the neck angle. A trigger point is noted at the origin of the left levator scapulae that refers pain to the cervical spine and to the superior aspect of the left shoulder. No other findings are noted on palpation.

### Range of motion
Range of motion of the cervical spine reveals limited right lateral bending (20/45) with a reproduction of the patient's neck and arm complaints. Complete left lateral bending of the cervical spine occurs (45/45), but it produces pain at the origin of the left levator scapulae without radiculopathy. Right rotation is within normal limits, but produces pain at the left upper cervical spine. The left rotation is full, but it produces pain along the lateral aspect of the cervical spine and paresthesias to the left shoulder but not into the arm and hand.

Range of motion of the left shoulder is within normal limits. The patient's paresthesias are recreated when the shoulder is abducted and rotated externally. The paresthesias are exacerbated only when the shoulder is tested in overpressure and not during simple placement of position.

### Orthopedic examination
Provocative orthopedic tests reveal an increase in the patient's complaints during the elevated arm stress test (EAST), the shoulder depression test, Adson's test, and Allen's maneuver. Provocative tests of the cervical spine are noncontributory.

### Neurologic examination
Sensory evaluation of the upper extremities is within normal limits. Deep tendon reflexes are scored +2 and are bilaterally symmetric; pathologic reflexes of the upper extremities are absent.

### Radiologic examination
Radiographs of the cervical spine reveal no bone abnormalities. Soft tissues do not indicate any pathology either.

- How does this information help you decide what is wrong with Jim?

### Case OBJECTIVES
1. Describe the boundaries of the thoracic outlet.
2. Describe the anatomy of the thoracic outlet. Describe the anatomy of the brachial plexus and its surrounding anatomic structures.
3. Describe the surrounding anatomy of the thoracic outlet. What anatomic structures can cause thoracic outlet symptomatology?
4. Describe the relationship of the cervical spine to the brachial plexus.
5. Describe the orthopedic provocative tests. Perform the test, describe what a positive finding is, and what anatomic structures are being tested by each procedure.
6. Describe the neurologic findings. Of what significance are the results?
7. Describe the organovisceral problems that can cause thoracic outlet syndrome. What would differentiate a mechanical presentation from a visceral presentation? Develop a list of differential diagnoses.

8. Describe a treatment and management protocol for this patient. What are the immediate, intermediate, and long-term goals?

## CASE 11

Patricia R., a 10-year-old girl, visits your office with her mother, with the complaint of right-sided lower back pain, which has been occurring for the past 3 weeks, and has been getting progressively worse. The pain is a moderate ache that occurs intermittently and is worse toward the end of the day and when she is doing somersaults during playtime. The pain does not radiate, nor does it disturb her sleep. She does not recall any trauma or any single event that may have initiated this problem. She was told to seek further medical attention when a routine physical examination by the school nurse revealed a curvature of the spine.

Patricia is one of three children (she has two brothers, aged 12 and 17). Her father also has a lateral curve of the lumbar spine and his x-ray films reveal spondylolisthesis of L5 on S1 caused by a defect in the right pars interarticularis (spondylolysis). Her mother has mild lower back pain, and radiographs of her lumbar spine reveal spina bifida occulta at L5. Patricia's mother states that Patricia had a brother who died as a neonate and who had hemivertebra with spina bifida vera. Patricia's 17-year-old brother has been diagnosed with os odontoidium.

- What could be happening to Patricia?

### Examination
Vital signs.
  Blood pressure: 110/72 mm Hg
  Pulse rate: 80 beats/min
  Respiration rate: 15 breaths/min
  Temperature: 98.9° F
  Height: 4'11''
  Weight: 50 lb

Examination of Patricia reveals a healthy 10-year-old girl. A static plumb-line evaluation (sagittal and back view) reveals a high right shoulder with a head tilt to the left. Her pelvis is high on the right. A right-sided curvature with the apex at T6 is noted in the thoracic spine, and a left-sided curvature is observed in the lumbar spine with the apex at L3. On the frontal plumb-line evaluation (side view), there appears to be an increase in lumbar lordosis. The cervical and thoracic spinal areas appear to have normal lordotic and kyphotic curvatures. Palpation reveals muscle tightness on the left side of her thoracic spine when compared to the right side.

### Provocative examination
Adam's test demonstrates a straightening of the spine in the lumbar area and no change in the curve in the thoracic area. There is no indication of a rib hump. Right lateral bending of the patient does not change the thoracic curve. All range of motion in the thoracic and lumbar areas are within normal limits.

### Neurologic examination

Sensory tests for the trunk and upper extremities are within normal limits. DTRs are scored +2 and are bilaterally symmetric for the upper extremity.

### Radiologic examination

X-ray examination of Patricia's spine reveals a 15-degree right-sided thoracic curve with the apex at T7 measured by Cobb's angle. The lumbar Cobb's angle measurement is 10 degrees. Slightly wedged vertebrae are noted from T6 to T9, with the wedge on the left. Risser's sign indicates no ossification of the iliac crest.

• How does this information contribute to determining what is wrong with Patricia?

### Case OBJECTIVES

1. Describe the embryologic development of the vertebrae.
2. Define scoliosis. Does the normal spine have a lateral curvature that is considered to be within normal limits?
3. Describe the different causes of scoliosis.
4. Describe the normal position of the spine during plumb-line evaluation in the anterior-posterior and the lateral views.
5. Describe the anatomy and biomechanics (osteo- and arthrokinematics) of the thoracic spine.
6. Describe the normal range of motion of the thoracic spine. What muscles cause these motions?
7. Describe Adam's test and the lateral bending test.
8. Describe the protocol for a serial x-ray examination for evaluation of scoliosis. How is the patient's position standardized? Describe Cobb's angle and Risser's sign.
9. Describe wedged vertebrae and the other bony anomolies found in this case. What causes their development? Can it be embryologic or developmental?
10. Develop a treatment and management protocol for this patient. What are the immediate, intermediate, and long-term goals for this patient? Is cotreatment necessary? What are the procedures used to determine when cotreatment is needed?

## CASE 12

Elizabeth H., a 78-year-old former pediatrician, visits your office complaining of pain in the middle back (two T10 to L2). She claims that the pain began that morning when, tending to her garden, she bent over to pick a weed and felt a "snap" in her back and was in immediate pain. She was able to straighten her back, but the pain was quite severe and made her catch her breath. The pain is a deep, dull ache that is well-localized. Putting ice on the area and laying on her back with a pillow over the involved area provided immediate relief, but she was unable to change this position because of the pain. Sitting and standing also worsen the pain. Elizabeth has not experienced pain such as this before. She knows that she has a spinal fracture and is seeking your help.

Her medical history is unremarkable, and consists of the usual geriatric complaints and discomforts. She has one younger brother who is becoming very senile, but she is unaware of his having any spinal fractures. Her parents have been deceased for the past 40 years.

### Examination

Vital signs.
    Blood pressure: 134/86 mm Hg
    Pulse rate: 70 beats/min
    Respiration rate: 14 breaths/min
    Temperature: 98.7° F
    Height: 5'4"
    Weight: 140 lb

Visual inspection of the patient's back reveals several senile nevi, but there are no other skin abnormalities. A lateral view of the patient's spine during a plumb-line evaluation reveals increased kyphosis at the thoracic spine and decreased lordosis at the lumbar spine. Point tenderness is located at the thoracolumbar junction from T10 to L2. There is no other referral or radiation of pain. Muscle spasm is located bilaterally from T8 to the sacrum.

Findings on inspection, auscultation, and palpation of the abdomen are normal.

### Range of motion

Active and passive range of motion tests of the thoracic and lumbar spine reveal a decrease in flexion, lateral bending, and rotation because of an increase in the patient's pain complaints. Extension with overpressure at the thoracolumbar junction gives the patient relief.

### Provocative examination

A slump test increases pain in the thoracolumbar area, and spinous percussion reproduces the patient's pain complaints. All other provocative tests for radiculopathy or neuritis are noncontributory.

### Neurologic examination

Sensory pin-prick evaluation is within normal limits from T8 to S1; L4 and S1 DTRs are scored +2 and are bilaterally symmetric; and, Babinski's reflex is not present. Romberg's test is within normal limits.

### Radiologic examination

A two-view series of radiographs is taken of the patient's thoracolumbar junction and lumbar spine areas. A vertebral compression fracture is noted at L1 on the lateral view and the anterior-posterior (A-P) view reveals a decrease in height at this level. A decrease in bone density is noted throughout the thoracolumbar and lumbar areas. Disc height appears to be within normal limits. No other bone abnormalities are present.

### Case OBJECTIVES

1. Define osteoporosis. How does it differ from osteopenia and osteomalacia?
2. Explain the physiology of osteoporosis in elderly women.
3. Describe the appearance of a patient with a compression fracture caused by osteoporosis.
4. Describe the difference in radiographic presentation between a compression vertebral fracture caused by osteopenia or trauma and a pathologic fracture.
5. Describe radiographic studies that would be necessary for further evaluation of the extent of this patient's osteoporosis.

**6.** Develop a list of differential diagnoses. Compare and contrast these diseases. What is osteomalacia?

**7.** Develop a treatment and management protocol for this patient. What are the immediate, intermediate, and long-term goals for this patient? What is the effect of exercise, hormonal therapy, and vitamin supplementation on osteoporosis? What is the role of the kidneys in this condition?

## CASE 13

Pearline M. is a 53-year-old woman who complains of left-sided lower back pain, with tingling extending into the left buttock and posterior thigh but not going below the knee. She is a trial lawyer for the law offices of Henry and Babcock. Pearline states that this episode of lower back pain began 3 days previously as she was straightening up from bending over to feed her cat. She immediately felt a sharp pain in her left lower back that sent a tingling sensation into the left buttock. The pain does not awaken her at night but leaves her with stiffness and soreness in the morning that are relieved with a hot shower. Her condition has not interfered with her daily activities. Pearline describes her lower back pain as a constant dull ache, not a shooting pain, that extends across the left buttock into the posterior thigh to her knee. The pain improves in the morning but worsens toward the end of the day.

Lying on either side with the hips and knees flexed helps to alleviate the pain. Wearing high heels and performing any movement involving reaching over her head aggravates the pain. On a 0 to 10 scale, Pearline rates the low back pain as a 2 in the morning and a 6 toward the end of the day (she gives a score of 10 to the pain after burning her hand with a hot iron). There is no change in urination or bowel habits.

Pearline's medical history reveals that she has been overweight most of her life and has been on numerous diets with no success. She has two brothers who are of normal weight and have no history of lower back pain. Both parents are still living, and neither have had any history of lower back pain. Her family clinician has indicated that she has no other medical problems.

• What could be happening to Pearline?

### Examination

Vital signs.
    Blood pressure: 126/88 mm Hg
    Pulse rate: 78 beats/min
    Respiration rate: 14 breaths/min
    Temperature: 98.8° F
    Height: 5'5''
    Weight: 165 lb

Postural analysis indicates that Pearline has an increased lumbar lordosis, but it does not reveal an antalgic position. Motion palpation demonstrates restriction of movement on extension, left lateral bending, and left rotation at the left and right L3 to L4 and L4 to L5 zygapophyseal joints. Palpation of the lower back reveals muscle splinting (guarding) throughout the left erector spinae muscle group from LI to L5 with numerous areas of point tenderness. A trigger point is found on the left side at L3. The iliopsoas is tight bilaterally.

### Range of motion

Range of motion tests in the lumbar spine reveal pain at L4 to L5 at a 45 degree-angle of active flexion, and she cannot bend further. Passive flexion produces pain at a 50-degree angle. Active and passive extension is limited to 2 degrees with reproduction of the patient's pain and tingling complaints. Lateral bending and rotation do not reproduce the pain complaints.

Active and passive ranges of motion for the thoracic spine, sacroiliac (SI) joint, and hip joint are within normal limits. Hip flexion beyond 90 degrees and extension beyond 40 degrees reproduce the patient's lower back pain complaints.

### Provocative examination

Provocative testing of the lumbar spine reveals no radiculopathy in the lower extremity during the straight leg raise. Valsalva's maneuver does not reproduce the patient's complaints. The sign-of-four test does not reproduce the patient's complaints or cause hip pain.

### Neurologic examination

Sensory examination for light touch, pain, and temperature, and 2-point discrimination is within normal limits. Reflexes of the lower extremities are scored +2 and are bilaterally symmetric. All muscle tests of the lower extremities are within normal limits (score of +5).

### Radiologic examination

X-ray examination of the lumbar spine does not show abnormalities. There is no indication of joint imbrication, osteophytic changes, or degeneration. Fergusson's sacral base angle is measured at 65 degrees, the gravitational line is anterior to the sacrum, and the patient's lumbar spine measures 53 degrees of lordosis.

### Laboratory examination

A CBC and UA are normal.

• How does this information help to determine what is wrong with Pearline?

### Case OBJECTIVES

**1.** Describe the anatomy and biomechanics of the lumbar spine and spinal cord.

**2.** Describe the histology, anatomy, and biomechanics of the lumbar facet zygapophyseal joint.

**3.** Explain and perform a static plumb-line evaluation. What do the results in this case indicate about the patient's posture? How does wearing high heels affect this patient's posture?

**4.** Describe kinematics and kinetics of lumbopelvic rhythm. Of what significance is this information to the clinician when the patient flexes at the waist during active range of motion?

**5.** Define hereditary, genetic, and familial conditions. How would Pearline's problem be labeled?

**6.** Define muscle spasm and muscle splinting. What are their similarities and differences? Describe the physiology of muscle strain. What is the difference between muscle spasticity and muscle spasm?

**7.** Explain the pain-spasm-pain theory. What significance does this theory have for the case?

**8.** Describe the radiographic findings. What is their significance in this case?

**9.** Describe the pathophysiology of Facet syndrome and lumbar sprain or strain. Develop a list of differential diagnoses.

**10.** Describe a treatment and management protocol for this patient. Explain the physiologic effect of adjusting or manipulating this patient. What are the immediate, intermediate, and long-term goals for this patient? Would Janda's protocol benefit this patient?

**11.** Describe the physiology of the relationship of joint motion to joint healing.

## CASE 14

Phil M., a 37-year-old truck driver, reports to your office with the complaint of sharp stabbing lower back pain. The pain feels like an electric shock coursing into his right buttock and down the posterior aspect of his thigh and leg to the bottom of his foot and the lateral side of the fifth toe. He is antalgic to the left. He states that this episode of pain began the previous day after a long drive from Dallas to Los Angeles. The pain, which began as a dull ache in his lower back, is now sharp and much worse. Similar episodes of lower back pain have occurred over the past 5 years. He has been a truck driver for the past 15 years and after long trips, he usually has some type of lower back pain. The current episode is the worst he has had and is also the first time that the pain has ever shot down his leg. The pain subsides if Phil rests on his back with his knees bent. Lengthy periods of sitting increase the pain, which becomes severe during coughing, sneezing, or straining during a bowel movement. He has not lost voluntary control of urinary or bowel functions.

Phil is one of four children (he has two older brothers and one younger sister) and is married, with three children. His father, now 62 years old, has a history of lower back pain, and had a laminectomy at the age of 51. According to Phil, he no longer has the problem. His oldest brother, Salvador, has a history similar to Phil of lower back pain and operates a jackhammer for the Jackson County road department.

• What could be happening to Phil?

### Examination

Vital signs.

Blood pressure: 124/84 mm Hg
Pulse rate: 74 beats/min
Respiration rate: 14 breaths/min
Temperature: 98.8° F
Height: 5'7''
Weight: 170 lb

As the patient enters your office you notice that he is antalgic to the left. Static palpation verifies the antalgia and also indicates the loss of lumbar lordosis. Motion palpation of the lower back reveals loss of flexion, right lateral bending, and bilateral rotation at L4 to L5 and at L5 to S1. Palpation of the lower back reveals muscle splinting and point tenderness

bilaterally throughout the lumbar spine. No other muscle tightness is present.

### Range of motion

Both passive and active motions of the lumbar spine produce pain in the lower back and the leg on flexion, and on left and right rotation. Flexion and rotation are limited to 5 degrees. Some relief of the pain is obtained on left lateral bending and extension.

### Provocative testing

Provocative tests reveal radiculopathy at 40 degrees of straight leg rise (SLR), the pain is exacerbated with −5 degrees of hip flexion and ankle dorsiflexion (Braggard's). Bowing of the leg occurs on waist flexion (Neri's bowstring); Valsalva's maneuver and bilateral knee extension with the patient in the seated position reproduce the patient's pain and radiculopathy.

### Neurologic examination

The patient has problems standing on his right toes. All other muscle tests are within normal limits. Sensory evaluation of light touch and pain produce a slight decrease in sensation over the S1 dermatome on the right side. Reflexes are scored +2 and are bilaterally symmetric except at the right Achilles tendon that scored +1.

### Radiologic examination

An x-ray examination reveals a decrease in disc height from L5 to S1. The gravitational line is located at the anterior one third of the sacrum, and Fergusson's sacral base angle is 49 degrees.

### Laboratory examination

The CBC and UA are within normal limits.

• How does this information add to the determination of what is wrong with Phil?

### Case OBJECTIVES

**1.** Describe the anatomy and biomechanics of the lumbar spine.

**2.** Explain the histology and biomechanics of the lumbar intervertebral disc.

**3.** Define vibration and resonance. What significance do these terms have with the case presentation? How does this information contribute to the understanding of Phil's disc problem?

**4.** Explain the palliative and provocative findings in this case. Compare and contrast these findings with a patient who has a lumbar Facet syndrome.

**5.** Describe and perform the orthopedic and neurologic procedures in this case. Describe (1) the anatomic structures being evaluated by the tests, (2) a positive result, and (3) the significance of this information to Phil's condition. Compare and contrast the results of a Facet syndrome with those of muscular strain.

**6.** Identify the muscles and the actions that cause lumbar rotation, flexion or extension, and lateral bending. What are the normal ranges of motion of the lumbar spine?

**7.** Define and explain the radiographic findings in this case.

**8.** Describe the biomechanics of the motion palpation and the static palpation findings in this case.

**9.** Explain the intervertebral disc pathophysiology that is relevant to this case. What is imbibition? What is disc degeneration?

10. Develop a list of differential diagnoses. Compare and contrast these diseases.
11. Describe the treatment and management protocol for this case. What is the role of manipulation or adjustment? What type of adjustive or manipulative procedures would be of benefit to this patient? What are the immediate, intermediate, and long-term goals for this case? Explain the role of the Melzak-Wall pain-gait theory in this case.
12. Develop an exercise program for this patient. What are McKenzie's protocol and William's flexion exercise? How would they benefit this patient? Would Janda's protocol help this patient? What is the physiologic role of motion in proper healing of a disc?

## CASE 15

Myra T. is a 27-year-old woman who complains of left-sided lower back and buttock pain. The pain occurs after prolonged bending at the waist and is an intermittent, dull ache that, at times, refers to her left hamstrings but does not shoot into the area. On a 0 to 10 scale, she rates the lower back and buttock pain as a 4 (the pain of childbirth being scored a 10). The pain is present when she sits or stands for prolonged lengths of time or bends at the waist (at the end of the range). She is an accountant by profession. She has had this pain for the past 4 years and has attributed it to childbirth. She has visited her primary physician several times over the past 2 years, but he has not been able to relieve her symptoms and has referred her to you. The primary physician has prescribed ibuprofen (Motrin; 400 mg tid) and physical therapy modalities, but this treatment has provided only temporary relief. The pain has not worsened over the past few months, but it is a nagging problem that she would like to take care of. Myra is an active young woman who enjoys bicycle riding, hiking, and swimming. She feels stiff and sore in the same areas after a long bicycle ride (she owns a mountain bike). Swimming relieves her pain for a short period of time, but she cannot do a frog-leg kick for too long because it triggers her lower back pain.

Her medical history and family history are unremarkable. She has had the usual childhood diseases and does not remember having lower back pain before childbirth. She is married and has two healthy boys, 4 and 6 years of age.

• What could be happening to Myra?

### Examination
Vital signs.
　　Blood pressure: 124/78 mm Hg
　　Pulse rate: 63 beats/min
　　Respiration rate: 12 breaths/min
　　Temperature: 98.0° F
　　Height: 5'2"
　　Weight: 137 lb
Inspection of the lumbar spine does not reveal any gross abnormalities. A high left scapula with corresponding shoulder unleveling is seen on plumb-line evaluation. The pelvis is slightly higher on the left. Palpation of the lumbar muscula-

ture shows muscle splinting on the left side when compared to the right. The gluteus maximus musculature is bilaterally symmetric. Elevation of the hips, knees, ankles, and feet from the floor is symmetric, and there are no valgus or varus deformities at the knees. The left hamstring muscles are supple on palpation and do not present any muscle spasm or splinting. Two trigger points are located at the piriformis and gluteus maximus musculature on the left. Point tenderness is located at the upper portion of the left SI joint. Motion palpation reveals restriction of the left SI joint at the superior aspect during flexion.

### Range of motion of the lumbar spine
Active and passive range of motions of the lumbar spine are within normal limits. The patient's pain complaints are elicited at the end of waist flexion and extension range. Rotation of the lumbar spine to the right elicits pain in the left SI joint area.

### Provocative testing
Provocative testing of the lumbar spine reveals pain at the end of lower extremity flexion (SLR). Iliac compression, Patrick's test, and Trendelenburg's test do not reproduce the patient's complaints. Further testing of the SI joint does elicit pain on the left side after Yeoman's and Gaenslen's tests are performed.

　　Muscle testing for strength and length reveals all the muscles of the lower back and hips to be of equal strength bilaterally. The left erector spinae muscles are shortened when compared to the right erector spinae muscles, because of muscle splinting. On gait analysis there is a slight rotary displacement of the trunk to the right during the right foot stance phase.

### Neurologic examination
Sensory evaluation of the lower back, buttocks, and lower extremities is within normal limits. Deep tendon reflexes of the lower extremities are scored +2 and are bilaterally symmetric. Romberg's sign and the finger-to-nose test are negative.

### Radiologic examination
Radiologic views of the lumbar spine do not reveal any abnormalities, and there is no indication of spondylolisthesis, spondylolysis, disc narrowing, or bone spurring. An anteriorposterior (AP) spot of the SI joints does not reveal any joint widening or inflammatory changes.

• How does this information help you decide what is wrong with Myra?

### Case OBJECTIVES
1. Describe the anatomy and biomechanics of the lumbar spine and the sacroiliac joints.
2. Explain the biomechanics of the results of the range-of-motion tests, provocative tests, and neurologic tests in this case. Compare and contrast these results to the Facet syndrome and lumbar disc cases.
3. Describe the orthopedic provocative findings. Include the test procedure, a description of a positive finding, and the anatomic structures being tested.
4. Describe the range of motion of the hip joint. Of what significance is this information in this case?
5. Describe the role of the hamstring muscles in this case. Why is it important that these muscles be evaluated in this case?
6. Explain the motion palpation and static palpation findings.

7. Explain the gait presentation in this case.
8. Compare and contrast the history and physical examination of a Facet syndrome, a lumbar disc syndrome, and an SI joint problem.
9. Develop a treatment and management protocol. What are the immediate, intermediate, and long-term goals for this patient?

## CASE 16

Sandra C., a 27-year-old secretary, has a complaint of right-sided lower back pain that radiates into the right buttock and down the thigh, into the leg and the foot. The lower back and the intermittent leg pain have been present for the past week. Over the past 3 years she has had two or three episodes of lower back pain, but all subsided with rest within 5 days. When asked to localize the area of complaint in the lower extremity, she implicates the entire aspect of the leg and the foot. The leg pain is a sharp, shooting sensation that occurs during attempts to bend over and pick up something or during prolonged periods of sitting. The lower back pain is a dull ache, and Sandra rates it as a 3 on a pain scale of 0 to 10 (10 being the score for the pain after a burn from a hot iron); the leg pain is rated a 6. She has no bowel or bladder problems and has little pain when she is asleep. In the morning, the lower back area is stiff and sore, and sometimes she feels the leg pain.

Her medical history and family history are unremarkable. She has not been hospitalized and has not had any surgeries.

• What could be happening to Sandra?

### Examination
Vital signs.
   Blood pressure: 120/78 mm Hg
   Pulse rate: 63 beats/min
   Respiration rate: 13 breaths/min
   Temperature: 98.6° F
   Height: 5'3''
   Weight: 125 lb
Inspection of the lower back and lower extremities is unremarkable. The abdomen is supple, and palpation of this area does not reproduce the patient's complaints. There is generalized muscle splinting at the lumbar spine and the range of motion in this area is full with lower back pain occurring only during bilateral rotation. Pain is elicited in the leg during hip flexion (SLR) at 25 degrees. The pain is located in the buttock area and radiates to the lower extremity. Patrick's test (fabere sign) does not reproduce the patient's complaints. However, internal rotation and adduction of the right hip does increase the patient's leg and foot pain. Point tenderness is located at the midbuttock area when the hip is supported in internal rotation and adduction.

### Neurologic examination
Neurologic testing of the lower extremities are within normal limits. There is no change in light touch, pain, or temperature sensations. All muscle tests of the lower extremities are within normal limits (scores of +5). The patient can walk on her toes and heels unassisted.

### Radiologic examination
X-ray examination of the lumbar spine does not reveal any pathology, congenital anomalies, or fractures. X-ray films of the hip are also negative.

### Laboratory examination
Laboratory examination is deferred at this time.

• How does this information determine what is causing Sandra's lower back, leg, and foot pain?

### Case OBJECTIVES

1. Describe the anatomy of the piriform muscle and its anatomic relationships to surrounding structures.
2. Describe the orthopedic provocative tests. How is the test performed, what is a positive finding, and what are the anatomic structures being tested?
3. Describe the significance of the findings in internal rotation and adduction of the hip.
4. Explain the neuroanatomy of the pain presentation in the lower extremity. How does this differ neuroanatomically with the intervertebral disc lower extremity radiculopathy?
5. Compare and contrast the findings in this case with the lumbar disc case and the facet case.
6. Develop a list of differential diagnoses. Compare and contrast these maladies.
7. Develop a treatment and management protocol for this patient. What are the immediate, intermediate, and long-term goals for this condition?

## CASE 17

Tom S. is a 36-year old-man who is seen at your office with a complaint of diffuse lower back pain and stiffness. The pain and stiffness began 3 months previously with no known provocative incident. The region of complaint consists of an area on both sides of the lumbar spine from L3 to S2 and both SI joints that are sore and tender to touch. Tom indicates that the pain and stiffness are much worse in the morning and that it takes him a very long time to get up and moving. A hot shower helps on occasion. Tom states that it is difficult for him to bend at the waist in the morning but he has no problems toward the end of the day. Although Tylenol provides some relief, he must sometimes take 5 to 6 tablets to feel better. It may take him 1 to 2 hours to recover after a severe bout of stiffness. He rates the stiffness as an 8 on a 10 scale (10 being the pain after dropping a cement brick on his toe) in the morning and at 3 in the afternoon. Moving around reduces the pain and stiffness, and by the end of the day he is feeling pretty good. Tom has no trouble falling asleep but during the night the back pain and stiffness seem to increase and wake him up. The pain has been progressing over time and Tom admits he has not felt good health; he feels fatigued and "run down." He has had intermittent episodes of lower back pain that have resolved without any treatment. Stiffness has been present on every episode. He does not complain of stiffness in any other joint; his problem has always been in his lower back.

Tom's medical history reveals that he has had the usual vaccinations and has had measles, chicken pox, and mumps. He has not had strept throat or rheumatic fever and has not noticed any joint swellings or unusual bumps on his elbows or hands. He is not a smoker, does not drink alcohol, and has no problems with bowel or bladder functions. No history of cancer, diabetes, high blood pressure, or cardiac problems is present.

His family history reveals that he has an older sister and a younger brother, neither of whom have problems similar to Tom's. His parents are alive and healthy and do not have a similar complaint.

• What could be happening to Tom?

### Examination
Vital signs.
  Blood pressure: 110/80 mm Hg
  Pulse rate: 69 beats/min
  Respiration rate: 14 breaths/min
  Temperature: 98.0° F
  Height: 5'8''
  Weight: 170 lb

A lumbar spine inspection does not reveal any hematomas or skin rashes. Point tenderness is exquisite over both SI joints. Plumb-line evaluation reveals a normal spinal curvature on the A-P view. A military spine is present on the lateral view, with loss of lordosis in the lumbar spine and an increase in kyphosis in the thoracic spine. The cervical spine is properly positioned in the lateral view, but, the lordotic curve is accentuated in the lower cervical area. The patient does not complain of neck pain. Static palpation reveals bilateral muscle splinting along the entire lumbar spine and the lumbar vertebrae appear to be very rigid, especially in flexion and extension motions.

### Range of motion
Active range of motion of the lumbar spine is full and uninhibited. The lumbar spine moves less than what is considered normal, but the patient is able to touch his toes. Passive range of motion reveals a lack of motion on flexion and extension with a hard end-feel on flexion. Motion palpation reveals a lack of joint play throughout the lumbar spine. Restrictions are noted in flexion and anterior glide at all levels of the lumbar spine. Other motions appear to be within normal limits. Other joints of the lower extremities function normally. Abdominal examination is unremarkable. There are no masses or abnormalities noted on inspection, auscultation, palpation, and percussion.

### Provocative testing
Provocative tests reveal negative SLR and Patrick's test. Testing of SI joint mobility reveals pain and tenderness (Gaenslen's test) and Schober's test indicates a lack of lumbar motion on flexion.

### Neurologic examination
All neurologic tests are within normal limits. There are no abnormal findings on pain and light touch evaluations. Deep tendon reflexes are scored +2 and are bilaterally symmetric and muscle tests of the lower extremity are scored +5. Romberg's test and tandem walk are within normal limits.

### Radiologic examination
A three-view lumbar spine evaluation is performed. The A-P lumbar view reveals sclerosing and joint widening at both SI joints. The zygapophyseal joints of the lumbar spine are normal, and no joint erosions or abnormalities are observed.

### Laboratory examination
A CBC, UA, thyroid panel, and arthritis profile are ordered. The results indicate a normal CBC and UA, negative findings for rheumatoid arthritis, an elevated ESR, and a negative test for uric acid. There is no indication of anemia and the thyroid panel results are within normal limits.

• How does this information help decide what is wrong with Tom?

### Case OBJECTIVES
1. Describe the functional anatomy, biomechanics, and neuroanatomy of the lumbar spine. What is lumbopelvic rhythm (flexion-relaxation phenomenon), and of what importance is it to this case?
2. Describe and perform the plumb-line, static palpation, and motion palpation findings. How do these results differ from the results found in other lower back problems?
3. Describe the normal anatomy, histology, and physiology of the SI joint.
4. Describe the orthopedic and neurologic tests performed on this patient. What anatomic structures are being evaluated, what is a positive test result, and how is the test performed?
5. Describe and perform the radiologic and laboratory evaluations. What are the typical results in ankylosing spondylitis (AS)?
6. Describe the pathophysiologic changes that occur in the SI joint in AS.
7. Compare and contrast the history and physical examination findings in a patient with AS, lumbar strain or sprain, lumbar facet syndrome, and lumbar intervertebral disc syndrome.
8. Compare and contrast the history and physical examination results (including x-ray findings and laboratory diagnosis) in a patient with AS and a patient with rheumatoid arthritis (RA).
9. Develop a list of differential diagnoses. Compare and contrast these diseases.
10. Develop a treatment and management program for this patient. What are the immediate, intermediate, and long-term goals for this patient? Discuss cotreatment options and develop a rehabilitation plan for cotreatment. Discuss medicinal treatments of AS.
11. Educate the patient about prognosis and exercise procedures for AS.

### CASE 18

Keith M., a 65-year-old pharmacist, complains of persistent, diffuse lower back pain that has been present for the past 3 weeks and has progressively become worse. Keith has taken Advil (two tablets tid), which provides slight temporary relief but does not rid him of the pain totally. He cannot find a position that is comfortable because the pain bothers him and seems to increase when he is sleeping. Taking a hot shower and letting the water run over the lower back provides mild relief but the pain returns once he gets out of the shower. There is no single position that leads to a change in pain. He claims that the pain does not travel into his hips or lower extremities and is only located in his lower back between L2 and L5 on either side. He has no problems with bowel or bladder functions. Keith gives a rating of 2 to the pain when it started 3 weeks previously, but he now rates it a 4 on a 0 to 10 scale (10 being the score for the pain on cutting his finger with a razor blade). His activities of daily living are disrupted, and he is always tired because he cannot sleep well at night.

Keith's family history and medical history are unremarkable. He has not been previously hospitalized and has had no surgeries. He is not presently taking any medication except for the occasional Advil.

- What could be happening to Keith?

### Examination
Vital signs.
   Blood pressure: 140/90 mm Hg
   Pulse rate: 80 beats/min
   Respiration rate: 15 breaths/min
   Temperature: 98.0° F
   Height: 5'10''
   Weight: 190 lb
The abdomen is normal: there are no abdominal masses, and it is not distended. Digital palpation of the prostate reveals a nodule located in the left posterior capsule; the median sulcus seems to feel obliterated.

### Range of motion
Palpation of the lumbar spine does not reveal any point tenderness. However, there is moderate bilateral splinting of the erector spinae musculature. The range of motion of the lumbar spine is full and does not provoke the patient's pain.

### Provocative testing
Provocative tests are negative, but the SLR reveals pain in the lumbar spine at 90 degrees in the area of L2 to L5 bilaterally.

### Neurologic examination
Neurologic examination of the lumbar spine and lower extremities is normal and reflexes have a score of +2 and are bilaterally symmetric.

### Radiologic examination
Radiographs of the lumbar spine reveal diffuse osteoblastic and osteolytic changes located in the entire lumbar spine area. A bone scan reveals increased radioisotope uptake in the lumbar spine and MRI reveals bony changes in the lumbar spine indicative of metastasis of prostatic cancer.

### Laboratory examination
Laboratory evaluation revealed elevated levels of prostate specific antigen (PSA) and acid phosphatase.

This patient was immediately referred to a urologist for further consultation and work-up for his prostatic cancer.

- What findings are presented in the history and physical examination that indicate that this patient does not have a musculoskeletal problem?

### Case OBJECTIVES
1. Describe the anatomy, including the vascular supply, of the prostate and compare this information to the anatomy of the lumbar spine.
2. Describe the venous supply of the prostate and its relationship to the lumbar spine. Of what significance is this information to this case?

3. Compare and contrast the findings in a patient with prostate problems that refer to the lumbar spine and a patient with musculoskeletal problems.
4. Describe and perform a prostatic examination. What laboratory tests are necessary for this case?
5. Describe the immediate, intermediate, and long-term goals for this case.
6. Educate this patient about his condition.

### CASE 19

Myra K., a 53-year-old secretary for a printing company, has a complaint of right shoulder pain. She states that the shoulder pain has been intermittent for the last 2 months, occurring especially during playing tennis, and has increased in intensity in the past week. She was painting her walls the previous week and felt sharp pains that prevented her from continuing. Her neck gets stiff if she sits at her computer for more than 2 hours. Myra discontinued tennis, aerobic exercises, and yoga 3 weeks previously because of the increased shoulder pain. Her family doctor diagnosed her with bursitis after an x-ray examination of her shoulder and prescribed anti-inflammatory medication (Motrin, 400 mg every 4 hours as needed) and put her arm in a sling. This treatment has provided some relief, but the pain has continued and she desires a second opinion. She has brought her radiographs.

Myra's medical history does not contribute any significant information to her presentation. Until 2 months previously she has never complained of shoulder pain. There is no history of previous accidents or trauma to her cervical spine or upper extremities.

- What could be happening to Myra?

### Examination
Vital signs.
   Blood pressure: 122/78 mm Hg
   Pulse rate: 73 beats/min
   Respiration rate: 12 breaths/min
   Temperature: 98.9° F
   Height: 5'1''
   Weight: 143 lb
Plumb-line evaluation reveals a normal contour of the spine without any abnormalities. An A-P plumb-line view reveals that the head and neck are in the midline of the body. Palpation of the lymph nodes and paracervical musculature is unremarkable. Both active and passive range of motion of the cervical spine is within normal limits. Resisted isometric muscle testing of the cervical muscles in all directions indicates the muscles to be strong and painless. Cervical compression tests in various directions are not painful nor does the compression tests refer pain to the right shoulder area (Spurling's and Lhermitte's signs). Intersegmental spinal palpation reveals tenderness at the C5 spinous and right C5 paracervical level with diminished end-feel on passive right cervical lateral bending and left cervical rotation at the C5 level.

Examination of the shoulder reveals a normal looking shoulder without skin lesions, bruises, or discoloration. There is a normal alignment between the clavicles, the sternoclavicular, and the acromioclavicular joints without any step deformity. A posterior view of the patient does not display any muscular atrophy or abnormal alignment. The scapulae are symmetric without winging. Palpation of the shoulder reveals tenderness at the insertion of the supraspinous muscle and the tendon of the infraspinous muscle.

### Range of motion

Active range of motion reveals normal ranges in all directions except for pain on shoulder abduction between 65 and 120 degrees and in external rotation between 40 and 60 degrees. There is pain and limitation of movement in elevation in the scapular plane at 150/160 degrees, and in forward flexion at 140/160 degrees. Passive range of motion of the shoulder is within normal limits except for pain at the end range in the coronal plane, forward elevation, and external rotation.

### Provocative testing

Resisted isometric testing of the shoulder and scapular muscles reveals pain and decreased strength in abduction (score of +4 on a 5-point scale) and external rotation (score of +3).

Tests for shoulder instability in posterior and inferior glide reveal normal motion and end-feel. The shoulder impingement test is positive on the right side.

### Neurologic examination

Sensory evaluation is within normal limits and the deep tendon reflexes of the upper extremity are +2 and bilaterally symmetric.

### Radiographic examination

Radiographs reveal a normal shoulder with no fracture or dislocation. Bone density is within normal limits.

- How does this information help determine what is wrong with Myra?

### Case OBJECTIVES

1. Describe the anatomy and biomechanics of the shoulder. What anatomic structures exist between the acromion and the head of the humerus?
2. Describe the biomechanics of the shoulder. Define and describe glenohumeral motion.
3. Describe the anatomy of the brachial plexus and its relationship to the shoulder.
4. Describe the three types of painful arcs. Which anatomic structures are involved in each arc?
5. Describe the principles of tissue testing and perform a selective tissue test of the shoulder.
6. Describe and perform the orthopedic and neurologic tests. Which are the anatomic structures being tested, what is a positive finding, and how is the test performed?
7. Describe the radiologic views taken to evaluate the cervical spine and shoulder. What special radiologic procedures would be needed to evaluate the structures of the shoulder further?
8. Develop a list of differential diagnoses for this patient's symptoms. Compare and contrast these diagnoses.
9. Develop a treatment and management protocol for this patient. What are the immediate, intermediate, and long-term goals for this patient?
10. Discuss the adjusting and manipulating procedures of the shoulder and cervical spine. Develop a protocol for the adjusting procedures for this patient.

### CASE 20

Steve L., a 27-year-old man has a complaint of a painful right elbow and sore right wrist. He states that this pain has been present for the past 6 weeks and is located on the lateral aspect of the epicondyle of his right elbow and on the radial side of his wrist. Mr. L. is a carpenter and recalls the wrist pain occurring after he slipped and fell on an open dorsiflexed hand. The pain was initially severe, but he applied an ice pack and felt relief in a few days. He does not remember any local swelling and although the wrist is painful at times he thinks it is getting better. He describes his elbow pain as a deep ache that was present intermittently for several weeks before he fell on his wrist. His usual work hours are from 7 am to 4 pm daily, but he has not been able to work a full shift because the elbow pain has increased. A forearm band provides him minimal relief. He has no history of previous elbow or wrist pain and is otherwise healthy. There is no spinal pain, radiating pain, or paresthesia in the involved upper extremity.

Steve's medical history reveals that he drinks about a six-pack of beer daily and he confides that, on occasion, he suffers from epigastric pain. He does not smoke tobacco or use any recreational drugs. He is single, has never been hospitalized or had any severe illness. His parents are in good health, and have never been hospitalized. His father is a carpenter and his mother is a housewife.

- What could be happening to Steve?

### Examination

Vital signs.

    Blood pressure: 132/84 mm Hg
    Pulse rate: 72 beats/min
    Respiratory rate: 12 breaths/min
    Temperature: 97.8° F
    Height: 5'10"
    Weight: 172 lb

The cervical spine is passively stressed in all directions to determine if there is a reproduction of pain in the right upper extremity. Motion palpation of the individual vertebral segments in all directions does not reveal any vertebral restrictions or tenderness, and the results are negative.

Inspection of the forearm and wrist reveal a normal carrying angle of the elbow, normal bone and soft-tissue contours of the forearm, wrist, and hand; no swelling or atrophy, especially of the thenar eminence, the first dorsal interosseous muscle, or the hypothenar eminence is present. Palpation of the right forearm and the volar and dorsal wrist reveal localized tenderness at the lateral epicondyle, in the area just proximal to the epicondyle, and at the anatomic snuff box.

### Range of motion

Active motions of the right elbow in flexion, extension, pronation and supination are painless and within the normal range. Active motion of the wrist is limited and painful in wrist flexion and radial deviation. Passive testing of the elbow in flexion, extension, pronation, supination, valgus, and varus are within normal range and painless except for pain at the lateral right epicondyle on passive pronation. Passive right wrist flexion is limited to 85 to 90 degrees compared to the left wrist, with minimal pain at the lateral right epicondyle. Passive right wrist radial and ulnar deviation is painful on the radial side of the wrist.

### Provocative examination

Resisted isometric testing of the wrist is painful on wrist extension and supination. Resisted supination of the wrist with the elbow extended aggravates the lateral elbow. Resisted flexion and extension at the elbow is negative. Mill's maneuvre and Finkelstein's test reproduce the patient's complaints. Point tenderness is located at the scaphoid.

### Neurologic examination
Sensory evaluation of light touch and pain are within normal limits. Deep tendon reflexes are +2 and bilaterally symmetric.

### Radiologic examination
Radiographic examination of the elbow and wrist is negative for fractures, dislocations, or soft tissue abnormalities. A hairline fracture is present at the scaphoid bone of the wrist.

- How does this information contribute to understanding what is wrong with Steve?

### Case OBJECTIVES

1. Describe the anatomy and biomechanics of the elbow and wrist.
2. Describe the anatomy of the radial, median, and ulnar nerves at the elbow and wrist.
3. Describe chronic inflammation. What importance does it have in this case?
4. Describe and perform the orthopedic tests at the elbow and wrist. How are the tests performed, what is a positive finding, and which anatomic structures are being tested?
5. Define the protocol and perform selective tissue tension tests at the elbow and wrist.
6. Describe the ranges of motion at the elbow and the wrist.
7. Describe the radiologic views of the elbow and wrist.
8. Develop a list of differential diagnoses. Compare and contrast these maladies.
9. Develop a treatment and management protocol for this case. What are the immediate, intermediate, and long-term goals? Develop a reactivation program for this patient.
10. Develop a protocol for adjusting or manipulating the elbow and wrist. Provide a scientific basis for the developed protocol. What are the goals for this protocol?

### CASE 21

Silvia S., a 27-year-old computer operator, is seen at your office with a complaint of right wrist pain and hand fatigue. She does not recall any trauma that could have caused her symptoms but states that the wrist pain began 6 months earlier. The hand fatigue is a more recent event that started about 4 or 5 days previously. The pain in her wrist has been getting gradually worse. It started as a dull ache and is now radiating into the thumb, the first finger, and the middle finger. The pain is of the sharp-shooting type and occurs only when Silvia puts her wrist in a certain position. The dull ache, at the volar aspect of the wrist, is still present. There is no pain on the radial aspect of the wrist. The wrist pain is least when she awakens in the morning and gradually increases as she works at the computer terminal. The hand fatigue does not show any temporal relationship. Silvia is very proud of her typing skills (100 words per minute) and is unhappy that her wrist and hand problems are slowing her down. Soaking her wrist and hand in hot water for about 20 minutes provides relief for about 2 hours. If she wraps her wrist the pain decreases slightly, but she is unable to type at her usual speed. On occasion, the right wrist pain awakens her during the night; however, the pain dissipates if she shakes her hands and wrists and she can go back to sleep. She wakes up about once or twice nightly. She has not been to any other physician for this problem.

Silvia has never had wrist or hand problems and has been working at her computer job for the past 2 years. Her previous job was in a printing bindery, and she did not have any wrist or hand problems at that time.

Her medical history is unremarkable. Her family history reveals that her husband passed away 1 year previously in an automobile accident, and she has two healthy sons, 9 years and 6 years of age, to take care of. Being the sole supporter of the family, Silvia cannot take time off from work.

- What could be happening to Sylvia?

### Examination
Vital signs.
  Blood pressure: 122/86 mm Hg
  Pulse rate: 80 beats/min
  Respiration rate: 14 breaths/min
  Temperature: 98.9° F
  Height: 5'4''
  Weight: 150 lb
Inspection of the right wrist does not reveal any gross abnormalities, effusions, or abrasions. Muscle atrophy of the thenar and hypothenar eminence of the hand is not present. Palpation of the palmar aspect is supple. The patient's dull ache pain is elicited over the palmar (volar) retinaculum of the right wrist.

### Range of motion
Gross active range of motion of the patient's right wrist is limited in flexion and extension because of the reproduction of her radicular pain complaints. All other ranges are within normal limits. Intersegmental motion palpation of the wrist reveals restrictions between the scaphoid and the trapezoid bones, and the capitate and the lunate bones. The metacarpal bones and phalanges move freely during passive motion palpation. A handshake of the right hand reveals overall weakness and reproduces the patient's pain complaints. During the handshake the patient also complains of a sharp, shooting type of pain into the thumb and first finger.

### Orthopedic examination
Right hand:
  Tinel's test (+)
  Phalen's test (+)
  Finkelstein's test (−)
  Froment's test (−)

### Neurologic examination
Sensory evaluation of pain in the right hand reveals dysesthesias and a decrease in sensation along the thenar eminence when compared to the left hand thenar eminence. DTRs are scored +2 and are bilaterally symmetric. Muscle testing reveals weakness (+4) during the thumb and first finger and the first and second finger opposition strength tests.

Muscle testing of thumb and fifth finger opposition reveals weakness in the thumb only. Muscle weakness is also revealed during thumb flexion and abduction. Thumb flexion reveals weakness at the metacarpophalangeal (MCP) and carpometacarpal (CMC) joints only, and not at the distal phalanx. Sylvia has difficulty making a fist, with the thumb, the first finger, and the second finger lagging behind.

### Radiologic examination
The A-P, lateral, and oblique radiographs of the patient's wrists did not reveal any bone abnormalities.

An electromyogram (EMG) and a nerve conduction velocity (NCV) study were ordered to further evaluate the muscle tests of the right hand. The EMG reveals a decrease in muscle activity of the flexor pollicis brevis and the opponens pollicis of the right hand when compared to the left. At rest, the EMG reveals spikes indicative of muscle denervation. NCV of the right median nerve reveals slowing within the carpal tunnel when compared to the NCV of the left median nerve.

• What does this information tell you about Sylvia's hand condition?

### Case OBJECTIVES

1. Describe the anatomy and biomechanics of the wrist.
2. Describe the anatomy of the carpal tunnel and the tunnel of Guyon. What is the relationship of these tunnels to wrist motion?
3. Describe and perform muscle tests of the hand. What is the grading system used to evaluate muscle strength?
4. Define NCV testing and electromyography (EMG). How are these tests performed and what anatomic structures are these tests evaluating? What do the results tell you about this case?
5. Describe the radiologic views needed to evaluate the wrist.
6. Develop a list of differential diagnoses. How would the case history differ if the cause of the problem is systemic?
7. Develop a treatment and management protocol for this patient. What are the immediate, intermediate, and long-term goals? What rehabilitative exercises would benefit this patient?
8. Develop a protocol for adjusting or manipulating the patient. What technique(s) would best benefit this patient?

### CASE 22

Alyssia T., a 34-year-old college registrar, comes to your office with a complaint of pain in the radial aspect of her right wrist. She states that this pain has been present for the past 6 weeks. Alyssia does not remember what exactly started the problem but has noticed that the pain increases after long periods of writing. She describes the problem as a well-localized deep ache that sometimes refers into the dorsum of her right thumb and the lateral aspect of the forearm. She is wearing a wrist band on the recommendation of a friend because it "helped her when she had wrist pain." The band provides some relief, but toward the end of the day she is in a lot of discomfort. She rates the pain as a 3 in the morning and a 7 in the evening on a 0 to 10 scale (10 being the pain after she broke her thumb). She has not had any wrist problems other than this complaint.

Alyssia's medical history reveals that she drinks a glass of wine daily and that on occasion she has epigastric pain. She does not smoke and does not use any recreational drugs. She is not married. Her parents, as far as she is aware do not have any medical problems. Her father is a carpenter and her mother is a housewife.

• What could be happening to Alyssia?

#### Examination
Vital signs.
  Blood pressure: 132/84 mm Hg

Pulse rate: 72 beats/min
Respiration rate: 12 breaths/min
Temperature: 97.8° F
Height: 5'1"
Weight: 134 lb

Inspection of the wrist reveals no discolorations, hematomas, or swellings. Exquisite point tenderness is located in the anatomic snuff box and when the area is palpated, pain radiates along the lateral forearm.

#### *Range of motion*
Range of motion of the right wrist is within normal limits in all ranges except ulnar deviation. Ulnar deviation is limited to 5 degrees and produces pain in the anatomic snuff box.

On motion palpation of the right wrist, flexion and extension produces normal translation and rotation motions; however, on ulnar deviation the patient complains of an increase of pain and the translation and rotation components cannot be properly evaluated. Radial deviation is within normal limits. Static and motion palpation of the elbow reveals a normal carrying angle, normal translation (gliding), and rotation on flexion and extension elbow motions. Supination and pronation motions are within normal limits as well.

#### *Orthopedic examination*
Right wrist
  Tinel's test (−)
  Finkelstein's test (+)
  Phalen's test (−)

Right elbow
  varsus (−)
  valgus (−)
  Mill's test (−)
  Tinel's test (−)

#### *Neurologic examination*
Sensory evaluation is within normal limits. Muscle testing of the elbow flexors with the forearm supinated and pronated reveals normal muscle strength. Muscle testing reveals slight weakness (+4 on a 5-point scale) on wrist extension and radial deviation in the right wrist when compared to the left wrist. This weakness may be caused by the patient's increase in pain. Deep tendon reflexes are +2 and bilaterally symmetric.

#### *Radiologic examination*
An x-ray examination of the right wrist does not reveal a fracture of the scaphoid bone. All other anatomic structures are within normal limits.

• How does this information add to the determination of what is wrong with Alyssia?

### Case OBJECTIVES

1. Describe the anatomy and biomechanics of the wrist and the hand.
2. Describe the anatomy of the anatomic snuff box.
3. Describe chronic inflammation. What significance does it have to this case?
4. Describe and perform the orthopedic provocative tests that are presented in this case. How are these tests performed, what is a positive result, and which anatomic structures are being tested?

5. Compare and contrast the history and physical examination of a patient with carpal tunnel syndrome, tunnel of Guyon syndrome, and de Quervain's disease.
6. Compare and contrast the history, physical examination, and radiologic interpretation of de Quervain's disease and scaphoid fracture.
7. Describe the radiologic views utilized in this case.
8. Develop a treatment and management protocol for this patient. What are the immediate, intermediate, and long-term goals that would help this patient? Is adjustment or manipulation necessary? If so, develop a protocol to evaluate the treatment's success.

## CASE 23

Esther P., a 61-year-old grandmother and retired bookkeeper, visits your office with a complaint of right midinguinal and anterior thigh pain. She states that the pain began 1 day after she was mugged and pushed to the ground by her assailant, an incident that had occurred 4 days previously. She remembers falling on her right side. She was able to get up after the assailant left with her purse.

She called her daughter who promptly took her to the emergency room where a brief history was taken and an examination was performed. Radiographs of Esther's lower back and hips were normal. She was sent home to rest and recuperate and instructed to contact her physician should any problems occur. Esther describes the pain as a consistent dull ache around her right hip. When she moves her lower extremity in a certain direction the pain becomes sharp and travels into the inguinal region and the anterior aspect of the right thigh. The only time that she feels the sharp pain is during walking (to the market) or standing for long periods of time (while doing housework). Lying down or sitting both alleviate the pain, with lying down providing greater relief. The area of greatest pain is located in the middle of the inguinal ligament and femoral triangle. She rates the pain during walking as a 6 on a 0 to 10 scale (a score of 10 being the pain of childbirth). Her pain has been getting worse and is now causing her to limp. She has been taking her sister's Motrin (two tables of 200 mg each, three times daily), but it has not been helping her very much. A heating pad and hot baths have both given her temporary relief. She has no bowel or bladder problems and does not smoke tobacco or drink alcohol.

• What is happening to Esther?

### Examination
Vital signs.
    Blood pressure: 135/84 mm Hg
    Pulse rate: 80 beats/min
    Respiration rate: 15 breaths/min
    Temperature: 98.7° F
    Height: 5'3''
    Weight: 120 lb
Point tenderness is located over the anterolateral aspect of the right iliac crest and the middle region of the right inguinal ligament. The patient has hematomas around the right but-

tock (in the area of the greater trochanter) and the proximal thigh. Abrasions are present over the right trochanter. Mrs. P. displays a limp towards the right side, and the plumb line, viewed from the right side, reveals an anterior lean of the upper trunk.

### Range of motion
Passive and active ranges of motion (ROM) of the lumbar spine are within normal limits. There is pain in the right lumbosacral area, the anterior iliac crest and midinguinal area at 60 degrees of flexion and 10 degrees of extension during active motion. The patient describes this pain as a dull ache located in the right SI and midinguinal areas.

### Orthopedic provocative examination
Provocative testing of the lumbar spine reveals negative SLR, Braggard's test, and Valsalva's manuever. Trendelenburg's test is questionable because the patient is not able to perform the test because of pain.

Range of motion of the right hip is limited with pain located at the midinguinal area during all motions. The patient is unable to put the right hip into a "figure 4" position (Patrick's FABERE test). Other provocative tests are not performed at this time because of the patient's pain complaints.

### Neurologic examination
All deep tendon reflexes of the lower extremities are rated +2 and are bilaterally symmetric. Babinski's reflex is not present. Pin-prick examination is negative over the lower back and the entire lower extremity. Muscle tests of the hip are not performed because of pain. Muscle tests at the knee and ankle joints are within normal limits.

### Radiologic examination
Radiographs of the right and left hips reveal a bilateral generalized loss of bone density with a slight ischemic necrosis of the right femoral head. An oblique fracture line (poorly defined line of sclerosis) is located at the subcapital region of the femoral neck on the A-P view of the right hip. Shenton's line is not interrupted bilaterally. The normal trabecular pattern in the femoral head and neck is greatly reduced in both the left and the right hips. There are no other bone abnormalities observed on the hip views.

### Laboratory examination
A CBC and UA are unremarkable.

• How does this information add to the determination of what is wrong with Esther?

### Case OBJECTIVES
1. Describe the anatomy and biomechanics of the hip joint.
2. Describe spiral, oblique, shear, three-point bending, and four-point bending fractures.
3. Describe the trabeculation of the hip joint. What causes the pattern seen in the hip?
4. Describe the inflammatory response when injury to bone occurs.
5. Describe the osteogenesis of healing bone. Of what significance is this knowledge for the treatment of this patient?
6. Describe the radiologic views that were taken in this case.

7. Describe the radiologic lines of mensuration used to evaluate the hip.
8. Describe the treatment and management protocols for this patient. What are the immediate, intermediate, and long-term goals for this patient?

## CASE 24

Sharon L., a 23-year-old woman, complains of right knee pain, which is of 3 months' duration. She states that the pain began during a long-distance run (7 miles). She is an avid runner who enjoys running 25 to 30 miles weekly. She participates in 10-kilometer running races monthly and has a time of 43 minutes. She has decided to train for a marathon and has recently increased her distance to 40 miles weekly. She has been training at this new distance for the last 3 months. Her pain is located on the medial inferior pole of the right patella and does not radiate into any other area. She scores the pain as a 1 on a 1 to 10 scale (10 being the pain resulting from a split toenail) during normal daily activity and as a 5 when she runs. The pain gradually increases during her run and reaches the rating of 5 at about the halfway mark. Uphill running does not increase her pain, but downhill running increases the pain rating to a 7. She has no recollection of having problems with any other lower extremity joint.

Sharon's medical history is unremarkable. Her parents are alive and well and have no history of knee problems. She has two sisters (both are younger) and they do not have knee problems either.

### Examination
Vital signs.
> Blood pressure: 110/78 mm Hg
> Pulse rate: 60 beats/min
> Respiration rate: 13 breaths/min
> Temperature: 98.4° F
> Height: 5'5"
> Weight: 110 lb

Inspection does not reveal any bruising, hematomas, or gross abnormalities. Palpation of the right knee reveals point tenderness at the medial inferior pole of the patella. The patellar tendon is supple and does not produce the patient's pain complaints when pressure is put upon it. The tibial tuberosity is not pressure sensitive either. Frontal plane plumb-line evaluation indicates a slight genu valgum of both knees; however, the Q angle appears symmetrically bilateral and within normal angular limits. Patella alta is not present in either knee. Gait analysis reveals the pain of the patient's chief complaint to occur between the flat foot and the midstance of the stance phase of gait. The patient's shoes show correct distribution of pressure and the foot does not seem to pronate excessively during gait.

### Range of motion
The right knee is limited in flexion with pain being produced at 125 degrees. Extension is within normal limits, and Helfet's test reveals normal motion of the tibia.

### Orthopedic examination
> Valgus/varus test (−)
> Apprehension test (−)
> Clark's test (−)
> Slocum's test (−)
> Pivot shift test (−)
> McMurry's test (−)

The patella moves easily during palpation. The quadriceps, hamstring, triceps surae, adductor, and abductor muscles are +5 on a 5-point scale and are bilaterally symmetric. The quadriceps are 40% stronger than the hamstring muscles. Muscle length testing reveals a tight iliotibial band.

Evaluations of the lower back, thigh, leg, ankle, and foot are within normal limits.

### Neurologic examination
All dermatomes of the lower extremity are within normal limits. DTRs are rated +2 and are bilaterally symmetric and muscle tests are +5 on a 5-point scale and bilaterally symmetric.

### Radiologic examination
A radiologic examination of the knee is deferred at this time.

### Case OBJECTIVES

1. Describe the anatomy of the knee (the patellofemoral and femorotibial joints).
2. Explain the gait cycle (kinematics and kinetics).
3. Describe the motions of the knee and patella during the gait cycle. How does patellar and knee motion differ during gait and passive and active ranges of motion evaluations?
4. Describe patellar tracking during gait evaluation.
5. Describe the location and type of pain the patient with a patellar tracking problem exhibits.
6. Describe the orthopedic tests. How are these tests performed, what is a positive finding, and which anatomic structures are being tested?
7. Describe the normal strength ratio between the quadriceps and the hamstring muscles. What information do the muscle tests provide about this patient's problem?
8. Develop a list of differential diagnoses. Compare and contrast these maladies.
9. Develop a treatment and management protocol for this case. What rehabilitative exercises would best benefit this patient? What are the immediate, intermediate, and long-term goals for this patient? Define and perform McConnell taping for patellar tracking problems.

## CASE 25

Tracy V. is a 25-year-old woman who is seen at your office with a very swollen right ankle. During a 3-mile run this morning, her right foot landed on a part of uneven pavement and she has twisted her ankle severely. She fell when it happened and, for several minutes, was unable to stand on the right foot because of ankle pain. She did not hear a rip or a tear, but the ankle became swollen almost instantly.

She walked home and immediately put her ankle and foot into a bucket of ice water. You decide that Tracy should go home and rest the ankle, apply ice to it with compression, and elevate it (R.I.C.E.) and return for a check up in 2 days.

Two days later, Tracy returns to your office. She claims that the ankle feels slightly better but is very swollen and black and blue. She now points to the pain as being located over the lateral malleolus, on the anterior aspect of the foot, and over the cuboid bone. It is still very difficult for her to walk on the ankle and she limps (away from the injured side).

She has no previous history of an ankle problem. Her medical and family history are unremarkable.

- What could be happening to Tracy?

### Examination

Vital signs.
    Blood pressure: 98/60 mm Hg
    Pulse rate: 58 beats/min
    Respiration rate: 12 beats/min
    Temperature: 98.6° F
    Height: 5'2''
    Weight: 105 lb

The right ankle is swollen at the lateral malleolus with a hematoma located at the lateral aspect of the heel pad of the foot. Point tenderness is located at the distal end and anterior aspect of the lateral malleolus. The foot is also tender to touch at the dorsal retinaculum and at the medial side of the cuboid bone.

### Range of motion

The patient's active range of motion is limited. Dorsiflexion is 20 degrees and reproduces the patient's pain complaints. Plantarflexion is 10 degrees and also reproduces the patient's pain complaints. The passive range of motion is painful and does not increase the active range of motion. Calcaneal inversion is limited (10 degrees) and produces pain at the lateral malleolus. Calcaneal eversion is limited (20 degrees) and reproduces the cuboid pain.

### Orthopedic examination

Anterior drawer (−)
Medial stability tests (?)
Kleiger test (−)
Tinel tap test (−)

### Neurologic examination

Responses to light touch, pain, and temperature are within normal limits. Reflexes of the lower extremity are +2 and bilaterally symmetric.

### Radiologic examination

Radiographs of the right ankle did not reveal any fractures, dislocations, or bone abnormalities. Ankle stress x-ray examination did not reveal any instability of the right ankle.

- How does this information help you decide what is wrong with Tracy?

### Case OBJECTIVES

1. Describe the anatomy and biomechanics of the ankle and the foot.
2. Describe the anatomy of the most common ankle sprains. When is the ankle most commonly injured during gait?
3. Describe the kinesiology (kinetics and kinematics) of human locomotion.
3. Define swelling, edema, and hematoma. What do these findings tell you about a soft tissue injury?
4. Describe and perform the orthopedic provocative tests. How are the tests performed, what is a positive result, and which anatomic structures are being tested?
5. Describe the radiologic views needed to evaluate the ankle.

What are ankle stress views and how do they help determine which anatomic structures are injured in this case?
6. Describe the sequence of soft tissue healing. How does this knowledge assist the clinician in developing a management program for this patient?
7. Describe the categorization of sprains. What sprain grade is this patient's presentation?
8. Develop a treatment and management protocol for this case. What physiologic therapy (for example, R.I.C.E.) and rehabilitative exercises would best benefit this patient? What are the immediate, intermediate, and long-term goals for this patient? Would patterned motion exercises (for example, a wobble board) help this patient?

## CASE 26

Christine J., a 37-year-old woman, arrives at your office complaining of inferior heel pain in her left foot. She first noticed her pain after a 6-mile run approximately 2 weeks earlier. She describes the pain as a burning sensation located at the bottom of her left heel. Christine continued to run (6 to 10 miles/day, 5 to 6 days/week) over the next 10 days without treatment. During this time she experienced morning pain and stiffness that would diminish after she took a few steps but then gradually increase during the day. Climbing stairs and running exacerbated her condition, and eventually the pain and burning progressed to the point where she stopped running 3 days earlier. At present, any weight-bearing activities lead to severe pain in the left heel and arch, causing her to walk on the lateral aspect of her foot.

Her medical history is unremarkable except for occasional lower back pain and a chronic right knee pain that was diagnosed as an iliotibial band friction syndrome by her family physician.

Christine is a high school English teacher and has been an avid runner for 15 years. During the past 3 years she averages approximately 50 miles each week and competes in 5- and 10-kilometer road races. She and her husband have been married for 5 years and have a 3½-year-old daughter.

- What could be happening to Christine?

### Examination

Vital signs.
    Blood pressure: 110/74 mm Hg
    Pulse rate: 64 beats/min
    Respiration rate: 12 breaths/min
    Temperature: 98.8° F
    Height: 5'1''
    Weight: 112 lb

Examination reveals a well-proportioned 37 year old woman who appears to be in excellent health. She walks with a limp, favoring her left foot.

The patient's involved foot is not swollen or discolored. Palpation reveals localized tenderness at the medial process of the calcaneal tuberosity of her left foot. This tenderness extends distally to the midarch. Slight tenderness is noted at the left Achilles tendon approximately 2.5 cm proximal to the attachment on the calcaneus.

### Range of motion

Passive dorsiflexion of the left ankle with extended toes cause extreme discomfort to the bottom of her foot. There is decreased left ankle dorsiflexion with the knee fully extended when compared to the right side.

### Neurologic examination

The neurologic exam is negative for motor and sensory deficits. Tinel's sign is negative for nerve entrapment.

Examination of joint play movements reveal restrictions at the left talocrural joint in long-axis extension (traction), subtalar rock, and anteroposterior glide of the tarsometatarsal joints.

### Radiologic examination

X-ray films of the left ankle and foot do not reveal any bone abnormalities. Slight soft tissue swelling is noted around the Achilles tendon and the origin of the plantar fascia. No other significant signs are present.

- How does this information add to determining what is wrong with Christine?

## Case OBJECTIVES

1. Describe the anatomy of the foot.
2. Describe the biomechanics of the foot during gait (kinematics and kinetics). What is the importance of the plantar fascia during gait (truss and windlass)?
3. Describe the relationship between the triceps surae and the plantar fascia.
4. Define joint play. What are the different types of joint play and of what significance are they to this case?
5. Explain the range of motion findings in the ankle.
6. Develop a list of differential diagnoses. Compare and contrast these maladies.
7. Develop a treatment and management protocol for this case. What rehabilitative exercises would best benefit this patient? What are the immediate, intermediate, and long-term goals for this patient? Would plyometric exercises help this patient?

# CHAPTER 2

# Neuroscience of the neuromusculoskeletal system

*KEY TERMS*

| | |
|---|---|
| *Spinal cord* | *Monosynaptic reflex arc* |
| *Brain stem* | *Myoneuro junction* |
| *Cerebellum* | *Muscle spindle* |
| *Basal ganglia* | *Golgi tendon organ* |
| *Cerebral cortex* | *Neuron and axon* |
| *Cranial nerves* | *Myelin sheath* |
| *Sensory and motor tracts* | *Somites: myotome,* |
| *Vestibular system* | *dermatome and sclerotome* |
| *Proprioception* | *Melzak-Wall pain-gait theory* |
| *Nociception* | |

The first step in understanding neurologic disease is to consider embryologic development of the neuromusculoskeletal (NMS) system. The components of this system are interrelated and functionally interdependent. In simple terms, a stimulus from the neurologic system causes muscle contraction that results in human motion. The proper embryologic development of these systems is of paramount importance in perceiving sensation and performing movements, and knowledge of this process assists the clinician in diagnosis of functional maladies.

## EMBRYOLOGIC DEVELOPMENT OF THE NEUROMUSCULAR SYSTEM

The science of embryology provides the clinician with the understanding of human development. This section will introduce basic concepts of the embryologic development of the structures of the neuromusculoskeletal system including the central, the peripheral, and the autonomic nervous systems.

This discussion of embryology will begin at the stage of development of the mesodermal cell layer. The fertilization process and the development of the blastocyst with the inner cell mass to form the trophoblast will not be discussed.

### Formation of somites (primitive body segments)

Tuan Tran

During the formation of the notochord and neural tube in the third week of embryologic development, the adjacent paraxial mesoderm organizes itself into longitudinal columns that segment into clusters or blocks that are called *somitomeres* in the cephalic region and *somites* in the occipital and caudal regions. Somites are responsible for the segmentation of the future neuromusculoskeletal system and the development of dermatomes, myotomes, and sclerotomes.[35,39] The organization of the somites begins at the cephalic region and proceeds toward the caudal region, with the first pair of somites being formed by the twentieth day of development. It has been estimated that about three new pairs of somites are formed each day, with a total of 42 to 44 pairs of somites formed by the end of the fifth week of intrauterine life[12,39] (Table 2-1).

Further organization of the mesodermal cells in the somites lead to the regression and disappearance of the first pair of occipital somites and the last few pairs of coccygeal somites. The remaining occipital somites form the structures of the cranium and head.[39,46] The cells of the somites are also precursors of most of the axial skeleton (spinal column, sternum, ribs, and some cranial bones) and related musculature, including the dermal layer of the skin.

**Differentiation of individual somites.** Individual somites undergo further morphologic changes and differentiate into three components: the dermatome, the myotome, and the sclerotome (Fig. 2-1). A central cavity, the myocele, is first formed, and the sclerotome, separating from the somite, migrates medially and surrounds the notochord and neural tube. The migrating sclerotomal cells develop an irregular shape and begin to produce chondroitin sulfate, proteoglycans, and other biochemical products that format the cartilage matrix. Eventually, the sclerotomal cells multiply rapidly to form the primordium of the base of the skull, the spinal column, and the rib cage. In the primordial spinal column, the

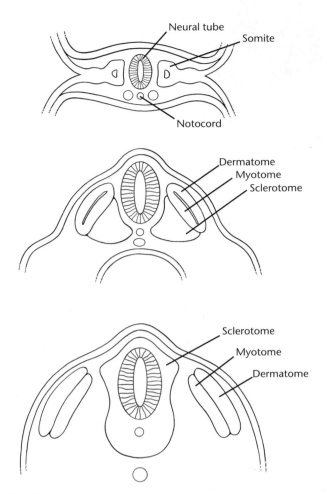

**Fig. 2-1** Embryologic development of the dermatome, myotome, and sclerotome from somite.

notochord is incorporated into the sclerotome and its remnant becomes the nucleus pulposus of the intervertebral disc.[12,35]

**Development of dermatomes, myotomes, and sclerotomes.** The cells remaining in the somite after separation of the sclerotome are referred to as the dermomyotome. The cells separate into a dorsal (external) layer called the dermatome and a medial (deep) layer of elongated cells known as the myotome. The cells of the dermatome will eventually migrate externally toward the ectoderm to form the dermis. The cells of the myotome represent the embryonic mesodermal cells that will differentiate into myoblasts and form the musculature of the body. These cells migrate medially as the epimere to form the muscles of the back, and laterally, as the hypomere to form the muscles of the trunk and limbs.[43] The head and neck musculature is formed from the branchial arches. The corresponding spinal nerves will also separate into dorsal and ventral components, entering the epimere and hypomere, respectively, for future innervation.

*Table 2-1*  Classification of the somites as they are formed

| |
|---|
| 4 pairs of occipital somites |
| 8 pairs of cervical somites |
| 12 pairs of thoracic somites |
| 5 pairs of lumbar somites |
| 5 pairs of sacral somites |
| 6-8 pairs of coccygeal somites |

## Development of the central nervous system

The wall of the neural tube consists of multipotential neuroepithelial cells derived from ectoderm. These cells multiply, migrate, and differentiate to establish the concentric layers of the neural tube.[44] Cell division occurs primarily in the innermost layer, which is the ventricular zone that consists of a single layer of pseudostratified epithelium. The marginal zone is located at the outermost layer of the neural tube and consists of the cytoplasmic processes of the cells of the ventricular layer. Between the ventricular and the marginal zones are the subventricular and intermediate zones (formerly called the mantle zone), the cells of which divide and migrate to the cortical plate, developing synaptic connections. The subventricular zone is a repository for the spongioblasts that give rise to astrocytes, oligodendrocytes, and ependymal cells.[43] The ependymal cells form the ependymal layer that lines the brain cavities, whereas the astrocytes and oligodendroglia migrate to all areas of the central nervous system (CNS). The astrocytes provide mechanical support and maintain the chemical environment for the neurons, and the oligodendroglia form the myelin sheaths by repeatedly wrapping layers of their cytoplasmic membranes around the axons. The cytoplasm then condenses to form myelin (Fig. 2-2).[44]

By the fifth week of embryologic life (day 25 to 30) the prosencephalon (forebrain), mesencephalon (midbrain), and rhombencephalon (hindbrain) form from the rostral portion of the neural tube. The telencephalon (endbrain) and diencephalon (interbrain) arise from the prosencephalon to form the cerebral hemispheres and the thalamus and hypothalamus, respectively. The rhombencephalon produces two structures: the metencephalon (afterbrain), which consists of the pons and cerebellum, and the myelencephalon or medulla.[32] The mesencephalon and the caudal portion of the neural tube remain undivided, with the latter becoming the spinal cord (Table 2-2).

**The spinal cord.** The spinal cord develops from the ectodermal layer of the neural plate. The neural plate lies along the dorsal midline of the embryo and through neural induction becomes committed to the formation of the CNS. The cells of the neural plate move toward the margins of the neural plate to form the centrally positioned neural groove, the closure of which forms the neural tube. The groove first closes in the neck area of the embryo; closure then proceeds in a caudal and rostral direction. The caudal, the intermediate, and the rostral portions of the neural tube develop into the spinal cord, the brainstem, and the hemispheres, respectively.[32,44] The cavity inside the neural tube will develop into the ventricular system of the brain.

Epithelial cells, called the neuroectoderm, lining the neural tube (the ependymal layer) develop into the neurons (neuroblasts) and glial cells (macroglioblasts) of the CNS. The cells of the neuroectoderm divide repeatedly and become the neurons and glial cells of the CNS gray matter.[3] Some of the neuroectodermal cells migrate to the mantle layer and provide scaffolding for this layer before proceeding to the marginal layer to develop the axonal processes that form the tracts of the brain and spinal cord.[4] The name of each tract is determined by the final destination of each bundle of axons (for example, the spinothalamic tract).[3]

The cells in the mantle layer of the embryonic spinal cord align into two columns: the alar plate (formed in the dorsal portion) and basal plate (formed in the ventral portion). Neuroblasts in the neural tube in the spinal cord area accumulate laterally and proliferate to form the dorsal and ventral regions. The plates are separated

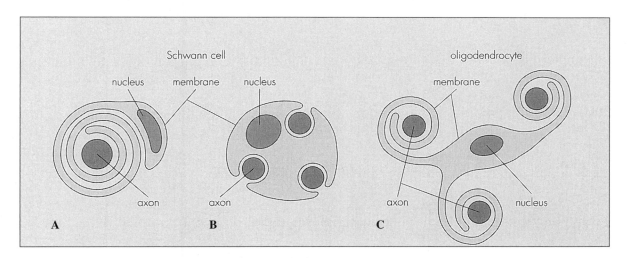

*Fig. 2-2* **A-C,** Wrapping of oligodengroglia, forming a myelin sheath. Note that the oligodengroglia encases the unmyelinated axon but does not wrap itself around it. (From: McMinn RM, Gaddum-Rosse P, Hutchings RT, Logan BM: *McMinn's functional and clinical anatomy,* St. Louis, 1995, Mosby, with permission.)

*Table 2-2*    Major anatomic structures of the adult nervous system derived from the neural tube

| Primary divisions | Level | Subdivisions | Major derivatives | Cavities |
|---|---|---|---|---|
| Prosencephalon | Supratentorial | Telencephalon | Rhinencephalon<br>Basal ganglia<br>Cerebral cortex | Lateral ventricles |
| | | Diencephalon | Thalamus<br>Hypothalamus<br>Optic nerves<br>Neurohypophysis<br>Pineal gland | Third ventricle |
| Mesencephalon | Posterior fossa | Mesencephalon | Midbrain | Aqueduct of Sylvius |
| Rhombencephalon | | Metencephalon | Cerebellum<br>Pons | Fourth ventricle |
| | | Myelencephalon | Medulla | |
| Primitive neural tube | Spinal<br>Peripheral | Neural tube<br>Neural crest | Spinal cord<br>Peripheral nerves<br>Ganglia | Central canal |

*Adapted from: Westmoreland B et al.: Medical neurosciences, ed 3, Boston, 1994, Little, Brown & Co.*

by a shallow groove called the sulcus limitans. The alar plate will mediate sensory input to the cord and become the posterior horn of the spinal cord. The basal plate will develop into the motor neurons in the ventral horn of the spinal cord (Fig. 2-3). Other neurons that do not align longitudinally and stay within the cord become the interneurons of the spinal cord.

**Growth of the spinal cord.** In the third month of embryologic development the spinal cord extends the entire length of the embryo (approximately 30 mm), and the spinal nerves pass through the intervertebral foramen.[39] As growth progresses, the vertebral column and dura lengthen more rapidly than does the spinal cord. At birth, the conus medullaris is located at L3. Further vertebral and spinal growth leads to the eventual position of the conus medullaris at T12 to L1 (Fig. 2-4).

## Development of the peripheral nervous system

Neurons whose cell bodies lie outside the CNS are derived from the neural crest located at the lateral margins of the neural plate. These cell bodies will form the dorsal root ganglia, the arachnoid, the pia mater, the chromaffin cells of the adrenal medulla, the postganglionic autonomic neurons, and the Schwann cells that form the myelin sheaths of the peripheral nervous system (PNS).

The axons from the cell bodies of the peripheral nerves develop in two locations: the dorsal root ganglia

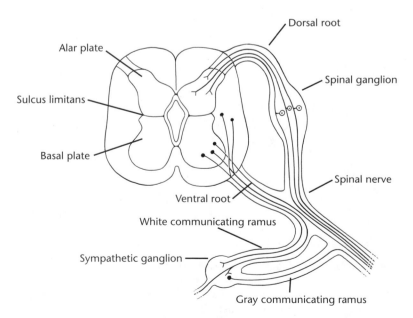

*Fig. 2-3*    Alar (sensory) and basal (motor) plates with axonal development.

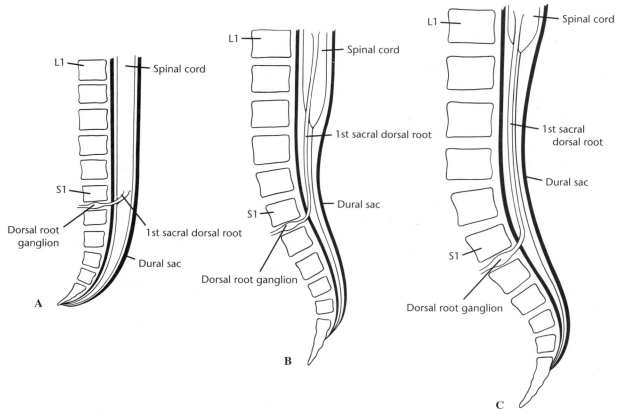

*Fig. 2-4*  Sequential growth of spinal cord. **A,** Embryonic cord extends entire length of vertebral column. **B,** Newborn infant, the spinal cord extends from L2 to L3. **C,** Adult, the spinal cord extends to L1.

and the basal plate. Sensory axons originate in the dorsal root ganglia, grow toward the alar plate, and then extend to the somites. The motor axons develop from the basal plate and grow distally to the somites. Growth of the axons occurs alongside the structures formed by the sclerotome, the myotome, and the dermatome of the corresponding somite. At the spinal level, these structures become the mixed spinal nerves. The neural processes of the spinal nerves are pulled along as the somites develop into the sclerotome, the myotome, and the dermatome, which differentiate into their corresponding anatomic structures.

Axons developing in the posterior fossa (brainstem) and at the supratentorial level become cranial nerves.[44] The motor axons join the corresponding myotome and the autonomic ganglia, whereas the sensory axons innervate the dermatomes, and the endodermal derivatives innervate the gut.

The dermatomal chart used by the clinician is correlated directly with embryologic development. The extremities develop from limb buds that twist at the seventh week of development. The upper limbs rotate 90° laterally and the lower limbs, 90° medially.[44] The twisting is also represented in the dermatomal map.

## Development of the autonomic nervous system

Neuroblasts located in the lateral horn of the future spinal cord begin to project into the ventral root to terminate in the sympathetic chain ganglia, or the prevertebral ganglia, where they meet with other cell bodies and terminate on glands (for example, the adrenal gland, which is formed by intermediate mesoderm) or smooth muscle of the vasculature supplying striated muscle.[3,35] The cell bodies of the motor efferents of the ANS originate from the basal plate of the mantle cells within the neural tube. Located in the sympathetic chain are other neuroblasts that are chemically drawn to the organs of innervation. These neurons originate in the neural crest and migrate to the chain ganglia. They then travel back to the spinal nerve, and as gray rami, travel within the ventral primary rami to the end organ.[3,44] On occasion, the gray rami do not accompany the spinal nerve but travel independently to the end organ, as is seen with the cardiac sympathetic nerves that travel directly to the heart.

Pre- and postparasympathetic neurons also originate from neuroblasts. These cells originate in the same areas as do the cranial nerves and the sacral area of the spinal cord. Some of the neuroblasts migrate with the end organ, whereas others remain in the neural tube.[44] Cytoplasmic extensions of the neuroblasts at the plate associate with those of neuroblasts in the end organ. Thus, as the developing end organs migrate to their destination, preganglionic extensions are developed.

## Embryologic development of the vertebral column
Tuan Tran

The vertebral column arises from the sclerotomal aspect of the somite. At the fourth week of gestation, the sclerotome migrates medially to surround the neural tube and notochord and to form a discrete series of neural arches.[46] Each neural arch sits on a group of sclerotomal cells called the centrum. The primitive vertebrae originate from the centrum and neural arches, which split into blocks that are divided by intersegmental arteries. The caudal portion of each neural arch and centrum condenses and joins the cephalic part of the underlying precartilaginous structure. Cells that migrate toward the notochord become the centrum primorium.

Between the neural arch and the centrum is a costal element that develops into a rib in the thoracic area, and in the cervical area, becomes part of the transverse process. In the sacral region, the costal element becomes part of the lateral aspect of the sacrum.

**Chondrification of the primordial blocks.** Each typical vertebra has three chondrification centers, one in the centrum and one in each neural arch. With further development, sites of ossification develop within the chondrified cartilage matrix. Secondary ossification centers are located in the spinous and transverse processes and the end plates of the vertebral bodies. Each typical vertebra therefore has three primary and five secondary ossification centers (Fig. 2-5).

Atypical vertebra differ in the number of ossification centers. An additional ossification center is located in the odontoid process of C2, which was originally the body of C1. The ossification center of the body of C2 fuses with the ossification center of the dens. The vertebrae form from a cartilaginous model in the first 3 months of in utero development. The model is formed by the vertebra body (centrum) that develops from the sclerotomal cells of a pair of somites that surround the notochord. The neural arches, which surround the neural tube, then fuse with the centrum to form a model of the whole vertebra. The three primary and five secondary ossification centers develop next. These centers are located at each vertebral arch (the lateral centers) at the transverse processes (TPs) and spinous processes (SPs) and at the centrum (the median centers). From the TPs and SPs, the ossification centers spread to produce the pedicles and other processes (articulating processes). The ossification of the vertebral arch begins in the seventh week of gestation and that of the centrum, at the eighth to tenth weeks.

The vertebral column is not entirely ossified at birth. In the newborn, each vertebra has three bony components: the centrum and the two halves of the ununited neural arch. The cartilaginous framework is present but calcification and ossification are not complete. By 1 year of age, the ossification centers will fuse, joining the neural arches with the centrum. The first area of the vertebral column to have the vertebral arches fused with the centrum is the cervical spine. This occurs by 3 years of age. Fusion in the lumbar spine is the last to occur and is completed by 6 years of age.

The five secondary ossification centers appear at 16 years of age. One secondary ossification center is located at each tip of the transverse process, one at the tip of the spinous process, and one each at the top and bottom of the centrum. On an x-ray film, the ossification centers at the top and bottom of each vertebral body can be seen to outline the epiphyseal plates. Complete ossification of the spine occurs at about 25 years of age; in women it occurs 2 years earlier.[14,34] This is why treatment for scoliosis must continue until the patient is 23 to 25 years of age. Ossification centers are present on x-ray films and should not be misconstrued as fractures. The age of spine can be determined by the presence of the secondary ossification centers located on the superior portion of the pelvis. At 13 years of age the lateralmost aspect of the pelvis begins to ossify. Ossification proceeds in a superior medial direction until complete fusion is achieved by 25 years of age. Risser's sign is used to determine bone age and development, and it reflects the progression of the secondary ossification center in the pelvis (see Case 11). If Risser's sign is present at an early age the clinician should consider the possibility of a preexisting physiologic problem (for example, a hormonal problem).

**Development of the intervertebral disc.** The intervertebral disc is derived from cells originating from the cephalic part of the sclerotome. The cells fill the space between the two precartilaginous bodies and form the annulus fibrosis. Mucoid degeneration of the notochord leads to the formation of the nucleus pulposus.

**Vertebral embryologic anomalies.** Several cases dealing with embryologic anomalies are presented in Chapter 1. A hemivertebra is a triangular malformation vertebra that is caused either by the failure of development of a primary ossification center, or by failure of one sclerotomal mass to migrate toward the notochord during early vertebral development. Consequently, only one side of the vertebra develops, resulting in a sharp lateral angulation that produces a severe vertebral scoliotic curve. If a hemivertebra occurs in the thoracic region, the associated rib is also absent.

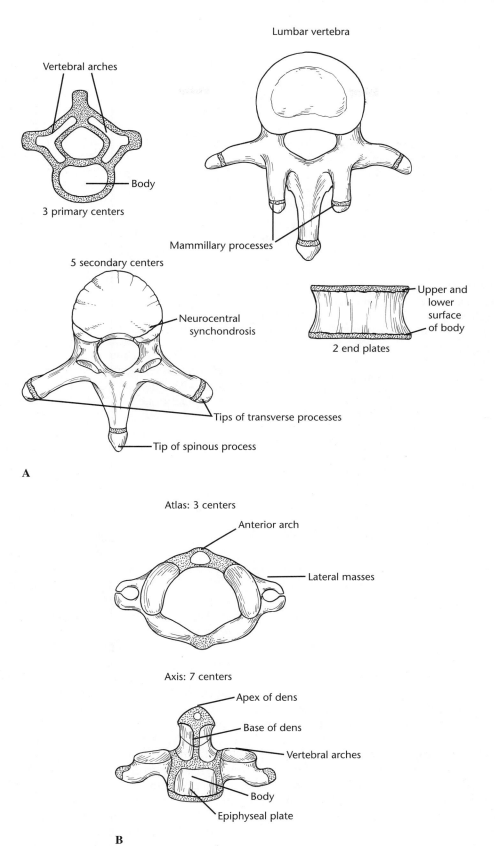

*Fig. 2-5*    Primary and secondary ossification centers of **A**, typical and **B**, atypical vertebrae.

Wedged vertebrae can be caused by either an embryologic anomaly or a mechanical problem. If there is incomplete formation of the sclerotomal blocks, a wedge may develop in the vertebral end plates. Another cause is improper growth of one half of a vertebra. This can be caused by unequal application of stresses and strains to the bone. The forces encountered by growing vertebrae play a major role in bone growth and development. Wolff's law states that bone responds to imposed demands. If the demand is too great, bone is reabsorbed, and, conversely, if the demand is low, the bone will not respond and therefore will not grow (Heuter-Volkmann's rule).

In early development, the somite is formed from paraxial mesoderm that migrates between the surface ectoderm that becomes a "flooring" for the early amniotic cavity and the neuroectoderm. Failure to migrate completely results in lack of the vertebral structures. These structures may not form at all, resulting in spinal bifida vera where the meninges and cord bulge out from the spinal column, leading to severe spinal and neurologic deformity. Another more common form of spina bifida is spina bifida occulta where the cartilaginous matrix is present but the ossification centers do not completely develop, leading to incomplete fusion of the posterior vertebral elements, as evidenced from x-ray films.

Spondylolysis can be caused by a developmental anomaly or by a fracture resulting from trauma. In its congenital presentation, marked flattening of the vertebral body and the lack of mesenchymal tissue of the vertebral arch at the lamina–articular process junction occurs. The lack of mesenchymal tissue prevents bone development and gives the appearance of a break or separation between the lamina and the articular process. The most common location of spondylolysis is at L4 and L5. Spondylolisthesis (see Case 11) may occur with spondylolysis when forces applied to the inferior articular processes are not dissipated, and the vertebral body is displaced forward.

## Embryologic development of long bone
Emile Goubran

Bone development (osteogenesis or ossification) occurs in two ways: By *intramembranous* ossification, in which bone develops in mesenchymal membranes (for example, the skull), and by *intracartilaginous* ossification, in which bone develops in a cartilage model (for example, long bones). Long bones develop by intracartilaginous ossification in the first trimester of in utero life, and this process occurs by the replacement of the cartilage model with bone. Intracartilaginous ossification will be discussed in this section.

The cartilage model closely represents the future bone in shape. The model consists of hyaline cartilage covered by perichondrium and grows in size by both interstitial and appositional mechanisms.

The process of ossification begins in the middle segment, in which the perichondrium assumes an osteogenic function because some of its cells differentiate to osteoblasts.[45] The cells then start to form bone of the intramembranous type and a ring of spongy bone surrounds the central segment of the shaft. This is the periosteal bone collar[41] that is now covered by periosteum. While the bone collar is developing, the central region of the diaphysis shows large, arranged cartilage cells. These cells are the oldest and are capable of producing the enzyme alkaline phosphatase that causes the cartilage matrix around the mature cartilage cells to calcify. Because of calcification, the cartilage cells are nutritionally deprived and consequently degenerate and die, leaving their lacunae empty. Sprouts from the periosteum over the periosteal collar, called periosteal buds, invade this central region of the diaphysis and fill the spaces vacated by the degenerating cartilage cells. These spaces, or cavities, become the primary marrow spaces.

The periosteal buds carry blood vessels, mesenchymal cells, and osteogenic cells to the cavities that become lined with a layer of osteoblasts. Osteoblasts then begin to deposit bone over the calcified cartilage matrix, first as osteoid, and then as calcified bone.

The center of the diaphysis constitutes the primary ossification center. The process of ossification spreads from the primary center toward the ends of cartilage in the same way that it developed in the primary ossification center. The periosteal bone collar also extends over the diaphysis in parallel with the spread of ossification toward the two ends of the cartilage model. The formation of the periosteal bone collar and ossification of the bone strengthens the cartilage model that has been weakened by the degeneration of the cartilage cells.[15]

Secondary ossification centers appear at the epiphyses of the developing bone at the time of birth. These secondary ossification centers are appropriately named apophyseal centers. From the epiphyseal centers, ossification spreads to replace the cartilage of the epiphysis, except for a thin shell of articular cartilage located at the most peripheral surface ends of the bone. A plate of cartilage also remains between the epiphysis and the diaphysis to constitute the epiphyseal cartilage plate or disc.

The first bone formed in the epiphysis and diaphysis of a long bone is cancellous bone. The bone of the epiphysis remains cancellous, its cavities become lined by endosteum, and it is filled with red (blood producing) marrow. The cancellous bone of the diaphysis undergoes the following changes: (1) Bone resorption occurs in the central portion of the diaphysis to open the primary marrow cavities into one big cavity. This occurs through the activity of osteoclasts that are capable of both demineralization of bone, as well as digestion of organic matrix.[15] Parathyroid hormone stimulates and calcitonin inhibits the osteoclastic resorption.[11] A definitive marrow cavity develops after bone resorption occurs in the center of the diaphysis; this cavity becomes lined with endosteum and filled with bone marrow. (2) Osteogenic activity occurs in the peripheral (outer) zone of the diaphysis where osteoblasts within the primary marrow cavities of the cancellous bone lay down concentric lamellae to convert these cavities to haversian systems and hence to develop compact bone around the definitive medullary cavity.

## PHYSIOLOGY OF THE NEURON
### GENE TOBIAS

In order to appreciate how the NMS system functions to control movement and posture, it is important to understand the role of the various chemical substances that comprise, surround, and interact with the fundamental cells of the system. These chemical substances provide the basis for two activities of NMS tissues: trophic interactions and electric events. Trophic interactions are particularly important during embryonic development of the nervous system and its target tissues. Trophic substances also help to maintain anatomic, biochemical, and physiologic characteristics of target tissues during childhood and adult life. These interactions are discussed further regarding fast- and slow-twitch skeletal muscle.

### The axon

An axon in the spinal canal (both sensory and motor) consists of neurofibrils surrounded by the pia mater, the arachnoid, and the dura mater (meninges). As axons join together to form a spinal nerve the pia mater becomes the endoneurium, the arachnoid becomes the perineurium, and the dura mater becomes the epineurium. A myelin sheath is deposited around the axon by Schwann cell membranes that first envelop the axon. The cell rotates around the axon many times, laying down multiple layers of sphingomyelin.[27] The myelin sheath often has a greater radius than the axon itself.

Every 1 to 3 mm the myelin sheath is interrupted by the node of Ranvier, which is a small area of unmyelinated axon that is only 2 to 3 $\mu$m wide. At this juncture, ions flow with ease between the axon and the extracellular fluid and produce an action potential.

The saltatory conduction of an action potential along an axon is greatly increased by the presence of the Schwann cell around the axon. The action potential jumps to each node of Ranvier, which greatly expedites nerve conduction. Axonal thickness is directly related to the amount of surrounding Schwann cell material. A higher nerve conduction velocity is seen in large myelinated axons when compared to unmyelinated axons (for example, unmyelinated nociceptive fibers have slower conduction velocities than do heavily myelinated fibers that transmit light touch) (Table 2-3). This is of significance to the clinician because with the stimulus of a light touch, pain stimuli can be blocked (the Melzak-Wall pain-gait theory).[33]

**Electric events (potentials).** Neurons and skeletal muscle cells can produce two kinds of electric events: *action potentials* and *graded potentials*. The production of these electric events is based on ion diffusion across cell membranes. All cells in the body have an external membrane made up of two layers of phospholipid molecules—a phospholipid bilayer—along with various inserted membrane protein molecules that are anchored in place by associated carbohydrate molecules. The phospholipid bilayer acts as a barrier to the diffusion of water and water-soluble substances (including ions) between the interstitial fluid outside the cell and the cytoplasm inside the cell and is, in part, responsible for the unequal concentrations of ions in the two fluids (Table 2-4). Based upon these concentration differences $Na^+$, $Ca^{2+}$ and $Cl^-$ would be expected to enter the cell by diffusion and $K^+$ to leave the cell by diffusion down their respective concentration gradients.[24,37]

The membrane proteins in nerve and muscle cells also influence electric events by serving as ion pumps and ion channels. Ion pumps use the energy from adenosine triphosphate (ATP) to move ions across the cell membrane up their concentration gradients. The two

**Table 2-3** Classification of axonal myelination and its relationship to the peripheral nervous system

| Myelination | Fiber diameter ($\mu$m) | Efferent fibers | Afferent fibers from cutaneous receptor | Afferent fibers from skeletal muscle and joint |
|---|---|---|---|---|
| Heavily myelinated | 20 | A alpha | | Type I (spindle) |
| Myelinated (spindle, GTO) | | A gamma (spindle fibers) | A beta (Merkel's and pacinian corpuscles) | Type II |
| Myelinated | 1–3 | B (preganglionic fibers of ANS) | | |
| Thinly myelinated | 1 | | A delta (thermoceptors and nociceptors) | Type III (nociceptors and mechanoceptors) |
| Unmyelinated | 0.2 | C (postganglionic fibers of ANS) | C (thermoceptors and nociceptors) | Type IV (nociceptors) |

**Table 2-4** Concentrations of ions in intracellular and extracellular fluids

| Ion | Ion concentration (mmole/liter) | |
|---|---|---|
| | Interstitial fluid | Cytoplasm |
| $Na^+$ | 150 | 15 |
| $K^+$ | 4 | 120 |
| $Cl^-$ | 115 | 10 |
| $Ca^{+2}$ | 2 | 0 |

most significant ion pumps in nerve and muscle cells are the $Na^+/K^+$ exchange pump and the $Ca^{2+}$ pump, which help to create and maintain the ion concentration differences for $Na^+$, $K^+$, and $Ca^{2+}$ and, therefore, the capability for ion diffusion. The difference in $Cl^-$ concentration is not due to a $Cl^-$ pump but rather to an electric balance between the negatively charged $Cl^-$ outside the cell with negatively charged protein inside the cell.

Ion channels are membrane proteins that determine ion permeability, namely, the ability of the ion to cross the membrane. There are three types of ion channels in nerve and muscle cells.[35] The resting channels, found throughout nerve and muscle cell membranes, are always open (they have no gates), are permeable mainly to $K^+$, and are responsible for the cell resting membrane potential (RMP). The RMP is the steady voltage difference across the membrane that exists when electric events (graded and action potentials) are absent. The RMP is $-70$ mV inside nerve cells and $-90$ mV inside skeletal muscle cells. The RMP is equivalent to the electromotive force of the cell because of the potential energy of the $K^+$ concentration gradient. A small percentage of the RMP (approximately 5%) is attributed to some ion pumps (for example, the electrogenic pumps) moving more positive ions (such as $Na^+$ and $Ca^{2+}$) out of cells than moving positive ions (such as $K^+$) into cells.[23]

The graded ion channels are located on the postsynaptic membranes of synapses between nerve cells and their target cells (such as other neuron cell bodies, dendrites, and skeletal muscle end plates). The graded ion channels have gates that open only when a neurotransmitter is present, allow permeability of $Na^+$ or $Cl^-$, and cause graded potentials. Graded potentials can be excitatory postsynaptic potentials (EPSPs) or inhibitory postsynaptic potentials (IPSPs) in neurons or end plate potentials (EPPs) in skeletal muscle cells (Table 2-5). Graded

potentials result in either decreasing the difference between the cell membrane potential and the threshold potential (causing depolarization) or increasing it (causing hyperpolarization). The threshold potential is typically 10-20 mV more positive than the RMP of the cell. The two action channel subtypes, the $Na^+$ and $K^+$ action channels are located along the axons of neurons and outside the end plate on skeletal muscle membranes. They have gates that open and close according to the level of the cell membrane potential: the $Na^+$ channels open at the threshold potential (the basis for the *all-or-none* law) and close at a cell voltage of $+30$ mV (the peak of the action potential) at which point the $K^+$ channels open. The $K^+$ channels close when the resting membrane potential is reached. These channel changes permit $Na^+$ to diffuse into the cell and $K^+$ to diffuse out of the cell, thus creating an action potential.

Because of the different membrane protein channels responsible for graded potentials and action potentials, these electric events have different characteristics and functions in nerve and muscle cells (Table 2-6). Graded potentials are created by a transformation of energy (transduction), have variable amplitudes, travel (propagate) short distances along cell membranes before disappearing, and can summate. They are used by cells to determine whether action potentials will be produced. Action potentials are created by an all-or-none phenomenon, have a constant amplitude (about 100 mV), travel long distances along cell membranes by being regenerated at each node of Ranvier or at a portion of the membrane, and are separate, individual events that do not add together.[27] Action potentials are especially useful in cells for long-distance, rapid relay of information.

The speed of action potentials is related to axonal morphology. Action potentials travel fast in larger diameter, myelinated axons (type A or type I); slow in smaller diameter, myelinated axons (type B or types II and III); and slowest in small diameter, unmyelinated axons (type C or type IV) and in muscle cells.

Case 2 presents a patient with possible damage to the oligodendrocytes (Schwann cells of the CNS) layering the axons in the central nervous system. The action potentials traveling along the axons have slowed and have become discoordinate, producing ataxic gait.

**Synaptic transmission.** Synaptic transmission allows information relayed by nerve cells in the form of action potentials to be transferred to the target cell, which can

**Table 2-5** Graded potentials and their neuronal effects

| Type | Location | Ion | Effect |
|---|---|---|---|
| Excitatory postsynaptic potential | Neuron cell body and dendrites | $Na^+$ | Depolarization |
| Inhibitory postsynaptic potential | Neuron cell body and dendrites | $Cl^-$ | Hyperpolarization |
| Endplate potential | Muscle endplate | $Na^+$ | Depolarization |

*Table 2-6*  Electric events in the neural system

| Characteristics | Graded potential | Action potential |
| --- | --- | --- |
| Creation | Transduction | All-or-none |
| Amplitude | Variable | Constant |
| Propagation | Dissipative | Regenerative |
| Summation | Yes | No |

be another neuron, a skeletal, cardiac, or smooth muscle fiber, or a gland cell. This process occurs at a synapse (Fig. 2-6) where the presynaptic axon ending (bouton) is in proximity to the postsynaptic membrane of the target cell. The space between the presynaptic axon and the postsynaptic membrane is called the *synaptic cleft* and is filled with interstitial fluid.

Synaptic transmission has two characteristics: (1) It is a one-way communication from the presynaptic neuron to the postsynaptic target cell and (2) it is chemically mediated via transversal of a neurotransmitter from the presynaptic neuron to the postsynaptic cell. The sequence of events that takes place during synaptic transmission is as follows: (1) the presynaptic neuron action potential arrives at the presynaptic ending and depolarizes the presynaptic membrane; (2) voltage-dependent gates on presynaptic membrane protein $Ca^{2+}$ ion channels open, causing an increase in presynaptic membrane $Ca^{2+}$ permeability; (3) $Ca^{2+}$ enters the cytoplasm of the presynaptic ending from the interstitial fluid by diffusion; (4) the $Ca^{2+}$ binds to membrane proteins on the

*synaptic vesicles* within the presynaptic ending causing the vesicles to migrate to the presynaptic membrane and to release their contents into the synaptic cleft by exocytosis; (5) the neurotransmitter diffuses across the synaptic cleft to the postsynaptic membrane of the target cell and binds to a specific postsynaptic membrane protein receptor; (6) the binding of the neurotransmitter to the postsynaptic membrane receptor triggers the opening of gates for $Na^+$ or $Cl^-$ on nearby postsynaptic membrane protein ion channels; (7) the permeability of the postsynaptic membrane for $Na^+$ $Cl^-$ increases, allowing these ions to enter the postsynaptic cell and create a graded potential, which can be an EPSP, an IPSP, or an EPP; (8) the neurotransmitter is removed from the synaptic cleft either by enzymatic degradation by a postsynaptic membrane protein enzyme or by reuptake by a presynaptic membrane protein transporter.

The type of graded potential produced depends upon the type of neurotransmitter, the ion-selectivity of the postsynaptic membrane ion channel, and the type of postsynaptic cell. A number of substances have been identified as neurotransmitters. Those most closely associated with the NMS system are listed in Table 2-7. Acetylcholine is released by alpha motor neurons that innervate skeletal muscle. Acetylcholine and dopamine are neurotransmitters associated with the basal ganglia. $\gamma$-Aminobutyric acid (GABA) and glutamic acid are responsible for triggering most of the IPSPs and EPSPs, respectively, in the central nervous system.

In Case 1 the binding sites located on the postsynaptic membrane have been changed or destroyed causing a decrease in usable receptor sites. The patient can produce an initial muscle contraction, but within a few seconds the contraction dissipates (myasthenia gravis). Treatment for this problem consists of administering antibodies to acetylcholine esterase. Preventing the breakdown of the acetylcholine allows the patient to sustain a muscle contraction for a longer period of time.

The myoneural junction is also directly affected in Lambert-Eaton myasthenic syndrome (LEMS), but in this disease acetylcholine production in the presynaptic membrane is low. With sustained muscle contraction, strength increases as more acetylcholine is released from the presynaptic membrane.

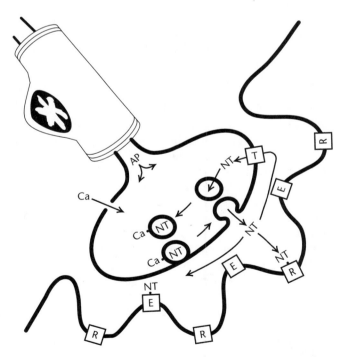

*Fig. 2-6*  Myoneural junction synapse. *Ca,* Calcium; *NT,* neurotransmitter; *AP,* axoplasm; *R,* receptor; *E,* enzymatic degradation; *T,* presynaptic neurotransporter.

*Table 2-7*  Neurotransmitters associated with graded potential events

| Neurotransmitter | Graded potential |
| --- | --- |
| Acetylcholine | EPP, EPSP |
| Dopamine | IPSP |
| $\gamma$-Aminobutynic acid | IPSP |
| Glutamic acid | EPSP |

## NEUROANATOMY OF THE PERIPHERAL AND CENTRAL NERVOUS SYSTEMS

GARY M. GREENSTEIN

Patients who exhibit pathologic conditions resulting in "awkward" human motions are presented in the first five cases. The change in a patient's coordinated motor movements assists the clinician in localizing the lesion to the PNS or to the CNS. Close observation by the clinician leads to a working diagnosis and the development of a treatment and management protocol. Spastic, discoordinated motion is usually exemplary of *upper motor neuron lesions* (UMNLs) located in the CNS. Muscle weakness or inability to move a joint because of muscle flaccidity (for example, foot drag during gait examination) is indicative of a *lower motor neuron lesion* (LMNL) in the PNS. The common findings of these different lesions are presented in Table 2-8.

A distinction between the anatomic structures of the CNS and PNS is needed in order to differentiate these lesion presentations.

The CNS consists of structures located in the brain and spinal cord (the motor axons located in the ventral horn are part of the peripheral nervous system). Lesions located in the cerebral cortex above the decussation of the tracts will display UMNL findings on the contralateral side of the body. UMNL located below the decussation and in the spinal cord will display ipsilateral LMNL signs and symptoms at the level of the lesion and UMNL findings below the level of the lesion. At the level of the lesion, the axons of the motor nuclei located in the ventral horn are usually affected, thereby eliciting LMNL signs.

The presentations of motor lesions of the PNS also depend upon the location of the lesion. If the lesion is in a peripheral nerve, all the muscles innervated by that nerve will display LMNL signs, whereas for lesions in the ventral nerve roots or spinal nerve signs of LMNL are seen only in the muscles innervated by that specific nerve root or spinal nerve.

The location of lesions within the sensory system is again determined by the relationship of the lesion to the decussation of the specific tract being evaluated. Lesions in the somatosensory area of the cerebral cortex (Brodmann's areas 3, 1, and 2) will cause changes in sensation (paresthesias, dysesthesias, and anesthesias) on the contralateral side of the body. In the spinal cord a lesion of the sensory tracts (for example, of the dorsal column-medial lemniscal pathway) will cause a loss (anesthesias), or change (paresthesias or dysesthesias) in sensation on the same side of the lesion. A lesion to the lateral spinal thalamic tract will produce a decrease or loss of pain (hypalgesia or analgesia) and temperature on the ipsilateral side at the level of the lesion and on the contralateral side below the lesion. Because of the somatotopic organization of the sensory tracts, a lesion located in the innermost portion of the cord in the thoracic or cervical areas will first have a loss of sensation at the level of the lesion and will then progress to *sacral sparing* (a loss of sensation in every area of the lower extremities except around the anal area).

Lesions in the periphery will produce ipsilateral paresthesias distal to the lesion. A peripheral lesion affecting the median nerve at the level of the carpal tunnel will display paresthesias at the thumb, the index and middle fingers, and in one-half of the ring finger (affects a multitude of dermatomes) (see Case 21). A lesion in a spinal nerve or nerve root will produce paresthesias along a dermatome (see Case 14).

Clinical neuroanatomic descriptions of the PNS and CNS are presented in this section. The discussion will begin with an introduction to the PNS and proceed to a discussion of the brain and the tracts and pathways of the spinal cord that convey messages to and from the periphery.

### The peripheral nervous system (PNS)

Human motion is a complex, fascinating interplay between the external environment and the human sensory and motor systems. Communication between the environment and the human system occurs through special receptors that receive external stimuli. These receptors send information to the cerebral cortex for interpretation, which in turn, directs striated muscle to respond (produce motion) to the stimulus. PNS is the neuroanatomic system that conveys information to and from the CNS. This information about the external environment is relayed via the receptor organs and axons of the PNS to the CNS. The several different types of receptors of the PNS are stimulus specific. They are located at the terminals of the axons of the dorsal root neurons and are the only part of the neuron that is sensitive to a stimulus.

All stimuli that can be interpreted by the PNS are conveyed by the *dorsal root ganglion neurons* and their axons (Fig. 2-7). By the use of labeled line codes, somatosensory modalities such as touch, limb propriocep-

**Table 2-8**   Objective findings for a lesion located in an upper motor neuron and a lower motor neuron

| |
|---|
| **Upper motor neuron lesion (UMNL)** |
| 1. Muscle spasticity, rigidity |
| 2. Pathologic reflexes (Babinski) |
| 3. Muscle hypertonicity |
| 4. Hyperreflexia |
| 5. Loss of superficial reflexes |
| |
| **Lower motor neuron lesion (LMNL)** |
| 1. Muscle weakness or flaccidity |
| 2. No pathologic reflexes |
| 3. Hypotonicity |
| 4. Hyporeflexia |
| 5. Loss of superficial reflexes |

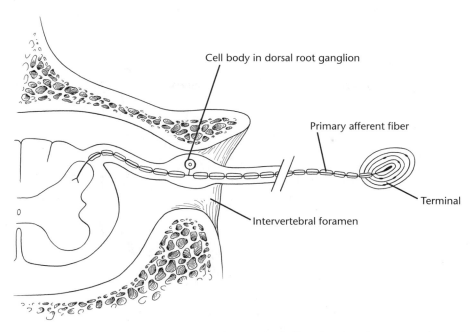

*Fig. 2-7*  Peripheral afferent and its pseudounipolar cell in the dorsal root ganglion. The dorsal root ganglion sits in the intervertebral foramen.

tion, temperature, and pain are mediated by separate receptors to the CNS.[29] The terminal branch is the only part of the dorsal root ganglion cell that is stimulus sensitive.

Dorsal root ganglion neurons are differentiated by the morphology of the peripheral terminal, its sensitivity to a stimulus, the diameter of the axon and cell body, and the presence or absence of a myelin sheath around the axon.[29] Each receptor terminal conveys a specific "message" to the CNS and is located in different areas of the skin, muscles, and joints (Fig. 2-8). Table 2-9 displays the different types of receptor terminals and the types of sensation they convey.

Nociceptive-stimulus receptors do not have specific terminals and this stimulus is conveyed by free nerve endings. Free nerve ending-stimulation is most often facilitated by a mechanical stretch stimulus. Other forms of nociceptive stimulation are chemical stimulation (mediated by substance P, histamine, or bradykinins from the inflammatory response) or thermal stimulation. Cutaneous and subcutaneous mechanoreceptors are stimulated by touch, vibration, pressure, or a combination of these stimuli. Proprioceptive stimulation comes from specifically designed receptors that are located in skeletal muscle, tendon, and joint capsules and are distinguished as muscle spindles, Golgi tendon organs, and joint capsule mechanoreceptors.

A different receptor end organ is located in hairy skin. Its mechanoreceptor is the hair-follicle receptor. In glabrous (hairless) skin the mechanoreceptor rapidly adapts to the Meissner's corpuscle as its end receptor, or it uses the slowly adapting Merkel's disk. These receptors are unique in that they receive input from a very small area, within 2 to 4 mm. The density of these receptors varies throughout the body. The palmar aspect of the fingers has the highest concentration of Merkel's disks and Meissner's corpuscles, which heightens the ability of the fingers to perceive and discriminate touch. The density of the Merkel's and Meissner's receptor organs in the palm of the hand is lower than in the fingers. A distance of 10 mm between two points is required for the palm to distinguish them as being separate. During a neurologic examination the clinician evaluates the function of these end receptors with the *two-point discrimination test* on the hand and compares the results to that in other parts of the extremity. Two points can be discriminated within 2 mm on the fingers, 10 mm on the palm of the hand, and 40 mm on the arm.[31]

Located in the subcutaneous tissue are the pacinian corpuscles, which are rapidly adapting receptors, and the Ruffini corpuscles, which adapt slowly. Both have large receptive fields making them poor for discerning spatial differences. They are located in all areas of the body and their activation contributes to the sensation of pressure. Both of these receptors are activated when a long-lasting stimulus is presented. It is a combination of different receptor stimuli to the CNS that causes the many varied sensations that are perceived by the body.

Any signal that stimulates a receptor travels along the afferent peripheral nerve. Anatomically, a peripheral nerve is a mixed nerve (contains both motor and sensory nerves) that receives sensory stimuli from the areas it

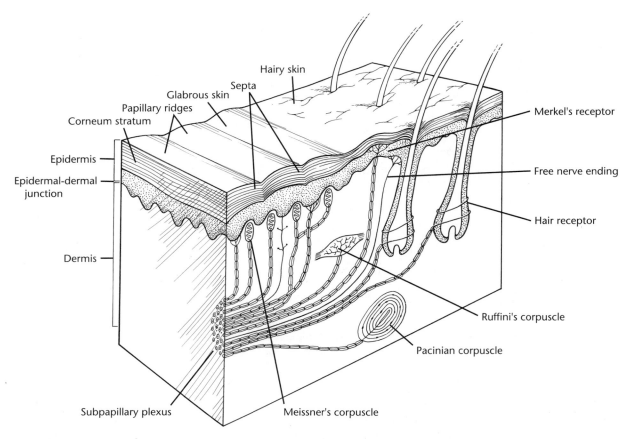

**Fig. 2-8**  Sensory receptor terminals and their location in the epidermis, epidermal-dermal junction, and the dermis. The most superficial receptor is the Merkel's receptor (disk).

innervates (for example, the brachial plexus receives stimuli from C5 to T1). Therefore, a lesion in a peripheral nerve will cause a loss in sensation in many dermatomes. Figure 2-9 illustrates the anatomic structures that combine to form a peripheral nerve. The nerve roots join to form a spinal nerve that bifurcates into ventral

*Table 2-9*  Characteristics of peripheral nervous system receptors

| Receptor type | Axon group | Type of sensation |
| --- | --- | --- |
| **Mechanical receptor** | A beta | Pain |
| Thermal and mechanothermal receptor | A or C | Sharp, pricking pain (axon group A) |
|  |  | Slow, burning pain (axon group C) |
| Polymodal receptor | C | Slow, burning pain |
| **Cutaneous and subcutaneous mechanoreceptors** |  |  |
| Pacinian corpuscle | A beta | Flutter, located in mesentery and interosseous membranes |
| Meissner's corpuscle | A beta | Touch |
| Ruffini corpuscle | A beta | Vibration |
| Merkel's disc | A beta | Steady skin indentation |
| **Muscle and skeletal mechanoreceptors** |  |  |
| Muscle spindle | Type I (primary) | Proprioception |
|  | Type II (secondary) |  |
| Golgi tendon organ | Type I |  |
| Joint capsule mechanoreceptor | Type III |  |

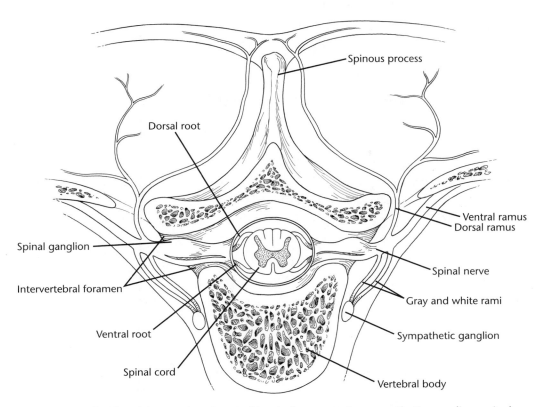

***Fig. 2-9***   The dorsal (sensory) and ventral (motor) nerve roots, sympathetic ganglion, spinal nerve, and ventral and dorsal rami in the thoracic spine.

and dorsal primary rami. The rami then join with other rami from different spinal nerves to form a peripheral nerve. This explains why a peripheral nerve can affect many levels of the spine (for example, the brachial plexus consists of the spinal nerves from C5 to T1).

## The central nervous system (CNS)

Anatomically, the structures of the brain (Table 2-10) are divided into those structures that lie between the

**Table 2-10**   Different levels of the brain

Telencephalon
   Cerebral cortex
Diencephalon
   Internal capsule
   Thalamus
   Basal ganglia
   Part of reticular formation
Mesencephalon
   Part of reticular formation
   Red nucleus and substantia nigra
   Midbrain (tegmentum and tectum)
Metencephalon
   Part of reticular formation
   Pons
   Cerebellum
   Vestibular appartus
Myelencephalon
   Medulla oblongata part of reticular formation

foramen magnum and the tentorium cerebelli (the posterior fossa level) and those structures that lie above the tentorium cerebelli (the supratentorial level). The anatomic structures of the posterior fossa are the brain stem (the medulla, the pons, and the midbrain), the cerebellum, and segments of cranial nerves III through XII.[44] (Fig. 2-10)

**The brain stem.** The brain stem is the transitional area between the brain and the spinal cord. It is the throughway for many of the tracts and pathways that mediate communication between the spinal cord and the cerebral cortex. Many of the anatomic features of the spinal cord and cerebral cortex are located in the brain stem. It contains descending and ascending pathways and tracts that communicate between the cerebral cortex, the cerebellum, the thalamus, the hypothalamus, the cranial nerves, and the spinal cord. The main structures of the brain stem are presented in Table 2-11. The brain stem also consists of 10 pairs of cranial nerves (nerves III to XII).

***The medulla.*** The medulla is the area of the brain stem where the transition from the spinal cord to the cerebral cortical structures begins. It extends from the foramen magnum to the caudal border of the base of the pons. The major ascending and descending pathways present in the spinal cord are also located in the medulla.

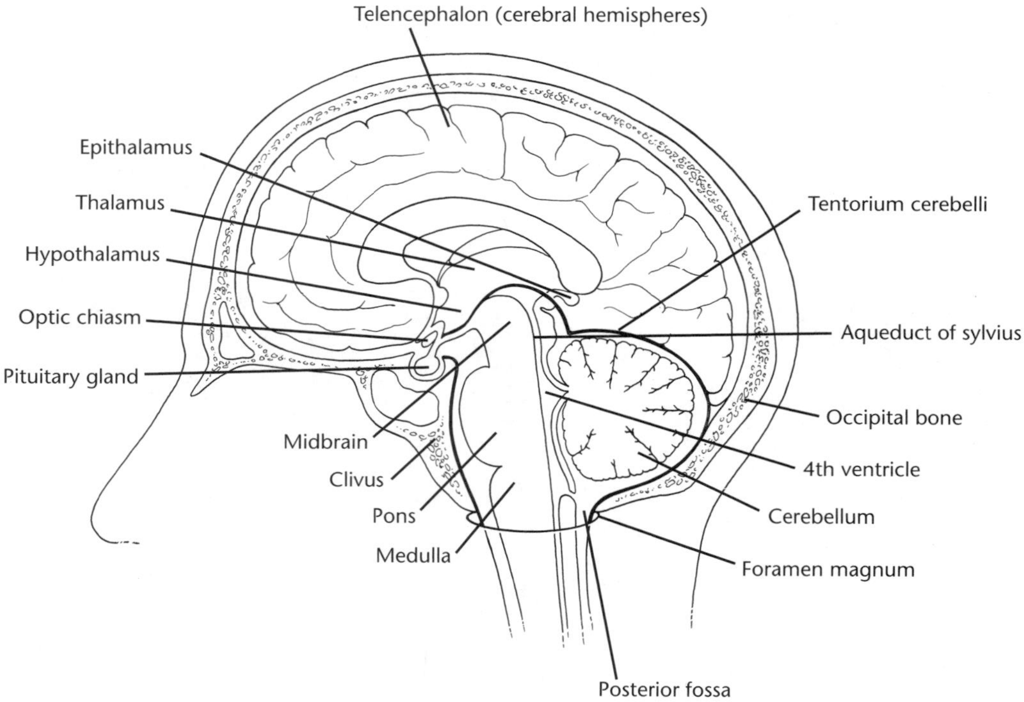

Telencephalon (cerebral hemispheres)

Epithalamus

Thalamus

Hypothalamus

Optic chiasm

Pituitary gland

Tentorium cerebelli

Aqueduct of sylvius

Occipital bone

4th ventricle

Midbrain

Clivus

Pons

Medulla

Cerebellum

Foramen magnum

Posterior fossa

**Fig. 2-10** Anatomical structures of the posterior fossa and telencephalon. The division line is the tentorium cerebelli.

Unique anatomic structures are also present in the medulla. The corticospinal tracts begin their descent and decussate at the lower end of the medulla; the fasciculus gracilis and the cuneatus terminate, and the medial lemniscus begins and decussates as the internal arcuate fibers in the medulla. The zone of Lissauer is replaced by the descending tract of the trigeminal nerve; the reticular formation replaces the central gray portion of the spinal cord; the dorsal spinocerebellar tracts enter the inferior cerebellar peduncle; the fibers of the inferior olivary nuclei discussate and travel to the opposite cerebellar hemisphere; and the central canal of the spinal cord is replaced by the fourth ventricle.

*The pons.* The pons consists of the basis pontis and the tegmentum. The ventral part of the pons (the basis pontis) contains the decussating pontocerebellar fibers, the pontine nuclei of the middle cerebellar peduncle, and the corticospinal, the corticobulbar, and the corticopontine tracts.

The tegmentum is dorsal to the basis pontis and ventral to the floor of the fourth ventricle. The spinothalamic tracts, the medial lemniscus, and the medial longitudinal fasciculi are located in this area. The acoustic and the vestibular divisions of CN VIII, the trigeminal nerve (CN V), the abducens nerve (CN VI), and facial nerve (CN VII) are all located in the tegmentum.

*The midbrain.* The midbrain lies between the pons and the diencephalon and consists of three regions: the tectum, the tegmentum, and the base. The base is the most ventral area, the tectum is the most dorsal, and the tegmentum is in between. The superior and the inferior colliculi are located in the tectum. The superior colliculus is associated with oculomotor control and the inferior colliculus acts as a relay station for the auditory fibers that pass to the thalamus. The aqueduct of Sylvius (a remnant of the neural canal) passes through the midbrain and is surrounded by a zone of periaqueductal gray matter.

The tegmentum lies ventral to the aqueduct and contains the nuclei and axons of CN III and CN IV, the red nuclei, and the decussation of the superior cerebellar peduncles. Other tracts that pass through the tegmentum are the lateral lemniscus, the spinothalamic tract, the medial lemniscus, the medial longitudinal fasciculus, and other pathways of the motor internal regulation system and the reticular formation.

Fibers from the dentate nucleus of the cerebellum decussate at the tegmentum and are grossly identified as the superior cerebellar peduncles. The red nucleus, located in the tegmentum, consists of cell bodies that synapse with the cerebral and cerebellar cortex and form the inferior olivary nucleus that project to the

*Table 2-11*  Anatomic structures of the brain stem

**Motor tracts**
 Corticospinal tract
 Corticobulbar tract
 Reticulospinal tract
 Rubrospinal tract
 Vestibulospinal tract

**Sensory tracts**
 Spinothalamic tract
 Medial lemniscus
 Spinocerebellar tract
 Descending tract of trigeminal nerve
 Trigeminothalamic tract
 Lateral lemniscus

**Other intersegmental tracts**
 Medial longitudinal fasciculus
 Oculomotor tract
 Auditory tract
 Vestibular tract
 Conscious and internal regulatory systems

**Nuclei of the tract of solitarius (visceral sensory relay)**

**Reticular formation (intermediate zone): nuclei of the reticular formation send axons to motor neurons controlling respiration and interneurons that project to preganglionic sympathetic neurons**

**Preganglionic parasympathetic neurons (CN III, VII, IX, and X)**

contralateral cerebral cortex; or synapse with the rubrospinal tract that decussates in the ventral aspect of the tegmentum and descends to the spinal cord.

The basis pedunculi forms the base of the midbrain and consists of the cerebral peduncles that contain the corticobulbar, the corticospinal, and the corticopontine tracts and the substantia nigra.

The location of the reticular formation is in the midbrain area. It surrounds the aqueduct of Sylvius with the *periaqeductal gray matter that is concerned with central modulation and control of pain.*

*Cranial nerves located in the midbrain.* The oculomotor nerve (CN III) is a mixed nerve that supplies both motor and parasympathetic fibers to the eye. Motor innervation is to the superior rectus, the medial rectus, the inferior rectus, the inferior oblique, the upper eyelid levator muscles, and the parasympathetic innervation (from the Edinger-Westphal nucleus) is to the pupil and the ciliary muscle of the lens of the eye.[48]

To evaluate the function of the cranial nerves that innervate the eye, both direct and consensual light reflexes (pupillary light reflex) are tested. In both tests, the sensory stimulus is supplied by a light directed at one eye, and pupillary constriction is observed either in the same eye (direct pupillary reflex) or in the opposite eye (consensual light reflex).

When light illuminates the eye, sensory fibers in CN II detect the light and transmit the stimulus to the optic nerve and to the optic chiasma where partial decussation occurs. The stimulus then travels along both optic tracts to the brachium of the superior colliculus of the pretectal area where the fibers pass to the Edinger-Westphal nuclei. The efferent portion of the reflex then continues along parasympathetic fibers with the oculomotor nerve (CN III) to the ciliary ganglion, synapses, and sends short ciliary nerves to the constrictor muscles of the pupil (Fig. 2-11). The normal response to light is pupillary constriction.

Sympathetic innervation to the eye arises from postganglionic fibers of the superior cervical sympathetic ganglion. The fibers ascend into the cranial cavity along the internal carotid artery and join CN III in the cavernous sinus. Damage to these fibers causes miosis; ptosis is caused by the loss of innervation of the smooth muscle in the upper eyelid (Muller's muscle).[44] Horner's syndrome develops when anhydrosis accompanies miosis and ptosis of the eye. Horner's syndrome can be caused by an apical lung tumor that presses against the superior cervical sympathetic ganglion. Anhydrosis is caused by the loss of sympathetic innervation to the sweat glands of the face.

The trochlear nerve (CN IV) innervates the superior oblique muscle of the eye and causes downward movement of the eye when it is in an adducted position. The trochlear nerve is unique in that it is the only completely crossed cranial nerve; it emerges from the dorsal surface of the brain stem.[44] All other cranial nerves located in the brain stem emerge from the ventral aspect. The major effects of damage to CN IV is diplopia on downward and inward gaze.

The trigeminal nerve carries sensory information from the face and provides motor input to the muscles of mastication. The sensory fibers mediate proprioception, touch, pain, and temperature but originate in different parts of the trigeminal nucleus. Proprioceptive fibers arise from cell bodies located at the mesencephalic nucleus. These cells lie along the lateral border of the fourth ventricle and aqueduct of Sylvius.[44] The peripheral axons of the first-order neurons innervate muscle spindle receptors in the muscles of mastication and synapse directly with the motor nucleus of CN V to produce the monosynaptic jaw-jerk reflex (Chovstek's test) (see Case 3).[44] The jaw jerk is the only muscle-stretch reflex that is elicited in the head and is mediated by the mandibular branch of CN V. The reflex is elicited by tapping the jaw, which causes a stretch in the muscle spindle leading to a contraction of the muscles of mastication.

Touch fibers form direct synapses on the main sensory nucleus of CN V. Second-order neurons ascend via both

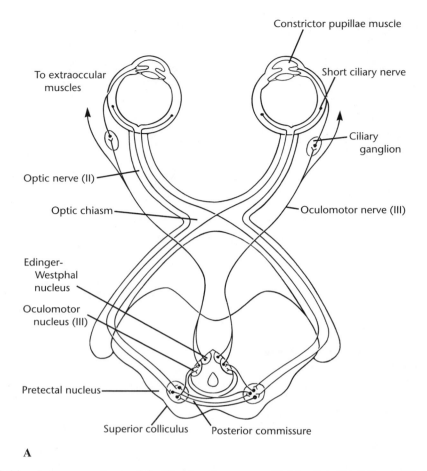

*Fig. 2-11* **A,** Neuroanatomy of the direct and consensual light reflex. The Edinger-Westphal nucleus contains the parasympathetic nuclei that travels with the oculomotor nerve (CN III) and produces pupillary constriction.

crossed and uncrossed pathways to the ventral posteromedial nucleus of the thalamus.

Sensory fibers of CN V carrying pain and temperature stimuli travel caudally to descend to the dorsolateral medulla and the upper three to four segments of the cervical spinal cord and form the spinal tract of the trigeminal nerve.[44] The sensory components of CN IX and X from the skin of the external ear, join the spinal tract of CN V when they enter the medulla. The second-order neurons immediately decussate and ascend as the ventral trigeminothalamic tract and terminate in the thalamus. Third-order neurons then ascend to the parietal lobe (Brodmann areas 3, 1, 2).

The three sensory divisions of the trigeminal nerve consist of the mandibular division ($V_3$) that exits the skull through the foramen ovale to innervate the lower aspect of the face; the maxillary division ($V_2$) that exits the skull through the foramen rotundum to innervate the midface; and the ophthalmic division ($V_1$) that pas-

ses through the superior orbital fissure to innervate the upper face (Fig. 2-12).

Located medial to the main sensory nucleus are the cell bodies of the motor nucleus of the trigeminal nerve. The motor root of CN V joins the sensory mandibular division, exits the foramen ovale just medial to the sensory root, and innervates the temporal, masseter, and medial and lateral pterygoid muscles, and the tensor muscle of tympanum. The temporal, masseter, and medial and lateral pterygoid muscles close the jaw; the lateral pterygoid muscle also causes lateral movement of the jaw and the tensor muscle of tympanum and other muscles help dampen the vibrations of the eardrum.

The location of the spinal nucleus of CN V and its innervation with cervical nerves from the occiput to C3 provides the clinician an anatomic basis for treatment of the cervical spine in the patient with a complaint of facial and head pain (see Case 6).[8] This disorder has been recognized as cervicogenic headache. The patient

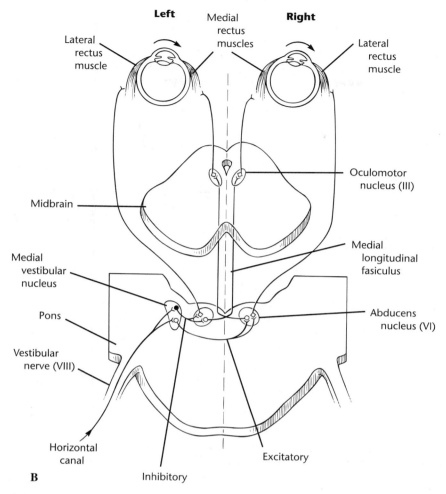

*Fig. 2-11* (*Continued*). **B,** Neuroanatomic tracts that produce lateral gaze of the eyes.

may display the symptomatology of any persistent type of headache.[7,8,9] Bogduk describes most headaches as having a neurologic cause that can be evaluated and treated by facetal injection into the first three cervical nerves.[21] The literature supports the contention that the clinician should examine the cervical spine in a patient with the symptomatology of persistent headache.

Also located in the pons is the facial nerve (CN VII). Case 3 discusses a patient who has complete facial paralysis on one side caused by a lesion of the lower motor neuron of CN VII (Bell's palsy). Not only does the facial nerve have five motor divisions that innervate the muscles of facial expression, but it also has components that send parasympathetic innervation to the submaxillary, submandibular, and lacrimal glands and to taste receptors of the anterior two thirds of the tongue. Anatomically higher centers innervate CN VII via the corticobulbar tracts. The descending corticobulbar fibers innervating the maxillary and mandibular parts of CN VII decussate just before innervating the nuclei. The

ophthalmic division of the facial nerve is doubly innervated by the corticobulbar tract, via decussated and unilateral fibers (Fig. 2-13). In Bell's palsy, a lesion located in the lower motor neuron (beyond the CN nuclei) results in total loss of facial expression on one half of the face and decreased lacrimation, salivation, and taste to the anterior two thirds of the tongue. The patient is unable to close the eyelid or display any facial expression on the affected side. The etiology of Bell's palsy is not known but the condition may be caused by inflammation of the facial nerve in the facial canal.[44] In contrast, a lesion located in the corticobulbar tract or anatomically higher cortical structures will produce facial paralysis in the maxillary and mandibular aspects of the facial nerve but not in the ophthalmic region, allowing the patient to be able to blink the eye (Case 4).

**The cerebellum.** The cerebellum is the largest structure of the posterior fossa. It develops from the metencephalon, associated with the rhombic lip of the alar plate. Its main functions are integration of unconscious

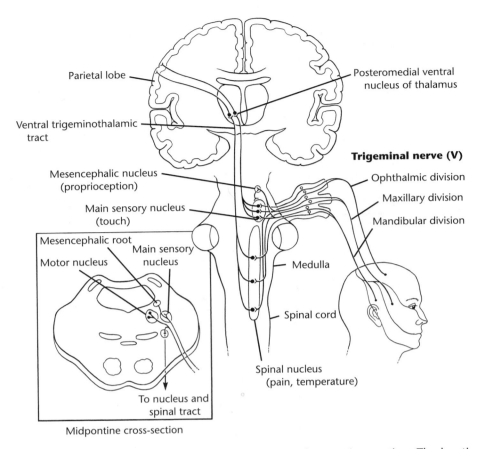

*Fig. 2-12* Trigeminal nerve (CN V) and its sensory and motor innervation. The location of the motor nucleus, which stimulates the muscles of mastication, is pictured in the inset.

proprioception, muscle coordination, and performing other motor function.

The cerebellum consists of two lateral lobes and the centrally located vermis. In transverse section, it is made up of the anterior and posterior lobes and the flocculonodular lobe. The vermis occupies an area in all the lobes along with the cerebellar hemispheres anterior to the primary fissure in the anterior lobe, the nodulus and flocculus in the flocculonodular lobe, and the cerebellar tonsils in the posterior lobe. The afferent spinocerebellar fibers are received in the vermis of the anterior and posterior lobes. This portion of the vermis controls the synergistic actions of the muscles necessary for walking. The lateral zone of the cerebellum coordinates ipsilateral limb movement. The flocculonodular lobe receives input from the vestibular system and is concerned with coordination of head and eye movements and the maintenance of equilibrium.[13,44]

The afferent and efferent pathways that synapse with the cerebellum travel through the cerebellar peduncles. The superior cerebellar peduncle contains the brachium conjunctivum (efferent fibers) and the ventral spinocerebellar tract (afferent tract). The brachium conjunctivum fibers join with the red nucleus and thalamus. Fi-

bers from the dentate nucleus cross in the superior peduncle and proceed to the contralateral red nucleus, the thalamus, and the inferior olivary nucleus. This connection, as in the middle cerebellar peduncle, sets up interconnections between the cerebral cortex, the pontine nucleus, and the cerebellum that are imperative for normal motor function.

The middle cerebellar peduncle (brachium pontis) is a relay station that carries afferent fibers from the contralateral pontine nuclei. The pontine nuclei receive afferent fibers from the ipsilateral cerebral cortex via the corticopontine tract. These pathways (corticopontocerebellar fibers) interconnect each cerebellar hemisphere with the contralateral cerebral hemisphere.

Information from the spinal cord, the medulla, and the vestibular nerve travels through the inferior cerebellar peduncle (restiform body). Unconscious proprioceptive sensory pathways (the ventral and the dorsal spinocerebellar and cuneocerebellar tracts) and others, along with the efferent pathways of the cerebellovestibular and cerebelloreticular tracts pass through the restiform body.

The role of the cerebellum is to coordinate willful muscular contractions.[20] Proprioceptive input that transmits positional information is received from the muscles,

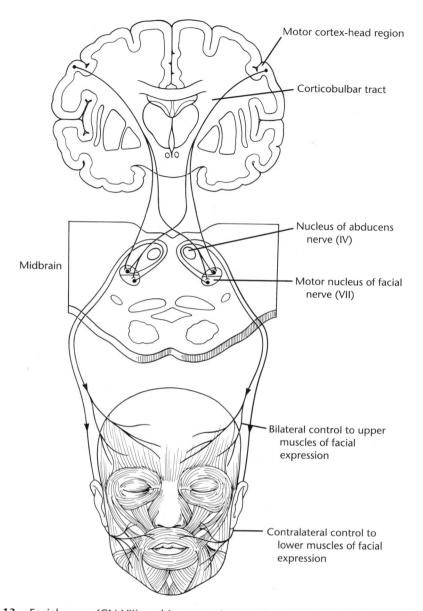

**Fig. 2-13** Facial nerve (CN VII) and its motor innervations. Note the dual innervation of the forehead. Differentiation of forehead motion helps the clinician determine if the patient has a lower motor neuron lesion (i.e., Bell's palsy) or an upper motor neuron lesion in either the cortex or the corticobulbar tracts (i.e., cerebral vascular accident).

the joints, and the vestibular system.[36] From this information the cerebellum coordinates the range, velocity, and strength of muscle contractions needed to produce steady volitional movements and steady volitional postures. The proprioceptive sensory stimulus for volitional movement and posture (unconscious proprioception) is transferred to the cerebellum from the muscle spindles and joint receptors via the spinocerebellar tracts. This information is interpreted by the cerebellum and is relayed through the Purkinje cell to the cerebro-cerebello-cerebral circuit and eventually is transmitted to the PNS by the spinal cord. Anatomically, the spinocerebellar

tracts are unilateral tracts (the ventral spinocerebellar tract decussates twice); the cerebro-cerebello-cerebral circuit allows the cerebellum to coordinate volitional movement by relaying information back to the motor cortex. The circuit crosses the midline two times, once at the level of the red nucleus and again, at the pons; with the lateral corticospinal tract crossing once at the pyramids of the medulla the cerebellar hemisphere has unilateral influence (Fig. 2-14). Therefore, a lesion located in the cerebellum causes unilateral motor signs.

The signs typical of cerebellar lesions are best observed in a person who is inebriated. The person cannot

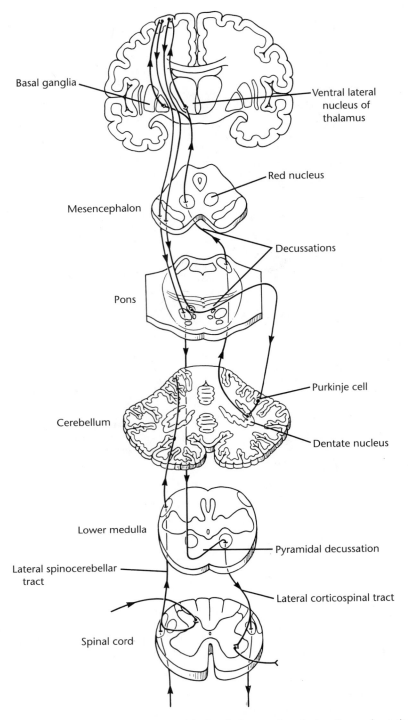

***Fig. 2-14***  Cerebellar interconnections with the thalamus, basal ganglia, and cerebral cortex. Intercommunication between the ipsilateral cerebellum, contralateral thalamus, basal ganglia, and cerebral cortex project to the skeletal muscle by the corticospinal tract. Decussation of the cerebello-cortico pathway occurs in the pyramids of the medulla. A lesion that is located in the cerebellum therefore causes ipsilateral signs.

coordinate any volitional muscular contractions and sways when standing, reels when walking (ataxia), slurs when talking (dysarthria), and has jerky eye movements when focusing (nystagmus).[20] Several neurologic tests mentioned in the case presentations evaluate cerebellar activity. Dysdiadochokinesia evaluates rapid motions of the extremities. Any jerky, inconsistent hand motions occurring during rapid pronation and supination of the hands is indicative of a unilateral cerebellar lesion. Other tests such as the Romberg's heel-to-shin, finger-to-finger, finger-to-nose, and Holme's rebound tests evaluate uncoordinated motion of the extremities and cerebellar integrity.

Lesions in the cerebellum may also present clinically as an intention tremor (in contrast with Case 5). An intention tremor is an irregular tremor of low-to-moderate amplitude that appears during intentional movements. The tremor is heightened during the finger-to-nose test and it may cause the patient to pass-point (dysmetria). Postural tremors are also indicative of disease in the cerebellum or its efferent pathways.[20]

### The supratentorium of the brain

The supratentorial region encompasses the areas of the brain located above the tentorium cerebelli—the dien-

cephalon and the telencephalon. The diencephalon consists of the thalamus, hypothalamus, and the epithalamus. The telencephalon consists of the basal ganglia, the basal forebrain, and the cerebral cortex.[44]

**The diencephalon.** The diencephalon is rostral to the brain stem and includes the third ventricle and its surrounding structures: the thalamus, the ventral thalamus, the epithalamus, and the hypothalamus.[23,44] The thalamus is the largest structure in the diencephalon and functions to integrate and relay information for the motor, the sensory, the limbic, and the conscious systems. It is anatomically divided into several groups of nuclei that consist of a narrow anterior nucleus and a broad posterior end containing the pulvinar and the geniculate bodies. The Y-shaped internal medullary lamina divides the thalamus into lateral, medial, and anterior areas. The lateral nuclei are arranged into a ventral and a dorsal layer. The ventral layer harbors the ventral anterior, ventral lateral, and ventral posterior nuclei. Within the dorsal layer are found the dorsolateral nucleus, the lateral posterior nucleus, and the pulvinar. The geniculate bodies extend from the pulvinar, and the midline nuclei are the intralaminar nuclei in the Y-shaped border (Fig. 2-15). Table 2-12 relates the thalamic nuclei and their major functions.

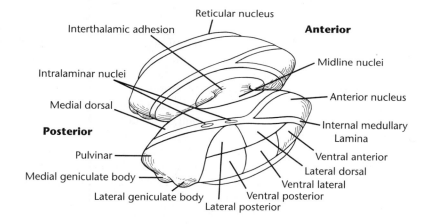

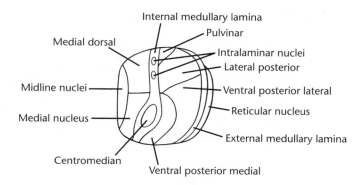

***Fig. 2-15*** Anatomical structures of the thalamus. Sensory and motor innervation most commonly involves the ventral posterior medial (VPM) and ventral posterior lateral (VPL) nuclei.

*Table 2-12*  Areas of thalamus directly related with sensory and motor systems

| Nuclei | Relay from sensory pathways and other brain areas | Internal capsule | Relays to cortex areas |
|---|---|---|---|
| VPL | Spinothalmic and medial lemniscal pathway (somatosensory information) | Posterior limb | Area 3,1,2 in cerebrum (somatosensory cortex) |
| VPM | Trigeminal thalamic pathways from head (somatosensory information) | Posterior limb | Area 3,1,2 in cerebrum (somatosensory cortex) |
| Ventral lateral | Cerebellar nuclei | | Area 4 in cerebrum (primary motor cortex) |
| Ventral anterior | Globus pallidus and substantia nigra | | Supplementary motor and premotor cortices |
| Intralaminar | Sensory system and consciousness system | | Basal ganglia |

VPL, *Ventral posterolateral;* VPM, *ventral posteromedial.*

The subthalamus, or the ventral thalamus, is a poorly defined area that includes the subthalamic nucleus, which is part of the basal ganglia. A lesion in this area leads to hemiballism, a movement disorder associated with uncontrollable flailing of an extremity.

The hypothalamus is the main control area of the visceral system. The major functions of the hypothalamus include regulation of water metabolism, food intake, reproductive function, and the sleep-wake cycle. It also exerts autonomic and neuroendocrine control and is involved in thermoregulation. The visceral system is under hypothalamic control.

**The telencephalon.** The anatomic structures that constitute the telencephalon are contained in the two cerebral hemispheres. The two hemispheres are located above the tentorium cerebelli and are separated by the falx cerebri. The cerebral hemispheres are divided into three anatomic regions: the basal ganglia, the subcortical white matter, and the cerebral cortex.

*The basal ganglia.* The basal ganglia consists of the caudate nucleus, the putamen, the globus pallidus, the subthalamic nucleus, and the substantia nigra. The putamen and the caudate nucleus constitute the neostriatum, or corpus striatum, which is the primary afferent receiving structure of the basal ganglia, collecting input from the cerebral cortex, the limbic system, and the thalamus.[13,44] The neostriatum relays this information to the prefrontal, premotor, and motor cortices of the cerebral cortex; this process is mediated by the frontal cortex. The basal ganglia is unique in that it has no neural connections with the spinal cord.[1,16]

The corticostriate projection contains afferent fibers from the entire cerebral cortex; it is topographically organized and projects to specific areas of the neostriatum. Afferent impulses from the sensory and motor cortex, from the prefrontal cortex, and from the limbic cortex and amygdala are received by the putamen, the caudate nucleus, and the ventral aspect of the striatum, respectively.[1] The putamen is primarily involved with motor control (sensory and motor cortex), the caudate

nucleus controls eye motion and certain cognitive functions (prefrontal cortex), and the striatum is related to the limbic area (limbic cortex and amygdala). The connections between the thalamus and the neostriatum (the centromedial nucleus connects the thalamus to the putamen) are also topographically organized and are another pathway used for communication between the basal ganglia and the cerebral cortex. The majority of cortical projections involved with sensation and motion are concentrated in topographically anatomically distinct organized areas in the striatum and project to the globus pallidus and the substantia nigra. Their organization appears to be similar to that of the motor cortex (homunculus).[1] These areas are critical for motor or cognitive behavior,[16] becoming active during passive joint movements or active motion. Neurons located in the putamen are involved with directing joint motion rather than with muscle actions, indicating that the basal ganglia is not involved in the initiation of stimulus-triggered movements nor with controlling the muscular forces needed to execute movement. The basal ganglia, however, is of considerable importance in the initiation of internally generated movements. This is consistent with the inability of a patient with Parkinson's disease to initiate movement (see Case 5).

The basal ganglia harbors several interconnecting pathways. Connections between the neostriatum, the globus pallidus, and the substantia nigra occur through the striatopallidal and striatonigral pathways. As with the corticostriatal pathways, these pathways are also topographically organized; therefore, specific sections of the globus pallidus act on particular areas of the substantia nigra and the neostriatum.

The major efferent pathways of the basal ganglia arise in the internal segment of the globus pallidus and a portion of the substantia nigra and project to three nuclei of the thalamus: the ventral lateral, the ventral anterior, and the mediodorsal nuclei.[1,16] Efferent pathways run from the thalamus to the prefrontal, the premotor, and the motor cortices, and the supplementary motor area. Through these connections the basal ganglia indirectly affects the corticospinal and the corticobulbar tracts of the spinal cord and the cranial nerves, respectively. Eye movements are also regulated by the basal ganglia through a projection from the substantia nigra to the superior colliculus.

The motor circuit of the basal ganglia is a subcortical feedback loop.[2,16] that projects from the supplementary motor area, the premotor area, the motor area, and the somatosensory cortex to topographically organized areas in the putamen. The motor circuit then projects to the supplementary motor and premotor cortices. This information is then transmitted to the spinal cord.

Cortical input to the basal ganglia is excitatory, with L-glutamine as the neurotransmitter. The inhibitory aspect of the basal ganglia is mediated by GABA and substance P and is found in the globus pallidus and the nondopaminergic portion of the substantia nigra. These areas tonically inhibit the thalamus, the superior colliculus, and other pathways.[44] Dopaminergic neurons modulate the activity of the circuits in the basal ganglia. Dopamine, produced in the substantia nigra, has an excitatory effect on the striatal neurons that inhibit the globus pallidus and, therefore, reverses the inhibition in the thalamus, the superior colliculus, and other pathways to allow movement.[1] A loss of the dopaminergic cells in the substantia nigra leads to loss of control of the globus pallidus and the thalamus and accounts for the hypokinetic and hyperkinetic movement disorders seen in diseases such as Parkinson's disease (Case 5) and Huntington's chorea.

Two subcortical loops exist between the basal ganglia, the cerebellum, and the cerebral cortex.[1,2] Both receive connections from the cerebral cortex, and, in turn, send projections back to the cerebral cortex by way of the thalamus. The connections between the basal ganglia and the cerebral cortex are different from those between the cerebellum and the cerebral cortex. The basal ganglia receives input from all areas of the cerebral cortex, whereas the cerebellum receives connections from areas associated only with sensorimotor functions of the cerebral cortex. Return communication from the cerebellum to the cerebral cortex is directed to the premotor and motor cortex, whereas the output from the basal ganglia is directed to the premotor, motor, and prefrontal association cortex. The cerebellum also receives somatosensory information directly from the spinal cord and has major afferent and efferent pathways with many of the brain stem nuclei directly connected with the spinal cord.[1,2] In contrast, the basal ganglia has very few connections with the brain stem and no direct tracts with the spinal cord.[16] These differences imply that the cerebellum directly controls the execution of movement and the basal ganglia are involved in the higher-order cognitive aspects of motor control.

In summary, the basal ganglia along with the cerebellum and cerebral cortex is involved in motor activity. The cerebellum directs joint motion through the putamen and plays a major part in patient initiated movement. The basal ganglia is not involved in the initiation of motion that is related to an external stimulus or with the control of muscular forces needed to execute motion. The most common manifestation of a lesion in the basal ganglia is Parkinson's disease (see Case 5). This patient with Parkinson's disease is unable to initiate the act of walking, an internal motivation. A resting tremor or stressful tremor of 3 to 6 cycles/sec with a low-to-moderate amplitude of the hands is also indicative of Parkinson's disease and is called a parkinsonian tremor. The tremor dampens during intentional movement. Intentional tremors are indicative of cerebellar disease. The rustling of the thumb against the pads of the fingers resemble a pill-rolling tremor and is caused by degeneration of the dopaminergic axons from the substantia nigra to the striatum.[20] Diseases of the basal ganglia are presented in Table 2-13.

*Subcortical white matter.* Located between the ventricles and the cortex are myelinated axons that connect multiple areas of the cerebral hemispheres. Three areas of axonal fibers make up the subcortical white matter. Projectional fibers travel between the subcortical nuclear structures and the cerebral cortex; commissural fibers interconnect similar areas of the two hemispheres; and the association fibers connect cortical areas within a hemisphere.

The *internal capsule* is the area traversed by the projectional fibers. The internal capsule is a V-shaped structure (in the horizontal plane) that is flanked laterally by the globus pallidus and the putamen and medially, by the thalamus. The axons of the projectional fibers are either afferent fibers, coming primarily from the thalamus (thalamic radiations) or efferent fibers traveling from higher cortical centers to the brain stem or spinal cord. The anterior portion of the internal capsule carries afferent information from the anterior and medial thalamic nuclei to the frontal lobe. The *corona radiata* is an extension of the internal capsule because the axons ascend and descend to different areas of the cerebral cortex, brain stem, and spinal cord. Efferent motor fibers travel through the genu of the internal capsule to the brain stem (the corticobulbar fibers) and the spinal cord (the corticospinal fibers). Other efferent fibers from the frontal lobe travel through the internal capsule and cerebral peduncles to the pontine nuclei and to the cerebellum. Afferent sensory fibers from the ventral posterolateral and posteromedial thalamic nuclei ascend through the posterior aspect of the internal capsule.[44] All axonal fibers that pass through the internal capsule are involved in the initiation of voluntary movement, integration of motor function, modifi-

*Table 2-13* Disorders of the basal ganglia

| Disorder | Pathophysiology | Chemical change | Clinical presentation |
|---|---|---|---|
| Parkinson's disease | Degeneration of nigrostriatal pathway, raphe nuclei, locus ceruleus, and vagus motor nucleus | Reduction in levels of dopamine, serotonin, and norepinephrine | Resting tremor, cogwheel rigidity, akinesia, bradykinesia, and postural reflex impairment |
| Huntington's chorea | Degeneration of intrastriatal and cortical cholinergic neurons and GABA-containing neurons | Reduction in levels of choline, acetyltransferatse, glutamic acid, decarboxylase, and GABA | Chorea, decreased muscle tone, and dementia |
| Ballism | Damage to one subthalamic nucleus often caused by CVA | | Severe involuntary movement disorder |
| Tardive dyskinesia | Alteration in dopaminergic receptors causing hypersensitivity to dopamine and its agonists | | Iatrogenic disorder with long-term use of phenothiazines or butyrophenones; abnormal involuntary movements of face and tongue |

*Adapted from Kaudel E, Schwartz J, Jessell T, editors:* Principles of neural science, *ed 3, New York, 1991, Elsevier.*

cation of reflex activity, modulation of sensory input, regulation of visceral function, and regulation of states of consciousness and attention.[44]

### The cerebral cortex

The cerebral cortex is divided into three layers: the neocortex, the paralimbic cortex, and the limbic cortex. The neocortex is the outermost part and contains sensory, motor, and associational areas. The neocortex is made up of a relatively thin mantle of gray matter (neuronal cell bodies) and consists of five lobes—the frontal, parietal, temporal, limbic, and occipital lobes—that are separated by two main sulci: the central sulcus and the sylvian fissure. The paralimbic cortex is located between the frontal and temporal lobes and connects the limbic system to neocortical regions. The limbic cortex is located on the medial aspect of the cerebral hemispheres and consists of the hippocampal formation and other hippocampal structures, a portion of the cingulate gyrus, and the primary olfactory cortex. Each lobe has specific functions in brain areas that are anatomically interconnected and also has connections with the deeper cortical structures and the spinal cord.

Brodmann devised a numbering system for the topography of the brain in which the human cerebral cortex is divided into 52 discrete areas. Some of the identified areas are important to our discussion. Areas 3, 1, and 2 are located in the postcentral gyrus where the primary somatosensory cortex is found. Area 4, the motor cortex, occupies most of the precentral gyrus, and area 6 is the premotor cortex. The prefrontal association cortex is located in areas 8, 9, 10, and 11; and the parieto-temporooccipital association cortex is areas 19, 21, 22, 37, 39, and 40. The major speech centers are located in areas 44 (Broca's area) and 22 (Wernicke's area); area 17 is the primary visual cortex and areas 41 and 42 are the primary auditory cortex. Figure 2-16 displays a map of the brain with its corresponding Brodmann areas. The next section will concentrate on the anatomic structures of the cerebral cortex involved with human motion.

**Motor function of the cerebral cortex.** The motor regions of the cerebral cortex are located in both cerebral hemispheres in the frontal lobe. They are located in three separate areas: the primary motor cortex (Brodmann area 4), the premotor cortex (Brodmann area 6), and the supplementary motor area (Brodmann area 8). The primary motor cortex is located in the precentral gyrus that extends from the lateral sulcus to the medial surface of the cerebral hemisphere. Its main function is to control skilled movement through the lateral and ventral corticospinal tracts. These tracts form synapses on motor neurons and interneurons. Rostral to the primary motor cortex are the premotor and the supplementary motor cortices, both located at Brodmann's area 6, with the premotor cortex at the lateral aspect, and the supplementary motor cortex at the medial aspect of this area. Both the premotor cortex and the supplementary motor areas are the higher order motor cortical regions and receive input from other areas of the brain. The primary motor cortex receive input not only from both the premotor and the supplementary motor areas but also from the cerebellum and the ventral lateral nucleus of the thalamus, which send major projections of axonal information. The basal ganglia, a midbrain structure, also sends projections to the supplementary motor area of the cortex.

Descending projections from the supplementary motor area project to the spinal cord and influence spinal motor neurons. The ascending projection from the premotor cortex is to the reticular formation, and this controls the actions of the girdle muscles and gives rise to the reticulospinal tracts.[32]

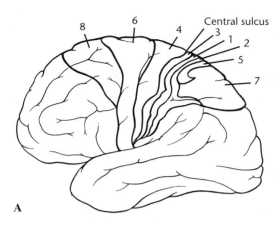

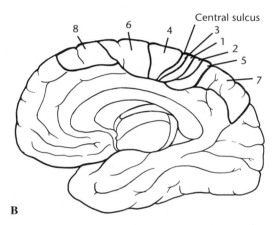

*Fig. 2-16* **A, B,** Brodmann areas of the cerebral cortex. Included are those areas most important to sensory and motor function. Sensory stimulation is interpreted most commonly by the postcentral gyrus (3, 1, 2, 5, and 7); motor function is most often relayed by the precentral gyrus (4, 6, and 8). The central sulcus is the dividing mark.

The motor function of the central nervous system involves four basic systems: (1) the precentral gyrus in the frontal lobe of the cerebral cortex, (2) the descending pathways of the cerebral cortex and spinal cord, (3) the interneuronal projections of the intermediate zone and the motor neurons of the ventral horn, and (4) the basal ganglia and cerebellum of the brain.

*Motor pathways in the spinal cord.* There are three types of descending motor pathways: (1) motor control pathways, (2) pathways that regulate sensory processing, and (3) pathways that regulate the functions of the autonomic nervous system.[13,32] Motor control pathways originate either in the cerebral cortex or in the brain stem and regulate voluntary motion or reflexes. Motor control of the head occurs via the cranial nerves that are located in the brain stem (CN III through CN XII).

Motor control areas of the limbs and trunk are located in the cerebral cortex in the precentral gyrus and other areas of the frontal gyrus.

Seven major descending motor control pathways in the spinal cord innervate motor neurons that project to the peripheral muscles. The *lateral corticospinal tract,* the *anterior corticospinal tract,* and the *corticobulbar tract* originate in the frontal lobe. The other four tracts— the *rubrospinal tract,* the *reticulospinal tract,* the *vestibulospinal tract,* and the *tectospinal tract*—arise from the brain stem (Fig. 2-17).

Each of the motor tracts have monosynaptic connections between the descending projection neurons and the motor neurons and polysynaptic interneurons. There are two types of interneurons involved with the motor pathways. Interneurons that have short axons and distribute branches in a single spinal cord segment are called intrasegmental neurons. Interneurons with long axons that project into several spinal cord levels are propriospinal (intersegmental) neurons. The interneurons are located primarily in the intermediate zone of the ventral horn. Segmental and propriospinal interneurons receive afferent information from mechanoreceptors, thermoreceptors, and nociceptors.[32]

The motor neurons located in the ventral horn of the spinal cord not only receive input from the motor tracts but also receive sensory input from the afferent nerves entering the spinal cord. These synapses can be direct (monosynaptic) or indirect (polysynaptic). The only afferent fiber that is monosynaptic with the motor neuron is the group Ia fiber from the muscle spindle. This makes up the monosynaptic reflex arc that produces the *deep tendon reflex.*[26]

The neurons of the motor pathways of the spinal cord are arranged so that the medial portion of both the white matter and gray matter of the spinal cord house the tracts, the neurons, and the interneurons that innervate the axial and girdle muscles. The lateral portion of the white matter, the gray matter of the lateral ventral horn, and intermediate zone house the tracts, the motor neurons, and the interneurons that innervate the distal limb muscles. Motor neurons that innervate the flexor and extensor muscles of the extremities are arranged so that the extensor muscle neurons are ventral to the flexor muscles.[2,32]

The *lateral corticospinal tract* and the *rubrospinal tract* are involved in voluntary limb movement. The lateral corticospinal tract originates in the precentral gyrus of the cerebral cortex.

The lateral corticospinal tract nuclei are found in three areas in the frontal lobe of the cerebral cortex: the primary motor cortex (Brodmann's area 4) the precentral gyrus, and the supplementary motor area (Brodmann's area 6). The parietal lobe contributes axons to the lateral corticospinal tract but, unlike the frontal lobe

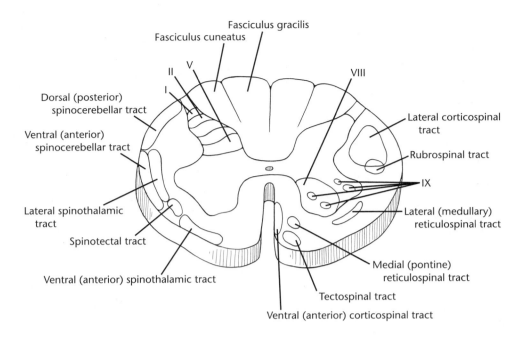

**Ascending tracts & rexed levels (sensory)**     **Descending tracts & rexed levels (motor)**

*Fig. 2-17*    Anatomical organization of the spinal cord. Rexed levels I, II, V, VIII, and IX are depicted.

axons, these axons terminate in the dorsal horn of the spinal column. The frontal lobe axons terminate in the intermediate zone or in the ventral horn.[2,4,32]

The lateral corticospinal tract descends from its neurons located in Brodmann's area 4 and 6 through the deeper structures of the cerebral hemispheres in the internal capsule and the basis pedunculi in the midbrain to the pyramids in the medulla. At the junction of the medulla and the spinal cord, the tract decussates and descends in the white matter of the spinal cord located in the lateral column. Decussation of this tract is the reason why Lou M. (see Case 4) has a lesion in the left hemisphere of the cortex but has problems in the right limbs. The corticospinal tract axons terminate at different levels in the spinal cord in the intermediate zone or the ventral horn gray matter.

The *rubrospinal tract* has fewer axons, is smaller in area than the corticospinal tract, and originates in the red nucleus of the midbrain. It descends in the same area as the lateral corticospinal tract, at the lateral aspect of the white matter. The tract decussates in the midbrain and descends in the dorsolateral portion of the brain stem and the dorsal portion of the lateral column of the spinal cord. It then terminates in the lateral portions of the intermediate zone and ventral horn. A lesion in this tract, above the midbrain, would again affect the contralateral limbs, whereas a lesion below the midbrain and after the decussation would affect the extremities ipsilaterally.

The four *medially descending pathways* that control axial and girdle muscles are the ventral corticospinal tract, the reticulospinal tracts, the vestibulospinal tracts, and the tectospinal tract. A characteristic feature of the medially descending pathways is bilateral control of axial and girdle muscles.[23,32] Because of this dual innervation of the axial and girdle muscles from both the right and the left cerebral hemispheres, a cerebral cortical lesion on one side will cause gross motor function changes in the contralateral upper and lower extremity but will have little effect on the axial and girdle muscles because of the dual innervation.

The *ventral corticospinal tract* originates in the primary motor and supplementary motor cortices. This pathway descends through the internal capsule, the basis pedunculi, the ventral pons, and the medullary pyramid. At the level of the pyramid the ventral corticospinal tract proceeds along the ipsilateral side of the spinal cord in the ventral column and terminates, with the neurons located in the medial aspect of the ventral horn and the interneurons located in the medial intermediate zone. The ventral corticospinal tract axons terminate on the ipsilateral and contralateral medial aspect of the ventral horn. The ventral corticospinal tract does not terminate any lower than the thoracic spinal cord and is, therefore, involved in the control of the neck, the shoulder, and the upper trunk muscles.[23,32]

The two *reticulospinal tracts* originate in different regions of the reticular formation. The *pontine reticulospi-*

*nal tract* originates in the pontine nucleus of the pons and the *medullary reticulospinal tract* originates in the medullary reticular formation of the medulla. These two tracts are involved in the autonomic, involuntary control of posture and locomotion. Their actual function is not well understood. Both tracts descend ipsilaterally to the medial intermediate zone and medial motor nuclei. The pontine reticulospinal tract descends in the ventral column, and the medullary reticulospinal tract descends in the ventrolateral quadrant of the lateral column of the spinal cord. Both tracts descend to the sacral cauda equina.

The *tectospinal tract* originates from the neurons of the superior colliculus (tectum) of the rostral midbrain. The tract forms synapses with the motor neurons in the ventral horn at the level of the cervical spine and is involved with the muscles of the neck, shoulder, and upper trunk. Because this tract begins in the superior colliculus, its close association with eye motion indicates that it is probably involved with the coordination of head and eye movements.

The *vestibulospinal tracts* originate from two of the four vestibular nuclei. The lateral vestibular nucleus (Deiters' nucleus; considered a medially descending pathway) leads to the lateral vestibulospinal tract that descends ipsilaterally to all levels of the cord and is important in maintaining balance and head position. The medial vestibulospinal tract descends on both sides of the cord to the level of the cervical spine.

**The primary somatic sensory cortex.** A sensory evaluation is performed on all patients that visit the clinician's office with a possible NMS problem. In many of the cases presented in this text, differences in sensory perception, after application of a stimulus such as pain, light touch, deep pressure, or vibration, are noted and recorded by the clinician. This information helps the clinician determine the location of the lesion that may be causing the patient's problem. The somatic sensory system is an integral part of motor function, as is the motor system.

Located in the postcentral gyrus and in the central sulcus of the anterior aspect of the parietal lobe is the *primary somatic sensory cortex (S-I)*. It consists of four functional areas: Brodmann's areas 1, 2, 3a, and 3b, with each area having a slightly different role in somatic sensation.[30] Lateral and posterior to the primary somatic sensory cortex and lying in the upper part of the lateral sulcus is the *secondary somatic sensory cortex (S-II)*. S-II receives input from S-I and projects to somatic fields in the insular region deep within the lateral sulcus. A higher order sensory cortex also exists within the posterior parietal lobe. Its role is to relate sensory and motor processing and integrate different somatic sensory modalities for perception.

Two major types of cells are located within the somatic sensory cortex: the pyramidal cells (output cells) and the nonpyramidal cells (interconnector cells).[30] The pyramidal cells, located in Brodmann areas 2, 3, 5, and 6, excite other neurons located within the somatic sensory cortex, the motor cortex, and the thalamus. The neurotransmitter used by the pyramidal cells is glutamate or aspartate. The nonpyramidal cells have several different classifications and include double bouquet cells, chandelier cells, and spiderweb cells. They use GABA as the neurotransmitter, and they function to inhibit neurotransmission.

The homunculus illustrates where the sensory afferents for each body part project to the primary somatosensory cortex (S-I) (Fig. 2-18). As is illustrated, there are many afferent axons in the hands, face, and lips. These axons occupy a large surface area of the sensory cortex and are extremely sensitive to sensory stimuli. Table 2-14 depicts the different areas of the brain and their relationship to sensation.

Many of the clinical presentations described in this text illustrate how the clinician tests for intactness of the sensory system. For example, the sharp and the dull end of a pin and a piece of cotton can be used to determine the ability of the patient to perceive pain and light touch, respectively. Dermatomes are located in the common areas tested on the extremities (Fig. 2-19). Clinicians use two dermatome maps (which have subtle differences) to determine if there is sensory change or loss at certain spinal levels. It is known that sensory afferents travel from specific limb areas to the dorsal horn of the spinal column by way of the peripheral afferents. Therefore, for example, the clinician uses a cotton swab and strokes the lateral aspect of the big toe to test the sensory dermatome of L4. The sensation felt by the patient is then compared to the same area on the opposite foot. Any difference would be noted by the clinician. The results can help clinicians determine whether the insult is in the CNS or located in a peripheral nerve, nerve root, or spinal nerve (PNS). Lesions to any one of these anatomic structures will cause a change in sensation. The general rule of dermatomal evaluation is that if only one dermatome is affected, a lesion in the dura, the dorsal root, or the spinal nerve is a consideration. If there are unilateral paresthesias in many dermatomes then the lesion is usually in a peripheral nerve. If the general sensory loss is bilateral and symmetric, then the consideration is systemic disease (for example, diabetes) or a lesion in the CNS.

### The spinal cord and its related somatosensory tracts

The somatic sensory system consists of *ascending* spinal pathways that involve five major modalities: touch discrimination (light touch, deep pressure, and two-point

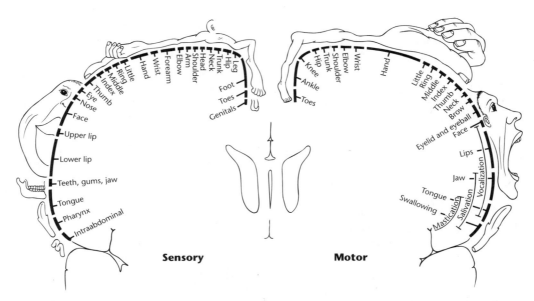

**Fig. 2-18** Homunculus of the sensory and motor cortex. Surface area is largest for sensory interpretation of the face, lips, and fingers. Motor nuclei surface area is largest for the hand and face.

discrimination), proprioception, vibration, nociception (pain), and temperature. Touch discrimination is defined as the ability of the system to recognize the size, shape, and texture of objects and their movement across the skin. Proprioception is the ability of the body to sense static position and dynamic movement, whereas vibration is the ability to detect oscillations. Nociception is the ability to signal the body that tissue damage, often perceived as pain, has occurred; pain is the psychosocial perception of a tissue lesion. Temperature is the sensation of warmth or cold.[30,40]

**Table 2-14** Anatomic relationships of the brain to sensation

| Area of the brain | Sensation |
|---|---|
| **Brodmann's areas** | |
| 1, 2, 3A, 3B | Sense of position; discrimination of size, texture, and shape |
| | Pain and temperature are altered if injury is present in Barens 3, 1, 2 |
| 3B (Hand homunculus) | Discrimination of texture, size, and shape of objects |
| 1 | Assessment of texture of objects |
| 2 | Differentiation of size and shape of objects |
| **Secondary somatic sensory cortex (S II)** | Discrimination of shape and texture; learning tactile discrimination based on the shape of an object |
| **Posterior parietal cortex (higher order sensory cortex)** | Perception of tactile stimulation |

Pathways that relay this type of information to the cerebral cortex from the external environment are the *dorsal column–medial lemniscal system* (for touch and conscious proprioception), the spinocerebellar tracts (for unconscious proprioception), and the *anterolateral system* (for pain, touch, and temperature).

**The dorsal column–medial lemniscal pathway.** The perception of touch is transmitted to the brain by four types of receptors located in the skin. The superficial skin has rapidly adapting Meissner's corpuscles and slowly adapting Merkel's cells.[31] Pacinian corpuscles and Ruffini corpuscles are located in the deeper tissues of the skin and respond to vibration (Pacinian corpuscles), and to rapid indentation of the skin (Ruffini corpuscles). These four receptors send Ib fibers to the spinal cord via sensory peripheral nerves whose nerve cells are located in the dorsal root ganglion (pseudo-unipolar cells). The central branch of a dorsal root ganglion cell enters the spinal cord at the dorsal lateral margin of the posterior horn.[4,32] The neurons are segregated in the horn depending on the sensory function they serve. Large-diameter tactile, vibrational, and proprioceptive neurons enter medially to the small-diameter axons (mediating pain and temperature). The large-diameter fibers enter the dorsal horn at the large-diameter fiber entry zone, and the small fibers enter at the zone of Lussauer. Once in the cord the sensory axons contribute to three different pathways: (1) They may become segmental branches that enter the gray matter of the spinal cord and form a synapse on interneurons or motor neurons (where they become part of the reflex arc) at that level. (2) They may become part of an ascending branch

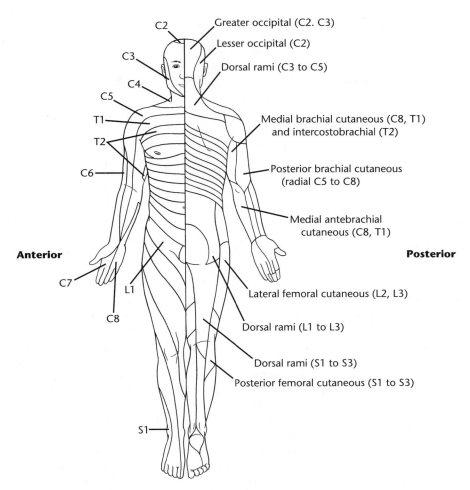

**Fig. 2-19** Dermatomal map (anterior view) and cutaneous nerve distribution (posterior view) of the human body.

where sensory information is transmitted to the brain. (3) They may form synapses on descending branches that, in turn, form synapses on the spinal cord interneurons that transmit information for intersegmental reflexes.[13,32,40,47] The usual path of the large-diameter fibers is to synapse in the dorsal horn of the spinal cord at Rexed's level III to VI in the intermediate zone and the ventral horn (Table 2-15).

**Table 2-15** Different schemes for nomenclature of the organizational areas in the spinal cord

| Nuclei | Rexed's lamina | Region |
|---|---|---|
| Marginal zone | I | Dorsal horn |
| Substantia gelatinosa | II | Dorsal horn |
| Nucleus proprius | III, IV | Dorsal horn |
| Clarke's nucleus | VII | Intermediate zone |
| Intermediolateral nucleus | VII | Intermediate zone |
| Motor nuclei | IX | Ventral horn |

The large-diameter fibers proceed up the spinal cord through the posterior columns by way of the *gracillis nucleus* or the *cuneate nucleus*. The sensory fibers coming from the lower extremities travel along the gracillis nucleus and those from the upper extremities travel along the nucleus cuneatus. As a signal ascends the cord in the dorsal columns contrast sharpening by lateral inhibition occurs.[44,47] Long ascending dorsal column afferent fibers contain L-glutamate as a neurotransmitter. L-glutamate excites interneurons that contain GABAergic neurotransmitters. These interneurons, through lateral inhibition, inhibit surrounding projection cells, thereby preventing summation of the signals from juxtapositional axons in the cord. The specificity of the signal allows spatial discrimination of a signal without interference from other areas.[40,44]

Decussation of the dorsal column–medial lemniscal pathway occurs in the medulla nucleus cuneatus or nucleus gracilis (second order cells), and by the internal arcuate dorsal column fibers travel to the medial lemniscus in the medulla. They proceed as the medial lemniscal pathway to the ventral posterior lateral nuclei and ventral posterior medial nuclei of the thalamus. These fibers then form synapses (third-order cells) and send their axons to the internal capsule and on to S-I in the posterior central gyrus of the parietal lobe of the cerebral cortex.[18,19]

In the primary somatic sensory cortex these fibers can travel to Brodmann areas 1, 2, 3a, and 3b. The majority of the somatic sensory fibers first project in areas 3a and 3b and then project to areas 1 and 2. Other fibers from the thalamus project to S-II, which also receives input from S-I.[29] Mishkin et al[29] found that the connections between S-I and S-II are required for the function of perception. If sensory cells have lesions in S-I, then the corresponding cells in S-II will not function; however, if there is a lesion in S-II, it does not have an effect on S-I. Other projections from the ventral posterior medial and lateral nuclei may go to the posterior parietal cortex (Brodmann's areas 5 and 7).

**Nociception and temperature pathways.** Nociceptors are free nerve endings (the least differentiated sensory receptors) that are activated by mechanical, thermal, or chemical stimuli and are located in many anatomic structures. Pain-sensitive structures of the spinal column and surrounding structures are innervated by the medial or lateral branch of the dorsal ramus, the recurrent meningeal nerve, the sympathetic trunk, or the gray rami communicantes.[17] The primary cell bodies of nociceptors are in the dorsal root ganglia and the trigeminal ganglia (CN V). Several different classes of nociceptive afferent receptors exist. Thermal or mechanical nociceptors have small-diameter, thinly myelinated A delta fibers that conduct at about 5 to 30 m/s.[29] The pain produced by the stimulation of these fibers is perceived by the patient as a very sharp well-localized pain of short duration. The sensation described by a patient who has received a blow is sharp initial pain that dissipates quickly and becomes more dull and diffuse over time.

Polymodal nociceptors produce dull aching pain. These fibers are activated by a variety of high-intensity mechanical, chemical, and hot or cold stimuli. They have small-diameter, unmyelinated C fibers that conduct slowly at 0.5-2 m/s.[29] Both A-delta and C fibers are widespread in skin and deep tissues. The mechanism that allows depolarization of the nerve endings to trigger an action potential in these fibers is not clear. It is believed that the transduction mechanism for each stimulus is distinct because each type of stimulus seems to produce a characteristic threshold potential.

Two possible mechanisms can produce hyperalgesia in peripheral tissues: a lowering of the nerve threshold or an increase in the magnitude of pain by suprathreshold stimuli.[29]

Both A-delta and C-peripheral fibers bifurcate upon entering the spinal cord. The branches of these fibers ascend and descend approximately three segments as part of the tract of Lissauer, whereas other axons synapse in the superficial dorsal horn.[17] Commonly mentioned areas in the dorsal horn that contain the nociceptive synapses are Lamina I (marginal zone), Lamina II (substantia gelatinosa), and Lamina V (primarily A-delta fibers). Controversy does exist as to which of the Rexed laminas are involved in nociceptive transmission. Laminas VI and VII are also known to be involved with nociceptive transmission to the spinothalamic tract. Laminas VII and VIII send nociceptive axons to the spinoreticular tract and laminas I and V transmit nociceptive fibers to the spinomesencephalic tract. Other laminas (III and IV) send nociceptive fibers to the spinocervical tract and the dorsal columns.[47]

***Neuroanatomy of the nociceptive pathways.*** Nociceptive afferents connect directly or indirectly with three major classes of neurons in the dorsal horn: (1) projection neurons that relay information to higher areas of the brain; (2) local excitatory neurons that relay stimuli to interneurons that relay information to higher areas of the brain; and (3) inhibitory interneurons that regulate the flow of nociceptive information to higher centers.[17,29]

Lamina I contains a high concentration of projection neurons that are specifically excited by nociceptors and are therefore termed *nociceptive-specific* neurons. Other projection neurons receive mixed information from nociceptors and mechanoreceptors and are called *wide-dynamic range nociceptors*. Wide-dynamic range nociceptors are also located in laminas IV and VI. A nociceptive stimulus can thus travel along three major and two supplementary projection pathways. The major nociceptive pathways are the spinothalamic tract, the spinomesencephalic tract, and the spinoreticular tract. The two supplementary pathways are the spinocervical tract and the dorsal column–medial lemniscal pathway.[29,42]

The spinothalamic tract is the most dominant nociceptive pathway. It originates from neurons located in Rexed laminae I and V to VII where all axons decussate to the contralateral anterolateral white matter and form synapses with neurons in the medial and lateral nuclear group of the thalamus. The pathway then travels in the internal capsule and corona radiata and terminates in the association sensory cortex and somatic sensory cortex. The nociceptive receptors of this tract are nociceptive-specific and wide-dynamic range neurons.[17]

The spinoreticular tract receive its axons from laminas VII and VIII. Most of the fibers of this tract decussate immediately at the cord level. Some of the fibers ascend ipsilaterally to send off branches that terminate in both the reticular formation of the brain stem and the midline (medial) and intralaminar (lateral) thalamic nuclei, and then proceed to the association cortex or the somatic sensory cortex. Located in the reticular formation of the brain stem is the *ascending reticular activating system* (ARAS). This system supplies neurologic circuitry for arousal and attentiveness that greatly affects a patient's awareness and psychologic attitude toward nociceptive stimuli.[29,42] The combination of the nociceptive stimulus, the psychologic attitude, and the awareness of the sensation is referred to as pain.

The spinomesencephalic tract receives axons from laminas I and V that decussate at the cord level and terminate in the mesencephalic reticular formation at the lateral periaqueductal gray region. The periaqueductal gray area is of significance to the clinician because of its role in blocking nociception. Descending fibers from the periaqueductal gray matter in the midbrain have been shown to block nociceptive input.[6,10] Stimulation of neurons from the periaqueductal gray area travel to the nucleus raphe magnus that is abundant in seritonin neurotransmitters.[5] Serotonergic fibers descend through the dorsolateral funiculus of the spinal cord by way of the raphe spinal tract and form synapses on laminas I and II. They form synapses with enkephalin- (an opioid peptide) containing inhibitory interneuron and nociceptive projection neurons. Activation of the opiod-peptide interneurons can inhibit nociceptive transmission by two mechanisms: by binding to receptors and blocking neurotransmitters and by directly forming synapses with the postsynaptic membranes of the spinothalamic tract neurons.[5,28]

Other nociceptive inhibiting pathways originate in the pons and contain norepinephrine as the neurotransmitter. These pathways inhibit nociception at the dorsal horn and also project to the raphe nuclei. Release of norepinephrine at this level results in tonic inhibition of the raphe neurons causing a constant release of serotonin and a long-term analgesic affects.[5]

Segmental control of nociception, located in the spinal cord, was first introduced by Melzack and Wall[33] in 1965. The gate control theory (pain-gait theory) contends that increased activity of large-diameter, low-threshold afferent fibers (for example, the Ia or Ib fibers) will inhibit small-diameter afferent fibers (A delta and C fibers) and will prevent transmission of nociceptive impulses to higher spinal and cortical centers. Inhibition of the nociceptive fibers occurs primarily in Lamina II (substantia gelatinosa). Interneurons in this area use enkephalin as the neurotransmitter. These interneurons synapse with large-diameter neurons and correspondingly inhibit the spinothalamic tract neurons (Fig. 2-20).

There are many physical modalities that the clinician uses to stimulate the large-diameter sensory afferent fibers that block nociception. Hand rubbing of the skin over the painful area partially decreases perception of the pain. Electric stimulation and ice also activate large-diameter afferent fibers that segmentally and supraspinally control nociceptive stimuli.

**Proprioceptive pathways.** There are two categories of proprioception in the human body: conscious and unconscious proprioception. Conscious proprioception is the ability of the CNS to determine the location of a limb in space. A typical example of conscious proprioception is a person moving a hand to some location with eyes closed, and being able to identify where that limb is located in space. Unconscious proprioception consists of balance and posture and is controlled by the cerebellum.

There are many neurologic mechanisms involved with proprioception in humans. The muscle spindle and Golgi tendon organ are important receptor organs that provide feedback to the brain about muscle length. Free nerve endings located in the joint capsule are other proprioceptive fibers that help the body determine joint position and joint motion. Incorporated within the conscious proprioceptive system are the vestibular system of the inner ear and the dorsal column–medial lemniscal pathway that relay messages to the somatosensory cortex and the cerebellum. These systems are jointly determined *kinesthetic sense.*

The muscle spindle is located in the muscle belly, primarily in the central portion of the muscle. The Golgi tendon organ is situated in the tendon along the myotendinous junction, and the joint receptors are located diffusely throughout the joint capsule. The vestibular system, along with the cerebellum, also plays a major role in balance, equilibrium, and posture. Conscious and unconscious proprioception can be used to describe the different neuroanatomic structures that provide the cerebellum or the postcentral gyrus of the cerebral cortex with valuable information about joint position, joint motion, muscle stretch, and gravitational pull and its effect on posture.

*The muscle spindle.* The muscle spindle is a complex proprioceptor that responds to both static muscle position (tonic response) and a dynamic change in the length of the muscle (phasic response). Muscle spindles are arranged in parallel within the extrafusal muscle fibers and slight variations in spindle morphology occur. Phasic muscles contain more spindles per area of muscle than do tonic (postural) muscles.

Generally, each muscle spindle consists of a fluid-filled capsule that is 2 to 20 mm in length and encapsulates 5 to 12 small specialized muscle fibers called *intrafusal fibers* (Fig. 2-21). Fibers that exist in striated muscle that are outside of the spindle are called *extrafusal fibers.*

The diameter of the intrafusal fibers ranges from one tenth to one fourth of the diameter of an extrafusal

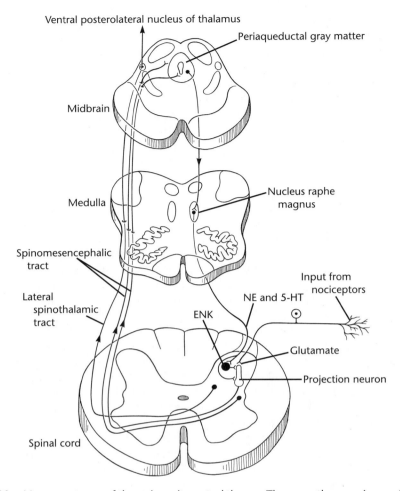

**Fig. 2-20** Neuroanatomy of the pain-gait control theory. There are three major nociceptive pathways: spinothalamic, spinomesencephalic, and spinoreticular pathways. The spinomesencephalic pathway (depicted here) plays a major role in pain modulation. *NE,* Norepinephrine; *5-HT,* Serotonin; *ENK,* Enkephalin. Glutamate is a facilatory neurotransmitter, *NE, 5-HT,* and *ENK* are inhibitory neurotransmitters that inhibit nociceptive transmission.

fiber. Each spindle contains one to three large intrafusal fibers and one to eight small intrafusal fibers. The large fibers are termed nuclear bag fibers because their nuclei are contained in the center with the appearance of a bag of marbles; in the smaller fibers, the nuclei are arranged in a chain at the equatorial region of the fiber and are called nuclear chain fibers. The chain fibers are contained within the spindle (intracapsular fibers) and connect to the inner surface of the capsular connective tissue. The longer, larger bag fibers project out of the spindle and connect to the endomysium of the extrafusal fibers (pericapsular fibers).[25]

The afferent innervation of the muscle spindle contains two types of nerve endings. The primary nerve ending is annulospiral that coils around the equatorial areas of all intrafusal fibers. The secondary nerve ending is flower-spray in appearance and terminates more toward the polar region of the chain intrafusal fibers. The axons of the primary nerve ending are large, heavily myelinated, fast-conducting group Ia fibers, whereas the axons of the secondary afferents are group Ib and/or II fibers. There is only one primary afferent axon that branches to all the intrafusal fibers, whereas there are one to five secondary afferent fibers that do not branch and that are located on the chain fibers only.[25] The primary afferent fibers have a lower threshold to stretch and respond to both phasic and tonic stretch. The secondary nerve endings have a higher threshold potential and respond to tonic length only.

During phasic muscle action the primary afferent fiber responds to the velocity of the change in length of the bag and chain fibers during stretch and changes its im-

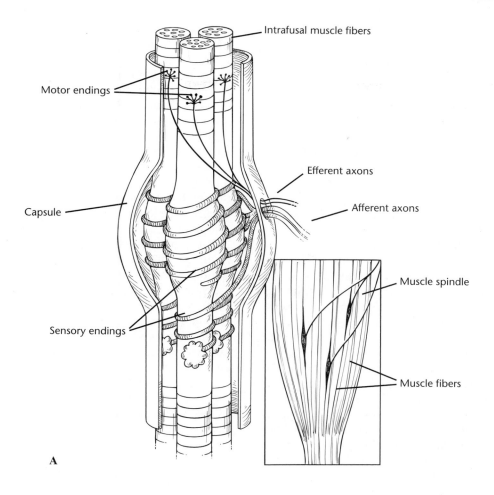

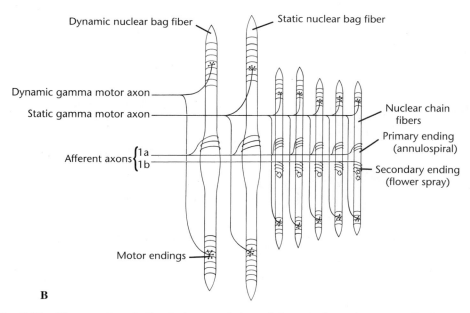

*Fig. 2-21* The muscle spindle. **A,** A general view of the spindle and its in-parallel location within striated muscle (insert). **B,** A detailed illustration of the anatomical presentation of the spindle with its nuclear bag and nuclear chain fibers. Annulospiral, flower spray, and motor endings are depicted.

pulse frequency accordingly. The impulse frequency of the afferents during tonic muscle activity is less than that during phasic muscle activity and remains constant.

Efferent innervation consists of both beta (or gamma II) and gamma motor neurons (fusimotor neurons) whose cell bodies are located in the ventral horn of the spinal column.[22] Each motor axon travels along its respective peripheral nerve to innervate the intrafusal (beta and gamma neurons) and extrafusal fibers (beta neurons).[22] In the intrafusal fibers, the motor axons terminate on the polar contractile regions of the bag and chain fibers. Each spindle receives seven to 25 efferent neurons. Stimulation of the efferent neurons cause the polar regions of the intrafusal fibers to contract, causing a concomitant stretch of the equatorial regions of the bag and chain fibers. The neurologic impulse of the beta and gamma motor neurons is equivalent to the alpha motor neuron stimulus to the extrafusal fibers. Stimulus from the muscle spindle also travels along spinal cerebellar pathways to the cerebellum and the dorsal column–medial lemniscal pathway and produces conscious and unconscious proprioception.

Neurologic tests that evaluate the integrity of the monosynaptic reflex are commonly known as deep tendon reflex tests (Fig. 2-22). By striking a tendon with a reflex hammer, the corresponding muscle is stretched, causing a stimulus to travel along the Ia afferent fiber of the muscle spindle. Only a few millimeters per second change in intrafusal fiber length is required to activate the Ia fiber. The stimulus then travels through the dorsal

horn to the ventral horn and synapses on the alpha, beta, and gamma motor neurons. Stimulation of the alpha motor neuron causes contraction of the extrafusal fibers, whereas stimulation of the beta and gamma fibers cause the muscle spindle intrafusal fibers to contract at the polar regions. Reciprocal inhibition of the antagonist occurs by stimulation of the Renshaw cells in the ventral horn that causes inhibition of the antagonist muscles or by presynaptic inhibition of the antagonist afferents to prevent the antagonist from responding to the initiated stretch.[25] Therefore, when a clinician tests the patellar deep tendon reflex, the hamstrings are reciprocally inhibited and the quadriceps muscle contracts just enough to relieve the spindle equatorial stretch.

The monosynaptic reflex arc is only one of several routes an afferent stimulus may take when the muscle spindle is stretched. The muscle spindle is one of the receptor organs of conscious and unconscious proprioception. Stimulus from the afferent fibers from the muscle spindle can travel through the dorsal column–medial lemniscal pathway for conscious proprioception. At the nucleus cuneatus or nucleus gracillis, the tract decussates along the arcuate fibers to the medial lemniscal pathway and to the ventral posterolateral or ventral posteromedial areas of the thalamus. The stimulus then proceeds by way of the internal capsule and corona radiata to the sensory cortex (postcentral gyrus, areas 3, 1, 2) of the cerebral cortex. Unconscious proprioception consists of the initial stimulation of the muscle spindle of the postural muscles. Stimulus from the afferents from the mus-

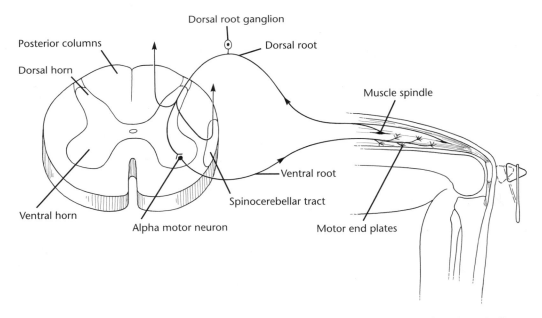

*Fig. 2-22* Neuroanatomy of the monosynaptic deep tendon reflex. Note that the spindle afferents are also part of the dorsal column medial leminscal pathway and spinocerebellar tracts that are responsible for conscious and unconscious proprioception.

cle spindle to the spinal cord then follows the cuneo, ventral, or dorsal spinocerebellar tracts and proceeds ipsilaterally to the side of stimulus (the ventral spinocerebellar tract decussates twice), and enters the cerebellum through the cerebellar peduncles. This information is then processed through the cerebellum, the basal ganglia, and the cerebral cortex. The message for correction of posture, sense of joint position, or sense of joint motion is then sent along the corticospinal tract or rubrospinal tract to stimulate and inhibit the peripheral muscles.

The muscle spindle is important for muscular adjustment to changes in posture. For example, standing in the erect posture causes slow changes in muscle length to occur because the shift of the center of gravity leads to a tonic response in the primary afferents of the spindle. A contraction of the stretched muscle will correct the gravitational shift and resume posture. At the ankle, the center of gravity lies just anterior to the malleoli, and it places a tonic stretch on the calf muscles (soleus). A forward lean at the ankle is corrected by the myotatic stretch reflex (monosynaptic reflex arc) that causes the soleus to contract by the necessary amount to counter the forward force and pull the body back over the base of support.

The muscle spindle is also involved in muscle stretch. The clinician attempts to lengthen a tight muscle by applying an external load. When a muscle is first stretched, the Ia afferent fibers fire at a rapid rate, with the frequency being directly related to the velocity of stretch (phasic response). When the muscle reaches a certain length, and this length is maintained, the frequency of impulse drops to a level that is appropriate to the new length (tonic response). It is believed that the bag and chain fibers also adapt to the new length by way of the inherent viscoelastic relaxation properties of the involved tissue. When a muscle is maintained at a new length, the equatorial areas of the bag and chain fibers initially resist the motion and respond by stretching (resistance is caused by the materials stiffness and relaxation properties). This correspondingly increases afferent output through the Ia fiber. Over time, the equatorial areas relax at the new length, causing the material stiffness to decrease, leading to less equatorial stretch, and concomitantly decreasing the Ia afferent stimulus.

The cortical signals for the programming of voluntary movements seem to reach the muscles over two pyramidal pathways. The first pathway consists of direct stimulus to the involved muscle group through the alpha and gamma motor neuron stimulation to the muscle spindle (alpha-gamma coactivation). The second pathway is described as the gamma loop and is an indirect pathway. Signals from the cerebral cortex travel to the gamma motor neurons causing intrafusal fibers to contract and putting a stretch on the equatorial area that activates the spindle afferent fibers. These afferent fibers transmit impulses back to the spinal cord and across the synapses to the alpha motor neurons of the muscle, which regulates the amount and rate of muscle shortening.[26]

***The Golgi tendon organ.*** The Golgi tendon organ (GTO) (Fig. 2-23) is an encapsulated structure located in the tendon of a striated muscle at the musculotendinous junction. It lies in series with the contractile muscle tissues and involves several muscle fiber tendons. The GTO is unique in that it has only afferent innervation; efferent innervation is absent. Activation of the GTO results in inhibition of its own muscle and activation of the antagonist. In instances where the neuronal activity of the muscle spindle decreases when its muscle decreases in length (concentric action), the GTO is highly sensitive to tendon stretch when concentric muscle stimulation increases. The GTO gives continuous feedback to the spinal cord about the active forces being produced by the muscle, and its actions are vital for a coordinated muscle response.[25]

The GTO is supplied by group Ib afferents that enter the cord through the dorsal horn and make di- or poly-

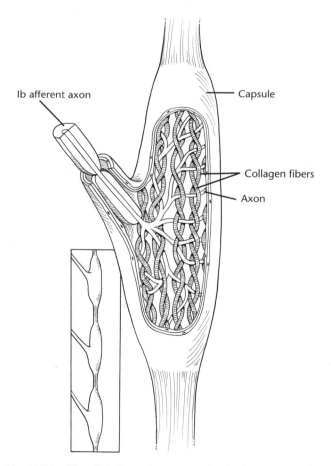

*Fig. 2-23* The Golgi tendon organ. It sits in series in the musculotendinous junction and within the tendon (inset).

synaptic connections with alpha and gamma efferents of their own muscle and to synergists and antagonists. Because these Ib efferent fibers act to inhibit their own muscle (autogenic inhibition) and the synergists, while facilitating the antagonists, the actions of the GTO can be considered to be opposite those of the muscle spindle. The exact mechanism of GTO action during voluntary motion is not well understood. Some type of inhibitory mechanism that affects the Ib afferent occurs during motion. Several examples of GTO reflex activity have been cited. The immediate relaxation of muscles after volitional movement ceases may by an example of the effect of inhibition by GTO. Inhibition of the Ib fiber occurs during motion; inhibition is reversed when motion ceases.[22] The GTO seems to participate in constant muscle contraction. Its afferent fibers supplies the cerebral cortex with information that helps maintain constant muscle strength. The GTO is also a protective mechanism that spontaneously shuts a muscle off when injury or rupture is possible. This is best seen in instances where an excessive load is applied to a muscle, which collapses to protect itself from injury (for example, arm wrestling). The occurrence of the clasp-knife phenomenon in patients with muscle spasticity can also be attributed to the GTO. As passive muscle stretching increases, spastic muscle tone also increases, causing the threshold of the GTO to be reached, with the muscle collapsing through inability to produce any further resistance. This is seen in patients who have suffered cerebral vascular accidents (see Case 4) and in other diseases that produce muscle spasticity. The lack of the clasp-knife phenomenon during a muscle stretch in a patient who has an upper motor neuron lesion is called muscle rigidity, with a lead-pipe muscle presentation. In a lead-pipe muscle presentation, the muscle is stretched but never relaxes reflexively leading it to move like a "lead-pipe."

## The vestibular system

The vestibular system assists in proprioception by providing the nervous system with information about gravity, rotation, and acceleration for the maintenance of balance and equilibrium.[44] Integration of sensory input with continual vestibular stimuli produces the normal sensory perception of motion. Any disturbance that leads to hypo- or hyperactivity of the vestibular system disturbs this synchrony and will produce the subjective complaint of vertigo. Vertigo is a specific form of disequilibrium that suggests a lesion of the vestibular system. Because of its intimate neuroanatomic involvement with the structures of the vestibular system described below, vertigo is accompanied by nausea, vomiting, ataxia, and nystagmus.

The vestibular portion of CN VIII is the neurologic pathway that transmits information about equilibrium and balance to the CNS. Numerous connections between the vestibular nuclei located in the medulla and the pons, the cerebellum, the reticular formation, the medial longitudinal fasciculus, the cerebral cortex, and the spinal cord integrate sensory information from the periphery with balance and equilibrium.

The vestibular receptors are enclosed in the vestibular portion of the labyrinth of the *utricle,* the *saccule,* and the three *semicircular canals* (Fig. 2-24). Hair cell receptors, bathed in endolymph, respond to mechanical movement and initiate impulses transmitted by CN VIII to the vestibular nuclei. Movement of the hair cells in the utricle and saccule produce action potentials that respond to positional and gravitational change. Hair cell motion is produced by otoliths, small calcified particles, that are present in the maculae and are located on the walls of the saccule and utricle. Head motion causes the gravitational pull on the otolith to change the distortion of the hair cells and initiate an action potential.

Each semicircular canal lies in a different plane, thereby allowing the receptors to respond to any motion around an axis. At one end of each semicircular canal is an enlargement called the ampulla. The *crista,* a specialized region of epithelium, is similar to the maculae and it projects into the lumen of the canal from the wall of the ampulla. When movement occurs, the endolymph, in the lumen of the canal, moves and distorts the crista. This motion, in turn, stimulates the hair cells, initiating an action potential.

Cell bodies of the first-order nuclei are located in the vestibular ganglion in the internal auditory meatus. They then travel along CN VIII to synapse in the superior medial, the lateral, and the inferior vestibular nuclei located in the floor of the fourth ventricle.[44] The third-order nuclei may converge on the inferior cerebellar peduncle to enter the cerebellum, whereas others may synapse on the inferior and medial vestibular nuclei then enter the cerebellum and terminate on the flocculonodular lobe. From this point, axons travel to the vestibulospinal tracts to regulate muscle tone in response to changing positions. Fibers from the vestibular nuclei travel along the longitudinal fasciculus and are involved in the coordination of head and eye movements. Where the fibers from the vestibular system terminate is not clear, but it is believed that the temporal lobe plays a major role in vestibular function.

## Clinical neurologic tests

Several clinical tests are typically used to evaluate the function of the NMS either during the physical examination of the patient or as special studies ordered by the clinician after the physical exam. These clinical tests are listed in Tables 2-16 and 2-17 and are all based on a chemical or structure associated with the NMS system.

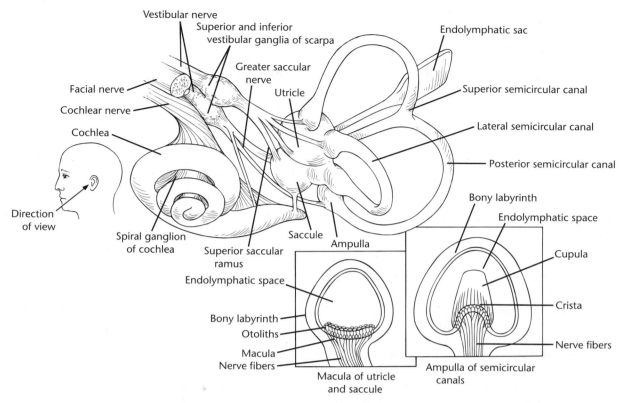

**Fig. 2-24** The vestibular system. Insets show the position of the otoliths of the macula in the saccule and the ampulla of the semicircular canals.

In each case presented in this book, neurologic tests, such as muscle testing, are used to determine whether a lesion is located in the PNS or the CNS. Noting the resistance of a muscle to allow joint motion helps the examiner record muscle rigidity or spasticity. Case 4 presents a patient with muscle rigidity and spasticity indicating that the lesion in this patient is in the CNS. Muscle weakness would be evidence that the lesion is located in the PNS.

Other neurologic tests are used to differentiate a lesion located in the cerebellum, the vestibular system, or the proprioceptive pathways (dorsal column disease).

**Table 2-16** Physical examination of the central nervous system

---

**Sensory functions tested**
Audition
Dermatomes
Nociception
Proprioception
Visual fields

**Motor functions tested**
Cardinal fields of gaze
Facial expression
Mastication
Muscle strength
Range of motion
Swallowing

**Reflexes tested**
Deep tendon reflex
Jaw jerk
Pathologic reflexes
Superficial reflexes

**Table 2-17** Special studies for evaluating of the central nervous system.

---

**Techniques measuring electric activity**
Electroencephalogram (EEG)
Electromyogram (EMG)
Nerve conduction velocity (NCV)
Sensory evoked potential (SEP)
auditory
somatosensory
visual

**Imaging techniques**
Magnetic resonance imaging (MRI)
Positron emission tomography (PET)
X-ray examination

The rule of thumb in differentiating lesions in these systems is that if a given task can be performed with the eyes open but not with the eyes closed then the lesion is located in the proprioceptive or vestibular systems. If the patient has difficulty performing the task with the eyes either open or closed, then the lesion is located in the cerebellum. Sight provides sense of joint position that is missing. Visualization of the structure being moved allows the patient to place it in the correct location. Finger-to-finger, finger-to-nose, and Romberg's tests are conducted in both the eyes-open and eyes-closed positions. Patients with proprioceptive problems can usually perform a task properly with the eyes open but not with the eyes closed. The patient's motion, however, is coordinated and not ataxic in presentation as is seen in cerebellar disease.

The heel-to-shin test is performed by having the patient run the heel of the foot along the opposite shin while in the supine position. If a cerebellar lesion exists, the patient will have difficulty bending the knee to contact the heel to the shin and will produce jerky motions during the attempt to move the heel along the shin.

Numerous neurologic tests are used to evaluate the function of the vestibular system. Caloric tests consist of irrigating the ear with either warm or cold water, which causes a convection current to occur within the endolymph, and observing for nystagmus either away or toward the stimulus, respectively. This is indicative of the integrity of the axonal attachments between the labyrinth, the vestibular nerve, the medial longitudinal fasciculus, and the oculomotor system in the brain stem. The Doll's eyes test examines the neurologic pathways located in the brain stem in the posterior fossa and tests the integrity of the semicircular canals. During rotary and flexion or extension movements of the head, the eyes should stay fixed and move in a direction opposite to that of head movement.

## Blood supply to the brain and spinal cord

Three main arteries supply the cerebral cortex: the anterior, the middle, and the posterior cerebral arteries. All three are extensions of the carotid or vertebrobasilar system. The carotid and vertebrobasilar arterial systems anastomose at the circle of Willis (Fig. 2-25). The internal carotid artery supplies the anterior and middle cerebral arteries, whereas the posterior cerebral artery is a branch of the basilar artery, which is a continuation of the vertebral arteries. The anterior cerebral artery supplies the medial and superior surfaces and the frontal pole of the cerebral cortex. The middle cerebral artery also branches off the internal carotid artery and courses laterally between the temporal and frontal lobes and emerges from the insula. Its branches spread over the lateral surface of the cerebral hemispheres and the temporal pole.[14,34,44] The basilar artery is formed at the caudal border of the pons by the anastomosis of the vertebral and the anterior spinal arteries. The basilar arteries branch off to form other arteries, as well as the posterior cerebral arteries, which are the sole arterial supply to the occipital lobe, the undersurface of the temporal lobe, the thalamus, the midbrain, the pons, the cerebellum, the medulla, and portions of the cervical spinal cord (namely, the inferior surface and the occipital pole).[34,44]

The blood supply of the brain stem is also derived from the vertebrobasilar arterial system. Paramedian branches from the vertebral and basilar arteries supply the midline region, and the larger circumferential branches supply the lateral area of the brain stem. The large posterior inferior cerebellar artery supplies the medulla, the inferior cerebellar artery supplies the pons, and the superior cerebellar artery supplies the midbrain.

Infarction of the paramedian region will involve the descending motor pathways, the medial lemniscus, and the nuclei of CN III, IV, VI, and XII.[44] In the event of infarction, the patient will not only have problems with motor function on one side of the body but will also have hypesthesias and problems with eye and tongue movement. Ischemia or infarction to the lateral region involves the cerebellum, the cerebellar pathways, the descending sympathetic pathways, the lateral spinothalamic tract, and the nuclei of CN V, VII, VIII, IX, and X.[44,48] Patients with a lesion in this location will have difficulties with unconscious proprioception, pain and temperature sensation, facial sensation and motion, balance, swallowing, and parasympathetic regulation. Depending on the location of the infarction, the patient's signs may be ipsilateral or contralateral to the location of the lesion. A lesion located after the decussation of the corticobulbar tract that supplies the involved nuclei or a lesion at the level of the nucleus will produce signs on the same side of the body as the lesion, whereas a lesion located before the corticobulbar decussation will produce signs on the side of the body opposite the lesion.

The veins of the brain course over the cerebral hemispheres and converge into the venous sinuses. The superior and inferior sagittal sinuses are the most prominent venous sinuses and are located in the dura mater. They course their way longitudinally in the falx cerebri between the hemispheres. These channels merge to form the transverse and sigmoid sinuses in the occipital region and exit the skull through the jugular foramen as the internal jugular veins.

The arterial supply to the spinal cord consists of one anterior spinal artery, two posterior spinal arteries, and the radicular arteries that anastamose with them. The anterior spinal artery is formed from two small branches of the vertebral arteries. The anterior spinal artery is

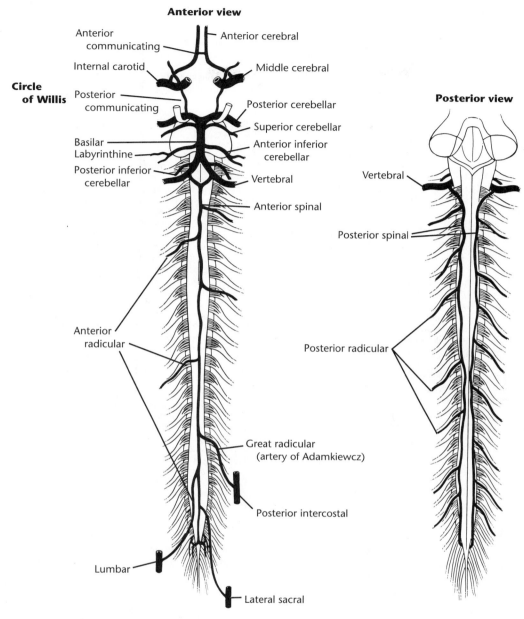

**Anterior view**

Anterior communicating

Anterior cerebral

Internal carotid

Middle cerebral

**Circle of Willis**

Posterior communicating

Posterior cerebellar

Superior cerebellar

Basilar

Labyrinthine

Anterior inferior cerebellar

Posterior inferior cerebellar

Vertebral

Anterior spinal

Anterior radicular

Great radicular (artery of Adamkiewcz)

Posterior intercostal

Lumbar

Lateral sacral

**Posterior view**

Vertebral

Posterior spinal

Posterior radicular

*Fig. 2-25* Vascular system of the spinal cord and the circle of Willis. The circle of Willis is a continuation of the basilar artery that is an extension of the anterior and posterior spinal arteries and vertebral arteries.

smallest in the T4 to T8 region and runs the length of the spinal cord in the anterior median fissure. It supplies the anterior two thirds of the spinal cord.

The posterior spinal artery originates in small branches of either the vertebral or the posterior inferior cerebellar arteries. The posterior spinal arteries anastomose frequently with the anterior spinal artery and supply the posterior one third of the spinal cord.

The anterior and two posterior spinal arteries provide a sufficient supply to the superior cervical aspect of the spinal cord.[34,38] A further supply from the radicular arteries helps feed the remainder of the cord. The radicular arteries originate from spinal branches of the vertebral, deep cervical, ascending cervical, posterior intercostal, lumbar, and lateral sacral arteries.[34,38] The radicular arteries enter the vertebral canal through the intervertebral foramen, divide into the anterior and posterior radicular arteries, which follow the ventral and dorsal nerve roots to the cord and anastamose with the anterior and posterior spinal arteries, respectively. They supply the vertebrae, the meninges, and the spinal arteries.

## REFERENCES

1. Alexander G, Crutcher M: Functional architecture of basal ganglia circuits: neural substrates of parallel processing, *Trends Neurosci* 13:266, 1990.
2. Alexander G, DeLong M: Central mechanisms of initiation and control of movement. In Asbury A, McKhann, G, McDonald W, editors: *Diseases of the nervous system: clinical neurobiology,* ed 2, Philadelphia, 1992, Saunders.
3. Bachop W: Development of the spine and spinal cord. In Cramer G, Darby S, editors: *Basic and clinical anatomy of the spine, spinal cord and ANS,* St Louis, 1995, Mosby.
4. Barr L, Kiernan J: *The human nervous system,* ed 5, Philadelphia, 1988, Lippincott.
5. Basbaum A: Cytochemical studies of the neural circuitry underlying pain and pain control, *Acta Neurochir Suppl* (Wein) 38:5, 1987.
6. Basbaum A, Fields H: Endogenous pain control mechanisms: review and hypothesis, *Ann Neurol* 4:451, 1978.
7. Bogduk N: Local anesthetic blocks of the second cervical ganglion: a technique with application in occipital headache, *Cephalalgia* 1:41, 1989.
8. Bogduk N, Marsland A: On the concept of third occipital headache, *J Neurol Neurosurg Psychiatry* 49:775, 1986.
9. Bogduk N, Marsland A: The cervical zygapophysial joints as a source of neck pain, *Spine* 13:610, 1988.
10. Bonica J: Anatomic and physiologic basis of nociception and pain. In Bonica J, editor: *The management of pain,* ed 2, Philadelphia, 1990, Lea & Febiger.
11. Borysenko M, Beringer T: *Functional histology,* ed 3, Boston, 1989, Little, Brown & Company.
12. Carlson B: *Human embryology and developmental biology,* St Louis, 1994, Mosby.
13. Carpenter M: *Core text of neuroanatomy,* ed 4, Baltimore, 1991, Williams & Wilkins.
14. Clemente C, editor: *Gray's anatomy of the human body,* ed 30 (American), Philadelphia, 1988, Lea & Febiger.
15. Cormack DH: *Essential histology,* Philadelphia, 1993, Lippincott.
16. Cote L, Crutcher MD: The basal ganglia. In Kandel ER, Schwartz JH, Jessell TM editors: *Principles of neural science,* New York, 1991, Elsevier.
17. Cramer GD, Darby SA: Pain of spinal origin. In Cramer GD, Darby SA, editors: *Basic and clinical anatomy of the spine, spinal cord, and ANS,* St. Louis, 1995, Mosby.
18. Darby S, Daley D: Neuroanatomy of the spinal cord. In Cramer G, Darby S, editors: *Basic and clinical anatomy of the spine, spinal cord, and ANS,* St Louis, 1995, Mosby.
19. Davidoff R: The dorsal columns, *Neurology* 39:1377, 1989.
20. DeMyer W: *Technique of the neurologic examination: a programmed text,* ed 4, New York, 1994, McGraw-Hill.
21. Dwyer A, Aprill C, Bogduk N: Cervical zygapophyseal joint pain patterns. I. A study in normal volunteers, *Spine* 15:453, 1990.
22. Enoka R: *Neuromechanical basis of kinesiology,* Illinois, 1988, Human Kinetics Books.
23. Gilman S, Newman S: *Manter and Gatz's Essentials of clinical neuroanatomy and neurophysiology,* ed 8, Philadelphia, 1992, Davis.
24. Gilroy J: *Basic neurology,* ed 2, New York, 1990, McGraw-Hill.
25. Gowitzke B, Milner M: *Scientific bases of human movement,* ed 3, Baltimore, 1988, Williams & Wilkins.
26. Granit R: The functional role of the muscle spindles: facts and hypotheses, *Brain* 98:531, 1975.
27. Guyton A: *Textbook of medical physiology,* ed 8, Philadelphia, 1991, Saunders.
28. Jessell T, Kelly D: Pain and analgesia. In Kandel E, Schwartz J, Jessell T, editors: *Principles of neural science,* ed 3, New York, 1991, Elsevier.
29. Kandel ER, Jessell TM: Touch. In Kandel ER, Schwartz JH, Jessell TM, editors: *Principles of neural science,* ed 3, New York, 1991, Elsevier.
30. Martin JH, Jessell TM: Anatomy of the somatic sensory system. In Kandel ER, Schwartz JH, Jessell TM, editors: *Principles of neural science,* ed 3, New York, 1991, Elsevier.
31. Martin JH, Jessell TM: Modality coding in the somatic sensory system. In Kandel ER, Schwartz JH, Jessell TM, editors: *Principles of neural science,* ed 3, New York, 1991, Elsevier.
32. Martin JH. *Neuroanatomy: Text and atlas,* ed 2, Stamford, 1996, Appleton-Lange.
33. Melzack R, Wall P: Pain mechanism: a new theory, *Science* 150:971, 1965.
34. Moore K: *Clinically oriented anatomy,* ed 3, Baltimore, 1992, Williams & Wilkins.
35. Moore K: The developing human: clinically oriented embryology, ed 4, Philadelphia, 1988, Saunders.
36. Norkin C, Levangie P: *Joint structure and function: a comprehensive analysis,* ed 2, Philadelphia, 1992, Davis.
37. Pansky B, Allen D, Budd G: *Review of neuroscience,* ed 2, New York, 1988, McGraw-Hill.
38. Romanes GJ: *Cunningham's textbook of anatomy,* ed 12, London, 1981, Oxford University Press.
39. Sadler, T. *Langman's medical embryology,* ed 7, Baltimore, 1995, Williams & Wilkins.
40. Schoenen J: Clinical anatomy of the spinal cord, *Neurol Clin* 9:503, 1991.
41. Stevens A, Lowe J: *Histology,* New York, 1992, Gower Medical Publishing.
42. Talbot J, et al: Multiple representations of pain in human cerebral cortex, *Science* 251:1355, 1991.
43. Tuchmann-Duplessis H, et al: *Illustrated human embryology,* vol 2, *Organogenesis,* New York, 1972, Springer-Verlag.
44. Westmoreland B, et al: *Medical neurosciences: an approach to anatomy, pathology, and physiology by systems and levels,* ed 3, Boston, 1994, Little, Brown & Co.
45. Wheater PR, Burkett HG, Daniels VG: *Functional histology,* Edinburgh, 1987, Churchill Livingstone.
46. Williams P, et al: *Gray's anatomy,* ed 37, Edinburgh, 1989, Churchill Livingstone.
47. Willis W, Coggeshall R: *Sensory mechanisms of the spinal cord,* ed 2, New York, 1991, Plenum Press.
48. Wilson-Pauwels L, Akesson E, Stewart P: *Cranial nerves: anatomy and clinical comments,* Toronto, 1988, Decker.

## SUGGESTED READINGS

Cramer GD, Darby SA: *Basic and clinical anatomy of the spine, spinal cord, and ANS,* St Louis, 1985, Mosby.

DeMyer WE: *Technique of the neurologic examination: a programmed text,* ed 4, New York, 1994, McGraw-Hill.

Westmoreland BF, et al: *Medical neurosciences: an approach to anatomy, pathology, and physiology by systems and levels,* ed 3, Boston, 1994, Little, Brown & Co.

# CHAPTER 3

# *The head and neck*

**CASE**

*Connection*

3, 4, 6, 7, 8, 9

## FUNCTIONAL ANATOMY OF THE HEAD AND NECK

J. PAUL ELLIS

The head and neck can display with a multitude of pain presentations as introduced in the cases in Chapter 1. The anatomic structures that cause the pain may, however, be ambiguous. It is necessary for the clinician to have a basic understanding of the functional anatomy and biomechanics of the head, neck, and cervical spine so that pertinent information is obtained from the history and physical examination. The information obtained can then develop an accurate working diagnosis that initiates treatment and management protocols necessary to improve the patient's health.

This chapter will focus on the functional anatomy of the head, neck, and autonomic nervous system and the functional anatomy and biomechanics of the temporomandibular joint.

### Bones of the cranial vault (calvaria)

Four bones make up the calvaria: (1) one frontal bone, (2) two parietal bones, and (3) one occipital bone. These bones are united by sutural synarthrodial joints that encapsulate and protect the brain and other soft tissues.

The base of the skull is made up of (1) the frontal bone, (2) the ethmoid bone, (3) the sphenoid bone, (4) the temporal bone, (5) the parietal bone, and (6) the occipital bone. These bones are fused together in the same way as the bones that constitute the cranial vault. The base of the skull is divided into three areas: (1) the anterior area, (2) the middle area, and (3) the posterior cranial bases. Each bone of the cranial base consists of foramina through which neuroanatomic and vascular structures traverse. Table 3-1 presents the foramina in the cranial base that are openings for the cranial nerves and important blood vessels that supply the brain. The bony protuberances and the muscular attachments of the six bones that make up the calvaria are presented in Table 3-2.

**The meninges.** The meninges consist of the three layers:

1. The dura mater is the outermost layer and is the toughest of the membranous coverings. It consists of two layers of collagenous connective tissue. The outer layer adheres to the skull and the internal layer is continuous with the dura of the cranial nerve and the dura of the spinal cord at the foramen magnum. The dura divides the cranial cavity into three interconnecting compartments, one subtentorial and two supratentorial compartments and provides support for the cerebral hemispheres and other structures.[35] Between the two cerebral hemispheres is the *falx cerebri*. The *tentorium cerebelli* separates the occipital lobes of the cerebral hemispheres from the cerebellum, and the *falx cerebelli* surrounds the cerebellum. Traveling within these three structures are the venous sinuses. The venous sinuses have no valves and no muscle in their walls, and their sole purpose is to drain blood from the brain.

2. The middle layer of the meninges is the arachnoid, which is delicate and transparent and composed of a weblike tissue. The subdural space separates it from the dura. The arachnoid is a thin covering over the brain and spinal cord that does not dip into the fissures or sulci of the brain.

3. The pia mater is the third and innermost layer. It is separated from the arachnoid by the subarachnoid space that contains cerebrospinal fluid (CSF). The pia mater is slightly thicker than the arachnoid mater and is highly vascularized. It is a loose connective tissue membrane that adheres to the surface of the brain and spinal cord. It dips into all the fissures and sulci of the brain and carries small blood vessels with it. The veins are located in the subarachnoid space.

## Bones of the face

There are seven different bones of the face: (1) two zygomatic bones, (2) one maxillary bone, (3) the nasal bones, including the inferior nasal concha, (4) one vomer bone, (5) two lacrimal bones, (6) two palatine bones, and (7) the mandibular bone (Fig. 3-1). In utero, each bone of the head and face develops from an intramembranous framework within which the bone develops from mesenchymal membranes.

## Muscles of the head and face

**The scalp.** The scalp extends from the superior nuchal line on the posterior aspect of the skull to the supraorbital margins and laterally to the temporal fossae at the level of the zygomatic arches. There are five layers of soft tissue that cover the calvaria. The scalp proper (consisting of three fused layers) is separated from the pericranium by loose connective tissue that allow movement of the scalp. Each letter of the word S C A L P is a key to its layers.[35]

Layer 1 consists of the skin, which is thin except in the occipital region. The skin has sebaceous glands, hair follicles, an abundant arterial supply (this leads to heavy bleeding when lacerations of the scalp occur), and venous and lymphatic drainage.

Layer 2 consists of connective tissue and is a thick subcutaneous layer that is richly vascularized, has fat lobules intermeshed with the connective tissue, and is well supplied with nerves.

Layer 3 is the aponeurosis epicranialis, a strong membranous sheet that is the membranous tendon of the belly of the epicranius muscle. The epicranius muscle consists of four parts and covers the superior aspect of the calvaria from the highest nuchal line to the supraorbital margins. The four parts consist of two occipital (occipitalis) muscle and two frontal (frontalis) muscle bellies. The frontalis has no bone attachments and causes the forehead to wrinkle; the occipitalis causes wrinkling in the occipital area of the scalp. All four

*Table 3-1* Foramina that contain cranial nerves (CN) and important arterial and venous supplies

| Foramina | Contents |
| --- | --- |
| **Anterior area: Frontal and ethmoid bones** | |
| Cribiform plate | CN I |
| **Middle area: Sphenoid, temporal, and parietal bones** | |
| Optic canal | CN II |
| Superior orbital fissure | CN V$_1$, CN III, CN IV, and CN VI; Sympathetic fibers |
| Foramin rotundum | CN V$_2$ |
| Foramin ovale | CN V$_3$; accessory meningial artery |
| Foramen spinosum | Middle meningeal artery and vein and CN V$_3$ meningeal branch |
| Foramen lacerum | Internal carotid artery, venous plexus; sympathetic nerve fibers |
| **Posterior cranial fossa: Small portion of the parietal and occipital bones** | |
| Foramen magnum | Spinal roots of CN XI; anterior and posterior spinal arteries, vertebral arteries; medulla, and meninges |
| Jugular foramen | CN IX, CN X, CN XI |
| Hypoglossal canal | CN XII |

*Modified from Moore, KL: Clinically oriented anatomy, ed 3, Baltimore, 1992, Williams & Wilkins.*

*Table 3-2*   Landmarks of the occiput, sphenoid, temporal, and mandibular bones with their respective muscle and ligament attachments

| Bony landmarks | Muscle or ligament |
|---|---|
| **Occiput** | |
| Supreme nuchal line | Occipitofrontalis (epicranius) (posterior belly) (O) |
| Superior nuchal line | Sternocleidomastoideus (I), splenius capitis (I), semispinalis capitis (I), trapezius (I) |
| Inferior nuchal line | Obliquus capitis (inferior and superior) (I), rectus capitis (posterior) (I) |
| External occipital protuberance (EOP) | Ligamentum nuchae (A) |
| Lip of foramen magnum | Anterior atlantooccipital ligament (A), posterior atlantooccipital apical ligament of the dens (A), alar ligament of the dens (A), cruciate ligament of the atlas (A), tectorial membrane (A) |
| Pharyngeal tubercle | Longissimus capitis (I), rectus capitis anterior (I), constrictor pharynges superioris (I) |
| Occipital condyle | Articular capsules (A) |
| Jugular process | Lateral atlantooccipital ligament (A) |
| **Sphenoid bone** | |
| Temporal fossa | Temporalis (O) |
| Medial pterygoid plate | Medial pterygoid (O), constrictor parrynges superior (O), pterygomandibular ligament (A) |
| Lateral pterygoid plate | Lateral pterygoid (O) |
| Scaphoid fossa | Lateral pterygoid (O) |
| Orbital surface of greater wing | Rectus muscles of the eye (O), superior oblique muscles of the eye (O) |
| | Spine of sphenoid, Sphenomandibular ligament (A) |
| **Temporal bone** | |
| Mastoid process | Sternocleidomastoideus (I), longissimus capitis (I), splenius capitis (I) |
| Superior nuchal line | Sternocleidomastoideus (I), longissimus capitis (I), splenius capitis (I) |
| Zygomatic arch | Masseter (superficial portion) (I), lateral temporomandibular ligament (A) |
| Temporal fossa | Temporalis (O) |
| Squamomastoid suture | Occipitofrontalis (epicranius; frontal belly) (O), auricularis posterior (O) |
| Styloid process | Stylohyoid (O), stylopharyngeus (O), styloglossus (O), stylomandibular ligament (A), stylohyoid ligament (A) |
| Carotid canal | Levator veli palatini (O) |
| Mastoid notch | Digastric (posterior belly) (O) |
| Mandibular fossa | Temporomandibular articular disc (A) |
| **Mandible** | |
| Coronoid process | Temporalis (I), masseter (I) |
| Anterior ramus | Temporalis (I) |
| Ramus of mandible | Temporalis (I), masseter (I), medial pterygoid (internus) (I) |
| Angle of mandible | Masseter (I), medial pterygoid (internus) (I), stylomandibular ligament (A) mandibular condyle, articular disc (A) |
| Neck of condyle | Lateral pterygoid (externus) (I), lateral ligament (A) |
| Alveolar process | Buccinator (O), constrictor pharynges superior (O), pterygomandibular ligament (A) |
| Pterygomandibular raphe | Buccinator (O) |
| Body of mandible | Platysma (O), depressor labii inferior (quadratus labii inferior) (O), depressor anguli oris (triangularis) (O) |
| Incisive fossa | Mentalis (O) |
| Mandibular symphysis | Mylohyoid (O), geniohyoid (O), genioglossus (O), depressor labii inferior (quadratus labii inferior) (O) |
| Mylohyoid line | Mylohyoid (O), constrictor pharynges superior (O) |
| Inferior genial tubercle | Geniohyoid (O) |
| Superior genial tubercle | Genioglossus (O) |
| Digastric | Anterior digastric (anterior belly) (O), platysma (inferior edge) (O), depressor anguli oris (triangularis) (O) |
| Mental foramina | Depressor labii inferior (quadratus labii inferior) (O) |
| Oblique line of mandible | Platysma (O), depressor anguli oris (triangularis) (O) |
| Lingula | Sphenomandibular ligament (A) |

*O, Origin; I, insertion; A, attachment of ligament.*

parts of the epicranialis are innervated by the facial nerve (cranial nerve [CN] VII).

Layer 4 consists of loose areolar tissue. This is the layer that allows free movement of the proper scalp. Being composed of loose connective tissue, it acts somewhat like a sponge and contains numerous spaces. Infection can spread easily in this area and can travel into the venous supply of the head (for example, to the emissary veins).

Layer 5 is the pericranium, which is a dense layer of specialized connective tissue.[2,35] Sharpey fibers attach the pericranium to the calvaria.

**Muscles of the face.** The muscles of the face contribute to the facial expression and lie in the subcutaneous

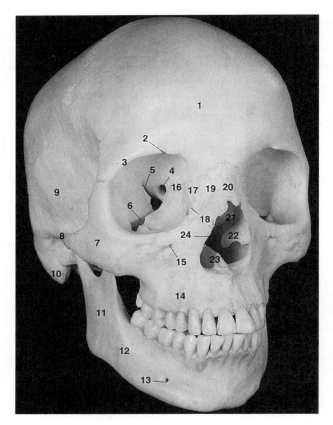

***Fig. 3-1*** Skull bones of the face. 1, Frontal bone; 2, supraorbital notch, sometimes a foramen, for the supraorbital vessels and nerve; 3, supraorbital margin; 4, optic canal; 5, superior orbital fissure; 6, inferior orbital fissure; 7, zygomatic bone; 8, zygomatic arch; 9, squamous part of temporal bone; 10, mastoid process of petrous part of temporal bone; 11, ramus of mandible; 12, body of mandible, bearing the lower teeth; 13, mental foramen, for the mental nerve; 14, maxilla, bearing the upper teeth; 15, infraorbital foramen, for the infraorbital nerve; 16, lateral wall of ethmoidal sinus, with air cells visible through the paper-thin bone (lamina papyracea); 17, lacrimal bone; 18, lacrimal groove, for the lacrimal sac; 19, orbital process of maxilla; 20, nasal bones; 21, middle nasal concha; 22, inferior nasal concha; 23, lower part of bony nasal septum; 24, margin of anterior nasal aperture (piriform aperture). (From: McMinn RMH, Gaddum-Rosse P, Hutchings RT, Logan BM: *McMinn's functional and clinical anatomy,* St. Louis, 1995, Mosby, p. 138, with permission.)

*Table 3-3* Muscles of facial expression

**Muscles of the scalp**
Epicranius
Auricularis
Temporoparietalis

**Muscles around the eye**
Orbicularis oculi
Corrugator (supracilii)

**Muscles around the nose**
Procerus (pyramidalis nasi)
Nasalis (compressor naris [transverse part])
Nasalis (dilator naris, [alar part])
Zygomaticus minor
Zygomaticus major
Buccinator
Depressor septi

**Muscles around the mouth**
Levator labii superioris alaeque nasi
Levator anguli oris (caninus)
Risorius
Depressor labii inferioris (quadratus labii inferioris)
Depressor anguli oris (triangularis)
Mentalis
Buccinator
Orbicularis oris

**Muscles of mastication**
Temporalis
Masseter
Medial pterygoid (internal pterygoid)
Lateral pterygoid (external pterygoid)

**Muscles around the eyeball**
Levator palpebrae superioris
Recti: superior rectus and inferior rectus
Recti: lateral rectus and medial rectus
Superior oblique
Inferior oblique

**Extrinsic muscles of the tongue**
Genioglossus
Hyoglossus
Styloglossus

**Intrinsic muscles of the tongue**
Longitudinalis linguae (superior and inferior)
Transversus and verticalis linguae

**Muscles of the palate**
Levator veli palatini (levator palati)
Tensor veli palatini (tensor palati)
Musculus uvulae
Palatoglossus (glossopalatinus)
Palatopharyngeus (pharyngopalatinus)
Tensor tympani
Stapedius

tissue with attachments to the skin. Most facial muscles are attached to bone or fascia and attach to skin to produce facial expression. All facial muscles are innervated by CN VII (Table 3-3).

Embryologically, the facial muscles are part of the subcutaneous muscle sheet in the head and neck that forms with the platysma and develop from the second branchial or pharyngeal arch.[2,8,35] The facial muscles and platysma are fused because of their common origin and are inner-vated by CN VII that develops along with the facial muscles. Muscles of mastication are innervated by CN V.

It is important to understand the gross facial changes that occur when a nerve lesion occurs in CN VII. A lower motor neuron lesion eliminates all facial motion on the ipsilateral side, whereas an upper motor neuron lesion of CN VII eliminates contralateral facial motion of the maxillary and mandibular branches of CN VII but not of the ophthalmic branch. In Case 4, facial expression is lost on the same side as the extremity involvement. This finding indicates that the lesion is located in higher cortical centers above the decussation of the corticobulbar or corticospinal tracts. A lesion of CN VII that occurs in the brain stem will cause loss of ipsilateral facial expression together with loss of function in the contralateral extremity. Ana-

tomically, a lesion in the brain stem will affect the CN VII nucleus, which is located higher in the brain stem than the decussation of the corticospinal tract.

Other findings of the face and head that help the clinician determine the location of a lesion are ptosis and eye movements (these signs indicate problems with accommodation and cardinal fields of gaze). A lesion to CN III or a lower motor neuron lesion of CN VII will cause ptosis (lidlag). The orbicularis oculi and levator palpebrae superioris raise the upper eyelid to open the palpebral fissure, and these muscles are innervated by CN VII and III,

***Table 3-4***   Cranial nerves: Muscles innervation and facial response

| Cranial nerve | Muscles innervated | Facial response |
|---|---|---|
| I | None (sensory function only) | |
| II | None (sensory function only) | |
| III | Medial, superior, and inferior rectus; inferior oblique | Moves eyes |
| IV | Superior oblique | Moves eyes |
| V | Temporalis | |
| | Masseter | Activates muscles of mastication |
| | Pterygoides | |
| | Tensor veli palatini | Tenses soft palate |
| | Tensor tympani | Tenses tympanic membrane |
| | Mylohyoid | Elevates hyoid bone |
| VI | Lateral rectus | Moves eyes |
| VII | Temporoparietalis | Tightens scalp |
| | Orbicularis oculi | Moves eyelids |
| | Corrugator | Forms wrinkles around eye |
| | Procerus | Wrinkles nose |
| | Nasalis | Compresses nostrils |
| | Zygomaticus | Raises angle of mouth |
| | Buccinator | Compresses cheeks |
| | Depressor septi | Narrows nostrils |
| | Levator labii | Dilates nostrils and draws upper lip upward |
| | Levator anguli oris | Elevates mouth angle |
| | Risorius | Retracts mouth angle |
| | Depressor labii Inferior | Depresses lower lip |
| | Depressor anguli oris | Depresses mouth angle |
| | Mentalis | Wrinkles skin of chin |
| | Orbicularis oris | Closes lips |
| | Stapedius | Draws the head of the stapes backward |
| | Platysma | Depresses lower jaw and lip |
| | Digastric | Elevates hyoid bone |
| | Stylohyoideus | Elevates hyoid bone |
| VIII | None (sensory function only) | |
| IX | Stylopharyngeus | Elevates pharynx and larynx during swallowing and speaking |
| X | Musculus uvulae | Raises uvula |
| | Glossopalatinus | Elevates back of tongue |
| | Pharyngopalatinus | Elevates pharynx |
| | Constrictor muscles | Constrict wall of pharynx during swallowing |
| | Parasympathetic response | |
| XI | Musculus uvulae | Raises uvula |
| | Glossopalatinus | Elevates back of tongue |
| | Pharyngopalatinus | Elevates pharynx |
| | Sternocleidomastoideus | Rotates head to opposite side |
| | Trapezius | Elevates shoulders |
| XII | Genioglossus | Protrudes, retracts, and depresses tongue |
| | Hyoglossus | Depresses tongue |
| | Styloglossus | Retracts and elevates tongue |
| | Linguae muscles | Modifies tongue shape |

respectively. Other muscles that are affected by a CN III nerve lesion are the superior rectus, inferior rectus, medial rectus, and the inferior oblique muscles. In Cases 3 and 4 the lesions are located in CN VII and not in CN III. Ptosis with eye motion problems is indicative of a CN III lesion. Ptosis alone indicates a lesion in the lower motor neuron of CN VII. Normal eye and eyelid function with a loss of facial expression, except in the ophthalmic area, is indicative of an upper motor lesion of CN VII.

### Cranial nerves

Anatomically, the muscles of the head and face are innervated by 12 pairs of CN (Table 3-4 describes their functions). The CN supply to organs provides four distinct functions: special sense, afferent sensory, efferent motor, and parasympathetic innervations. Certain CN supply direct innervation to skeletal muscle; others supply cardiac muscle and smooth muscle in the viscera and glands; and others receive sensory stimuli only.

Innervation to skeletal muscles of the head and neck is supplied by the CN. Innervation to cardiac, smooth muscle, and glands occurs through preganglionic fibers to autonomic ganglia for peripheral relay to the organs concerned. The sensory nuclei of the CN are secondary neurons that receive stimuli from the cell bodies (ganglia) of first sensory neurons from outside the central nervous system (for example, the otic ganglion sends sensory stimuli to the trigeminal ganglion).

The CN are numbered according to their anterior to posterior locations in the brain (Fig. 3-2). CN I is located in the telencephalon; CN II is in the diencephalon; CN III and CN IV are in the midbrain; CN V is in the pons; CN VI, CN VII, and CN VIII are in the area between the pons and the medulla; CN IX, CN X, CN XI (cranial root), and CN XII are located in the medulla.[8,35]

As is seen in case presentations pertaining to this chapter, the eyes, ears, nose, and throat are examined when a patient complains of head or neck pain. Infection in these areas can cause many of the musculoskeletal signs and symptoms commonly seen. A clinician must conduct a thorough examination of the head and neck to rule out infection, tumors, or other masses that may cause the patient's complaints. A major difference between musculoskeletal injury and infection is that in infection the patient usually displays the consitutional signs of fever, malaise, and fatigue indicating that the patient is ill. At all times the clinician is trying to reproduce the pain, either by asking the patient to move a structure or by palpating the involved area to exacerbate the patient's pain. Patients who display signs that indicate an increase in intracranial pressure (for example, an eye examination showing papilledema) or changes in hearing, speaking, swallow-

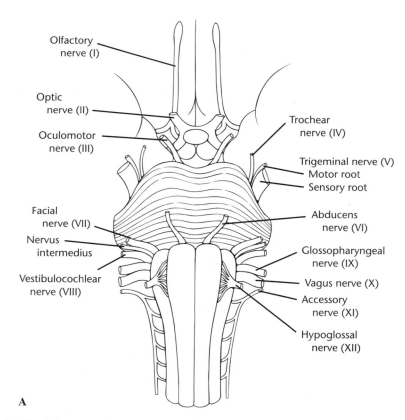

**A**

*Fig. 3-2* Cranial nerves. **A,** Location of the cranial nerves in the brain stem and telencephalon.

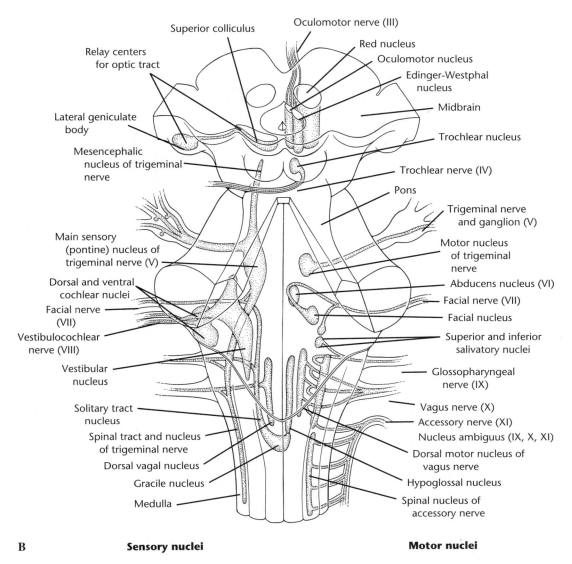

Labels on figure:

Superior colliculus
Oculomotor nerve (III)
Relay centers for optic tract
Red nucleus
Oculomotor nucleus
Edinger-Westphal nucleus
Midbrain
Lateral geniculate body
Trochlear nucleus
Mesencephalic nucleus of trigeminal nerve
Trochlear nerve (IV)
Pons
Trigeminal nerve and ganglion (V)
Main sensory (pontine) nucleus of trigeminal nerve (V)
Motor nucleus of trigeminal nerve
Dorsal and ventral cochlear nuclei
Abducens nucleus (VI)
Facial nerve (VII)
Facial nerve (VII)
Facial nucleus
Vestibulocochlear nerve (VIII)
Superior and inferior salivatory nuclei
Vestibular nucleus
Glossopharyngeal nerve (IX)
Solitary tract nucleus
Vagus nerve (X)
Accessory nerve (XI)
Nucleus ambiguus (IX, X, XI)
Spinal tract and nucleus of trigeminal nerve
Dorsal motor nucleus of vagus nerve
Dorsal vagal nucleus
Hypoglossal nucleus
Gracile nucleus
Spinal nucleus of accessory nerve
Medulla

**B**          **Sensory nuclei**                    **Motor nuclei**

*Fig. 3-2* (*Continued*). **B,** A midcoronal view. Note the separate nuclei for motor and sensory distribution of the cranial nerves. Also note the location and area of the trigeminal nerve (CN V).

ing, or vision need to be referred immediately to a neurologist for a proper work-up.

The sensations of the face and scalp are divided by a coronal plane located just anterior to the ear (auricle) (Fig. 3-3). Sensory innervation to the face and scalp, anterior to the auricle of the ear, is derived from CN V; the postauricular area is innervated by cervical nerves (C2 to C4). Irritation by mechanical (trigger point) or chemical means of C2 to C4 will produce dermatomal pain to areas on the scalp, neck, and shoulders.

## Head pain

Head pain can have many different pain presentations (for example, dull ache, throbbing, shooting, and stabbing). Cases 6, 7, and 8 describe patients with common head pain presentations. The patient's pain presentation

and the pain's location informs the clinician about the anatomic structures involved (for example, pain of muscular origin has a specific pain pattern). The most common types of head pain symptoms described by the patients are throbbing pain (vascular or neurologic), aching pain (muscular), pain referred from a trigger point, and sharp-shooting, shocklike pain that travels to a dermatome (neurologic). Anatomically, there are three distinctive types of pain presentations that are attributed to the neuromusculoskeletal system. *Myotogenous* pain is described by the patient as a dull, diffuse ache and originates from a muscle or tendon. *Sclerotogenous* pain is described as a deep, dull, more localized ache that may refer to other areas. Its origin is most commonly in bone or ligament (for example, from the capsule). *Dermatomal* pain is a sharp, shooting, shocklike distribution of pain

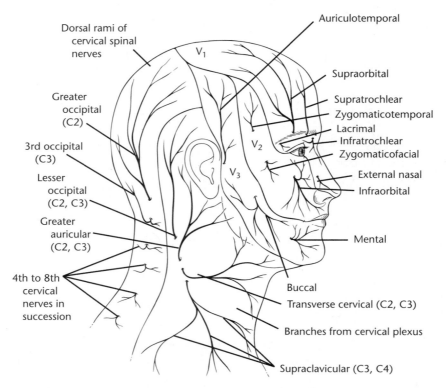

**Fig. 3-3** Sensory innervation to the face and skull. Sensory innervation to the face, anterior to the ear, is by CN V. Sensory innervation posterior to the ear occurs by Cervical nerves I, II, and III.

that travels to a dermatome. The pain originates from a nerve root, a spinal nerve, or the dura. If more than one dermatomal pattern is involved then the lesion may be located in a peripheral nerve.[2,35]

Patients who are involved in whiplash injuries can have head pain that occurs immediately after the accident or weeks later. A common presentation is the patient with suboccipital headache following a whiplash injury. The bilateral suboccipital headache occurring after a rear end motor vehicle accident described in Case 8 is a common occurrence. Similar types of head pain presentations may occur weeks after the insult. The postconcussion syndrome consists of persistent head pain that is described as a bilateral achy, tight feeling. Pressure and acceleration of the head are the determining factors, and head trauma is not required.[43] The pressure produced by the brain hitting against the skull and the acceleration of the brain causing the pressure to increase in the skull cavity are the determinants of the syndrome. The temporal and frontal lobes are the most commonly affected areas of the brain. The patient may complain of migraine headaches that may occur weeks after the initial injury. The migraine may occur daily and is associated with nausea, vomiting, light and noise sensitivity, dizziness, vertigo, and fatigue.[53] Other neu-

rologic signs are associated with the postconcussion syndrome. Visual symptoms and insufficiency of eye convergence are the more common findings of the syndrome.[43] These signs are caused by palsy of the trochlear nerve. CN IV is located at the dorsal aspect of the brain stem. Upon forced rotational motion of the head and neck, the nerve is traumatized, producing visual problems. Psychologic complaints can appear 3 months after the original whiplash injury. Minor depression and fatigue are the most common findings.[41] Cognitive symptoms can occur 4 weeks after injury. The most common findings are memory attention loss, reduced processing speed,[16] reduced attention,[28] increased reaction time[48] and reduced memory for new information.[11] Other findings may be benign positional vertigo caused by labyrinthine concussion, hearing loss, and tinnitus.

Trigger points are commonly observed in the patient with head pain. Trigger points and tender points are common occurrences in patients with neuromusculoskeletal maladies; yet, there is little understanding of the pathophysiology of these findings. The discussion that follows will present the current theories on these presentations.

**Trigger points and tender points.** Many of the cases described in Chapter 1 present patients who have trigger points or tender points. The pathophysiology of a trigger point is a question that has concerned clinicians since Travell first described trigger points in the 1940s.[51] In the following introduction its anatomic, physiologic, and neurologic bases are introduced. The difference between a tender point and a trigger point is that digital compression (of approximately 4 kg) on a trigger point will refer the pain to another area whereas compression of a tender point only causes local pain without referral. A trigger point is described as a hyperirritable region within a taut band of skeletal muscle fibers that has one or more minute loci and is characterized by spontaneous end-plate electric activity.[38] The specific criteria for a trigger point, as described by Travell and Simons are (1) a palpable firm area (taut band) in a muscle that has a localized spot of exquisite tenderness to manual pressure, (2) a characteristic pattern of pain, tingling, or numbness in response to sustained pressure on the trigger point (a referred pain pattern), and (3) a local twitch and jump sign when the trigger point is transversely distorted.[23]

Histologically, a trigger point reveals an increase in temperature, impaired local circulation with tissue hypoxia, and electromyographic evidence of spontaneous electric activity.[23] There are two theories that attempt to explain the formation of the trigger point: the muscle spindle hypothesis and the sensitive loci theory. The muscle spindle hypothesis states that spontaneous electric activity originates within a muscle spindle leading to the formation of the trigger point. Hubbard further states that the muscle spindle's surrounding sac has nociceptive[22] and sympathetic innervation. Sympathetic stimulation of the muscle spindle can cause intrafusal muscle fiber contractions. When sympathetic nerves are stimulated a 10% to 20% increase in tension in nonfatigued fast twitch (FOG) muscle, and an increase in muscle spindle excitability and spindle afferent discharge occurs.[22] The sensitive loci theory states that multiple sensitive loci in the trigger point produce their own local twitch response with referral of pain.

What is the theoretical evidence for pain referral from trigger points? Currently, there are three theories: convergence-facilitation; convergence-projection; and peripheral branching of axons. The convergence-facilitation theory proposes that the normal background activity of sensory afferent fibers is facilitated by abnormal visceral or skeletal stimuli coming from the trigger point and is registered as pain. The convergence-projection theory states that cutaneous afferent fibers from the referral areas converge on the same area of the spinal cord, thalamus, and cerebral cortex as the irritated skeletal muscle and that the stimulus then projects to the referral area (see Chapter 2). The peripheral branching of axons is caused by the stimulation of one branch of an axon that is interpreted as coming from

**Table 3-5** Criteria for fibromyalgia and myofascial pain syndrome

**Fibromyalgia**
- widespread and symmetric aching and pain of at least 3 months' duration
- 11 or more tender points out of 18 characteristic sites
- defined by digital palpation at approximately 4 kg pressure with the thumb pulp over the sites
- sleep disturbance

**Myofascial pain syndrome**
- typical and consistent referral pain patterns in each specific trigger point of an individual muscle
- a sensitive and irritable spot on a palpable taut band
- palpable or visible local twitch responses of the taut band
- restricted range of motion of the involved muscle
- muscle weakness without atrophy

another branch of the same axon causing the referral pattern.

Another common musculoskeletal malady is the presence of tender points. Tender points display the same findings as trigger points but lack pain referral.[44] The presence of multiple tender points is associated with a syndrome that is present most often in women. It consists of aching pain that is most commonly located in the proximal limbs and the girdle area, sleep disturbance (usually caused by a lack of stage 4 sleep), and psychological stress that worsens the condition. There are usually 13 to 19 tender points located in the area of chief complaint. This syndrome is called fibromyalgia[44] (Table 3-5).

Other theories on the causes of head pain have focused on vascular changes (for example, in migraine and cluster headaches) and neurologic involvement. Recent literature[12] has proposed that the nerves of the upper cervical spine participate in headache pain. Case 6 describes a patient with headache that is aggravated by motion of the cervical spine. Anatomically, the cervical nerves of C1 to C3 have rootlets that intermingle with the trigeminal nucleus. The headache has been exacerbated and sent into remission by injections of hypertonic saline and analgesics into the upper cervical spine. Bogduk has suggested that there is a combination of the cervical neurologic supply with the trigeminal nucleus, the trigeminocervical nucleus.[12] This gives the clinician a rationale for examining the upper cervical spine in patients who suffer from headache.

## LOCAL, REGIONAL, AND CORRELATIVE ANATOMY OF THE TEMPOROMANDIBULAR JOINT APPARATUS
DARRYL CURL

The temporomandibular apparatus (TMA) consists of (1) the teeth and supporting structures, (2) the skeletal components (mandible and temporal bones), (3) the paired temporomandibular joints, (4) the muscles of mastication, and (5) the associated cervical musculature. A disorder in any of these components can, and will, alter the normal behavior of the head and neck. Therefore, there is a compelling rationale for the clinician to have a working knowledge of the local and regional anatomy of the temporomandibular system.

## Teeth and supporting structures

The adult dentition consists of 28 teeth (32 if the "wisdom" teeth are present) while the pediatric dentition consists of only 20 teeth (all of which are shed by about 12 years of age). Each tooth has a crown (that portion above the bigingival collar that is covered by enamel) and a single or multiple root (molars generally have multiple roots).

Each tooth is held in its alveolar socket (a gomphosus joint), in the maxilla or mandible, by thousands of microligaments collectively called the periodontal ligament. The periodontal ligament has many important functions. It serves to anchor the teeth in the alveolus, dissipate the impact and grinding forces along the surface of the root, and, through specific mechanoreceptors, provide for proprioceptive input governing the activities of chewing, swallowing, and possibly speech.

Under optimal conditions, the 28 to 32 teeth in the adult are equally divided between the maxillary and the mandibular arches, so that the 14 to 16 teeth of one arch contact their mates on the other arch. The maxillary arch is slightly larger than the mandibular arch allowing the maxillary teeth to overlay the mandibular teeth when the teeth are in full contact. This anatomic arrangement is considered a normal occlusion and is designated a Class I angle.[15] A Class I angle occlusion is deemed to be the most efficient form of occlusion meaning that muscular effort required during mastication and speech is as minimal as possible.

When the teeth are in full occlusion, the 28 to 32 teeth meet against each other in a cusp-to-fossa relationship. This cusp-to-fossa relationship is a complex one and involves the principle of tripodization (Fig. 3-4). Tripodication is a term used to describe the highly stable three-point contact area in that portion of a tooth that is in occlusion (opposing tooth-to-tooth contact). Optimally, the adult dentition has approximately 138 to 144 contact points that strike simultaneously during full occlusion. Various references have been made throughout the dental literature that irregular contact patterns (premature contact points or eccentric contact points) create problems for the teeth, their supporting structures, and the muscles of mastication.[20,25,27] The molar teeth are normally highly contoured surfaces that form cusps and fossae. It is the interdigitation of the cusps and fossae of the teeth that allow for an efficient chewing surface. Because of interdigitation food is easily chewed with minimal muscular effort.

Irregular contact patterns have been proposed as one of the contributory factors to TM disorders.[40,42] Some researchers believe that the irregular contact areas stimulate the mechanoreceptors in the periodontal ligament and cause an irregular firing pattern in the motor neurons of the muscles of mastication.[17,33] It is further argued that the cumulative effect of this irregular muscular activity induces muscular fatigue and inappropriate

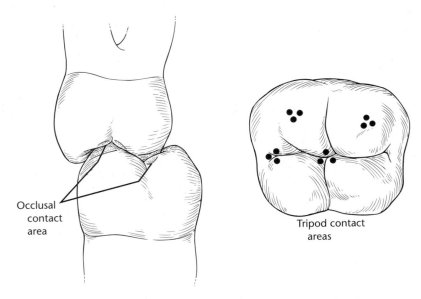

Occlusal contact area

Tripod contact areas

*Fig. 3-4* Cusp to fossa relationship displaying tripodization.

mandibular movement patterns and precipitates TM dysfunction.[4,5,29]

Teeth can lose their cusp-fossa relationship as a consequence of wearing of the occlusal surface; this problem is easily detected because the surfaces of the teeth appear flattened and smooth when the oral cavity is examined (See Case 7). Teeth whose surfaces are excessively worn cause a significant decrease in chewing efficiency and lead to an overloading of the muscles of mastication. This condition is particularly troublesome in patients who habitually grind (brux) their teeth. Bruxers frequently complain of headache, especially headache brought on by chewing. This is because the muscles of mastication are overworked from the bruxing habit and from the decreased chewing efficiency resulting from flattened teeth (see Case 7).

## Skeletal components

The TMA consists of three major skeletal components: the maxilla, the mandible, and the temporal bone. There are two maxillary bones, two temporal bones, and one mandible. These components are developmentally, structurally, and functionally different from each other.

The adult maxilla is normally thought of as being a single bone. However, although this is true functionally, the maxilla is composed of two maxillary bones, which fuse at the midpalatal suture during development. The superior portion of the maxilla forms the floor of the orbit of the eye and the floor of the nasal cavity. Inferi-orly, it forms the hard palate and the alveolar ridges. The maxilla is the stationary component of the masticatory system.

The adult mandibular bone is suspended from the skull by muscles and ligaments. The posterior portions of the mandible form the ascending ramus that gives rise to the condyles (which are part of the TM joint) and the coronoid processes (which provide attachment for the temporalis muscles). The mandible is a dense bone and, contrary to popular opinion, is in a dynamic state of change from birth to death. Abnormal muscle forces can, and do, deform the mandible, especially in the area of the condylar head.[47] It is believed that the earliest change in patients with degenerative joint disease of the TM joint is a shortening of the condylar neck and not, as once believed, a flattening of the condylar surface.[24]

There are two condylar heads of the mandible, one on each side. Each head is an ellipsoidal structure in which the medial pole is generally larger than the more functional lateral pole. A line through the medial and the lateral poles will form an oblique posteriomedial angle to the sagittal plane of the skull. The typical condyle is 15 to 20 mm wide from the medial to the lateral pole. The anteroposterior width is generally 8 to 10 mm. The condyle is convex in its anteroposterior dimension, with a slight convexity in the mediolateral dimension.

The temporal bones are paired and form the superior (cranial) articular surface with the mandibular condyle and its disc (Fig. 3-5). The condyle actually articulates

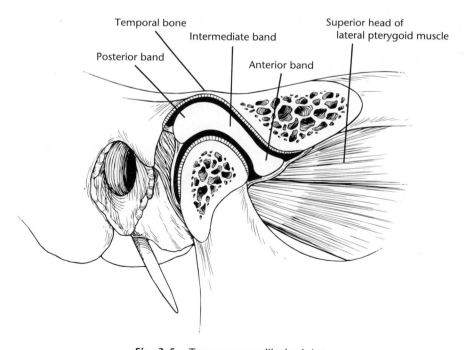

*Fig. 3-5* Temporomandibular joint.

with the squamous portion of the temporal bone midway into the concave mandibular (glenoid or articular) fossa. Posterior to the fossa, the squamotympanic fissure extends lateral-to-medial to divide into the petrosquamous fissure anteriorly and the petrotympanic fissure posteriorly. This fissure is of importance when mechanisms of middle and inner ear problems that occur in association with TM disorders are being considered. It is believed that this fissure serves as the conduit for inflammatory products formed in the TM joint in the course of TM disorders, thereby disturbing the normal function of the ear.[34]

The posterior roof of the articular fossa is very thin and is not designed to withstand heavy forces. This thin cortical plate separating the TM joint from the cranial vault has been incorporated into the current concept of condylar position in reference to the temporal bone. It was once believed that the condyle functioned while firmly seated in the articular fossa, and only left its modified ball-and-socket position during the translatory phase of mandibular movement. It is now well accepted that the condyle lies out of the articular fossa and ideally functions midway along the articular eminence (Fig. 3-6).

Anterior to the fossa is the articular eminence (AE) located at the root of the zygomatic arch of the temporal bone. The AE is a thick, dense bone indicative of a load-bearing area. Although there are various theories regarding ideal condylar position,[14,19,32] with each having some logical premise, patients can function well without the condyle in this supposed ideal position. The clinical significance of the relationship of the condyle and the AE is related to the slope or steepness of the AE.[46] The degree of convexity of the AE is highly variable and clinically important. The steepness of its surface dictates the pathway of condylar motion. A steep slope of the AE predisposes an individual to anterior disc dislocations. A flat slope allows the patient a greater degree of freedom from internal derangements. The increase in the slope of the AE may be part of the cause of acute disc dislocation. This problem is commonly referred to as acute closed lock in which a patient hears a loud sound coming from the TM joint. The sound is followed by pain and a locking of the joint, and the patient's forceful attempts to open the joint are to no avail. In other cases, patients with chronically blocked nasal airways become chronic mouth breathers. In mouth breathers, the capsular structures of the TM joint may become lax as the jaw adapts to an open-mouth habitus. These lax capsular structures are less capable of keeping the articular structures in their proper relationship. The medial and lateral collateral ligaments hold the articular disc on top of the mandibular condyle. As these ligaments loosen, the ability of the disc to remain on top of the condyle during movement is compromised. After a period of time, it is not uncommon to see a spontaneous dislocation of the disc from its condylar position. The anterior dislocation of the disc prevents the condyle from translating during opening of the jaw.

### Articular disc

The TM joint is a compound joint (that is, it requires at least three bones in articulation). This definition is fulfilled by considering the articular disc to be nonossified bone. Interposed between the condyle and the articular eminence is a dense fibrous connective tissue structure (the disc) that permits the complex motions of the TM joint. The TM joint moves in a hinging motion (ginglymoid) during the first 12 to 15 mm of opening, followed by a gliding motion (arthrodial) up to the maximum normal opening of 60 mm. Therefore, the TM joint is properly termed a compound ginglymoarthrodial joint.

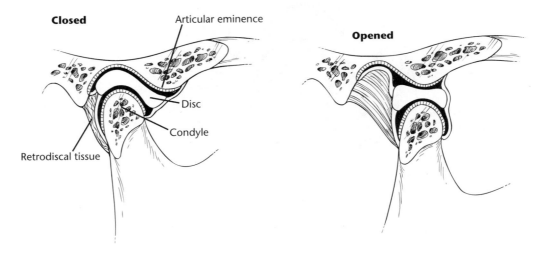

**Fig. 3-6** Position of the condyle of the temporomandibular joint.

The *biconcave* articular disc consists of dense fibrous connective tissue and is devoid of blood vessels and nerves. In the sagittal plane the disc has three distinct thicknesses that are divided into regions: (1) the anterior band, which is slightly thinner than the posterior band; (2) the intermediate zone, which is the thinnest region and is the area of greatest articular function. In the normal joint, the articular surface of the condyle rests in this central region; and (3) the posterior band, which is the thickest region (see Fig. 3-5).

The disc is thicker medially than laterally, corresponding to an increased joint space medially. This thinner lateral portion of the disc is, paradoxically the area bearing the greatest functional load. It is, therefore, the portion of the disc most likely to experience perforations and tears.

The precise shape of the disc is dependent upon the morphology of the condyle and articular eminence. Although disc morphology is, to a certain extent, adaptable to the functional demands of the articulating surfaces, the overall morphology (biconcavity) of the disc is maintained unless pathology or long-term faulty joint dynamics irreversibly alters it.

The disc's adaptable contour, therefore, results in an automatic self-centering effect. When the disc is compressed (as during bruxing or clenching) a rotation of the disc brings the thinner intermediate portion between the articular surfaces. Conversely, when the interarticular pressure is decreased (as during the power-stroke of chewing), the disc rotates, via the action of the superior head of the lateral pterygoid, so that the thicker portion lies between the articular surfaces to temporarily fill the widened joint space and maintain articular contact.

In addition, the disc contour prevents linear sliding motion (in the sagittal plane) between the disc and the condyle but allows rotatory motion. This important feature of disc morphology permits the disc and the condyle to translate together as a functional complex without disc displacement. Linear displacement of the disc is almost impossible unless there is an appreciable loss of disc contour or direct trauma. Linear displacement may occur immediately (from acute trauma, for example, mandibular "whiplash" or gradually (as a result of functional abuse) from the loss of disc contour at the posterior band.

A bilaminar zone of retrodiscal tissue (RDT) attaches from the disc posteriorly to the superior retrodiscal lamina of the Typanic plate, and to just below the posterior aspect of the condylar articular facet to the inferior retrodiscal lamina of the tympanic plate. The body of the RDT is a large venous plexus that fills upon forward movement of the condyle. The retrodiscal tissue is also innervated and can cause intracapsular pain.

Trauma to the RDT, either direct (for example, by direct posterior impact to the mandible) or insidious (for example, by condylar encroachment as a result of occlusal deficiency or discal displacement) can result in inflammation and swelling (retrodiscitis), pain, and even acute malocclusion simulating mandibular fracture. This acute malocclusion is a condition in which the patient describes the teeth as not touching on the ipsilateral side when full occlusion is attempted.[9] This occurs as a result of intracapsular edema.

The disc is attached anteriorly in two ways. Superiorly it is attached to the anterior capsular ligament and inferiorly to the margin of the articular surface of the condyle. Between these superior and inferior attachments, the disc is also attached by tendinous fibers to the superior lateral pterygoid muscle.

Recent microdissection studies give evidence of clinically significant indirect discal attachment (via the lateral capsular wall) by the fibers of the deep masseter muscle.[1] This is an interesting finding and may help explain some discal malpositions, for example, a "lateral" disc.[30]

## Articular cartilage

The articulating surfaces of the condyle and mandibular fossa are covered with dense fibrous connective tissue, not with hyaline cartilage. Dense fibrous connective tissue is less likely to break down from the effects of aging and has a much greater ability to repair and remodel than does hyaline cartilage. This is significant, radiographically, because the condylar head may appear as an uneven bony surface when actually it is covered by a smooth fibrocartilaginous tissue.

## Ligaments

The mandible is suspended from the skull by a network of ligaments and muscles. The complexity of this suspension mechanism is remarkable, considering that the mandible can withstand tremendous biting forces (in excess of 900 psi) while moving with exquisite control and precision.

The ligaments are important to the function of the TM joint as they serve to stabilize, limit motion, shift the axis of rotation, and provide proprioceptive information. Laxity of the ligaments may predispose the individual to disc dislocations and retrodiscal damage (retrodiscitis) as well as other TM disorders.

The discal collateral ligaments attach to the articular disc along its medial and lateral borders. They assist in dividing the TM joint into two distinct and noncommunicating joint spaces—the superior and the inferior joint spaces. These ligaments allow the disc to rotate on the articular surface of the condyle and at the same time prevent subluxation or dislocation of the disc from the condyle.

The capsular ligament (fibrous capsule) surrounds the joint and resists medial, lateral, and inferior forces that tend to dislocate the mandibular condyle from the articular eminence. The capsular ligament functions to contain the synovial fluid in each of the upper and lower joint spaces. It is highly vascularized and innervated with nociceptive fibers and is the structure most likely to cause capsulitis-type pain. Trauma to this ligament is likely to cause bleeding into the TM joint. This is significant because the presence of blood or blood products within the capsule is believed to initiate the formation of intracapsular adhesions. Discal adhesions of the TM joint are one of the most common causes or cofactors of internal derangement disorders of the TM joint. The patient with this problem usually complains of a clicking sound every time the jaw is opened or closed.

The TM ligament reinforces the lateral aspect of the capsular ligament and functions to limit the extent of mouth opening during the rotational phase of mandibular movement. This ligament is composed of two bands that extend from the lateral surfaces of the articular eminence and zygomatic process to attach to the condylar neck.

The outer oblique band of the TM ligament travels posteroinferiorly from the zygomatic process to attach to the lateral surface of the condylar neck. It functions during the initial opening phase of mandibular movement, becoming taut at nearly 12 to 15 mm of opening. Tightening of the outer oblique band of the TM ligament brings about a change in the opening movement from rotation about a fixed point to translation forward and down the articular eminence. Forward translation is a unique feature of the TM joint found only in humans, and it functions to protect the submandibular and retromandibular structures from compression by the mandible.

The important inner horizontal band of the TM ligament travels posterior to the lateral pole of the condyle and to the posterior aspect of the articular disc. This band limits the posterior movement of the condyle, protects the RDT from trauma, and restrains posterior condylar movement during pivoting motions of the condyle when lateral mandibular excursions are made. A serious consequence of inadequate posterior dental support (for example, after loss of teeth or excessive attrition) is inevitable and progressive elongation of this ligament until it no longer restrains the condyle from damaging (compressing) the RDT. This, typically, is one of the causes of a painful condition called retrodiscitis.

The sphenomandibular ligament extends from the spine of the sphenoid bone to the lingular process of the medial surface of the mandible. Clinicians from the dental field[37] report that this ligament serves no significant limiting function in mandibular movement. Other clinicians[26] claim that the sphenomandibular ligament serves as a main suspensory ligament during wide mandibular opening. Alternatively, as reported by Okeson[37] the TM ligament serves this function during moderate mandibular opening.

The stylomandibular ligament extends from the styloid process to the angle of the mandible and to the posterior border of the ramus of the mandible and, in doing so, separates the masseter and medial pterygoid muscles. This ligament, reportedly, functions to limit excessive protrusion of the mandible.

The existence of the mandibular-malleolar (Pinto's) ligament is controversial.[39] It supposedly travels through the petrotympanic fissure and connects the neck and anterior process of the malleus to the medioposterior part of the joint capsule, disc, and sphenomandibular ligament. If it does exist, then it may explain many of the middle ear complaints associated with TM dysfunction.

When attempting to understand the relationship between the TM joint and the ear one needs to note that the TM joint is, phylogenetically, a recently developed structure and is peculiar to mammals. (It is also the last joint to develop in the human embryo). An interesting developmental structural relationship exists between the ear and the TM joint. The primitive jaw articulation of lower vertebrates is homologous to the articulation between the malleus and the incus in mammals. Hence, one can readily understand that the structures of the ear and TM joint are intimately related in mammals.

In addition to the structural relationship there is an interesting neurologic intimacy between the ear and the trigeminal nerve that innervates the mandible. The following structures are important for ear function and are innervated by the trigeminal nerve: the tensor tympani muscle (attaches from the cartilaginous Eustachian tube to the malleus); the tensor palatini muscle (attaches from the sphenoid and Eustachian tube wall to insert in the soft palate aponeurosis); dilator tubae muscle (dilates the Eustachian tube); and the mandibular-malleolar ligament (Case 7).

### Kinetics of the temporomandibular joint

Many muscles act upon the mandible to control or participate in the TM joint's varied functions. These muscles were identified years ago and early anatomic efforts were focused on defining the function of this complex muscle group with the consequence that understanding of the natural biomechanics of the head and neck region suffered. Recently, a new understanding has been reached in regard to the complex activity of this muscle group.

The temporalis muscle has three divisions based on fiber direction and function (Fig. 3-7). The fibers of the anterior division run vertically and act to raise the mandible in a vertical manner. The fibers of the middle division run obliquely in a posterior direction and act

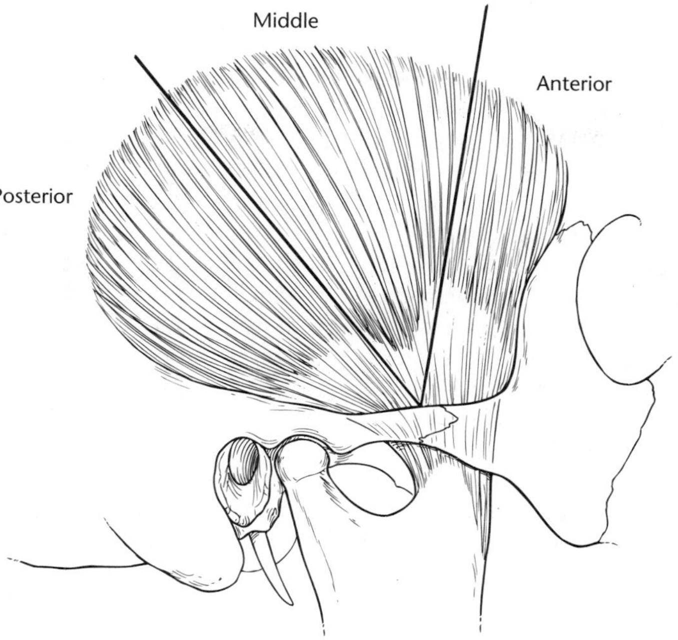

*Fig. 3-7*  Temporalis muscle and its three divisions.

to elevate and retrude the mandible. The fibers of the posterior division run horizontally and their function may be to retrude the mandible. However, some researchers maintain that only fibers below the root of the zygomatic process are significant in the temporalis function, and, therefore, this posterior division would function in elevation and act minimally in retrusion. Because of the multidirectional nature of the fibers the temporalis muscle is capable of coordinating closing movements and is therefore a significant positioning muscle of the mandible.[4]

The masseter muscle has two heads: (1) the superficial head, whose concentric action causes mandibular elevation and protrusion and (2) the deep head, which stabilizes the condyle against the articular eminence when a biting force is applied with the mandible protruded (for example, biting through a sandwich).

During the act of chewing the superficial portion of the masseter muscle is more active on the side that the bolus of food is located compared to the superficial portion of the contralateral masseter.[5] Hence, differentiation of activity within the masseter muscle may be relevant to the examination process of a patient complaining of pain in the masseter area.

It has been reported recently that the deep fibers of the masseter muscle that deviated 30 degrees from the vertical fibers insert into the lateral portion of the anterior band of the TM disc. This finding is of potential importance for explaining the unusual phenomenon of

a laterally subluxated articular disc. In this situation, muscle fibers attaching to the lateral aspect of the disc may account for this lateral dislocation if the contractile force is sufficient in either strength or duration. This muscle attachment may be of clinical importance in treating entrapped lateral plica.[36]

The medial pterygoid muscle originates from the medial surface of the lateral pterygoid plate and the pyramidal process of the palatine bone. It travels lateral, inferior, and posterior to insert on the medial surface of the ramus and angle of the mandible. It functions to elevate the mandible and is active in protrusion of the jaw.

The inferior lateral pterygoid and superior lateral pterygoid muscles have been described as having a common tendon and function in an identical manner.[18] A recent report described the functions of the two bellies to be nearly opposite.[52] Some modern texts describe the two bellies as two distinct muscles.[3,37]

The inferior lateral pterygoid muscle extends from the lateral surface of the lateral pterygoid plate and travels posteriorly, superiorly, and laterally, to insert into the neck of the condyle of the mandible. Concentric contraction of this muscle on each side of the jaw protrudes the mandible and assists the mandibular depressors during jaw opening.[54] A unilateral contraction of the inferior lateral pterygoid muscle produces mediotrusive movement of the jaw. Cocontraction of the inferior lateral pterygoid muscle and the posterior fibers of the temporalis muscle maintains sharp contact of the articular surfaces during translatory motions.

The superior lateral pterygoid muscle extends from the infratemporal surface of the greater sphenoid wing horizontally and travels posteriorly and laterally to insert into the articular capsule, disc, and neck of the condyle. Some authors[3,31,37,52] state that it is inactive during jaw opening and is active in conjunction with elevators, especially during power strokes to stabilize the disc and condylar head against the articular eminence.

The digastric muscle also has two bellies. The anterior belly originates from the digastric fossa on the lingual surface of the mandible. The posterior belly originates from the mastoid notch of the temporal bone. The anterior and posterior bellies descend toward the hyoid bone and are united by an intermediate tendon at the lesser horn of the hyoid bone. The posterior belly is innervated by the facial nerve (CN VII) and acts to depress the mandible when the hyoid bone is fixed. When the mandible is fixed during swallowing, the digastric muscle (with the suprahyoid muscles) elevate the hyoid bone.

The accessory muscles (suprahyoids) of the mandible are the stylohoid, geniohoid, and the mylohoid muscles. These act to stabilize or move the hyoid as necessary during mandibular movement. They are also involved in maintaining the mandibular rest position and tongue postural position. Disturbances in function of this muscle group can negatively impact the patency of the oral airway via either a disturbed mandibular rest position or a faulty tongue postural position.

The infrahoid muscles (the sternohoid, omohyoid, sternothyroid, and thyrohyoid muscles) act in the stabilization and depression of the hyoid, thereby allowing the suprahyoids to act upon the mandible. These muscles are integral for maintaining mandibular rest position, depressing the larynx and hyoid bone, and fixing the hyoid bone in order to provide a stable base on which the tongue and mandible can be moved. This muscle group has been described as a cervical continuation of the rectus abdominus muscle and therefore provides an intermuscular continuum from the mandible to the pubis symphysis.[6]

The omohyoid muscle (omo = shoulder, Fig. 3-8) is an interesting muscle. It attaches to the hyoid and to the superior border of the scapula just medial to the scapular notch. The omohyoid muscle is attached midway to the deep cervical fascia. This fascia, in turn, is attached to the apices of the lungs and to the jugular vein. Therefore, one function of the omohyoid is to render the lower portion of the cervical fascia tense, thereby lessening the inward pull of the soft parts that would otherwise compress the jugular vein and lung apices during sustained inspiratory efforts.[8]

The omohyoid muscle also serves as an important kinematic link between the shoulder girdle and the TM apparatus. A greater incidence of shoulder disorders in populations with TM disorders has been reported.[13]

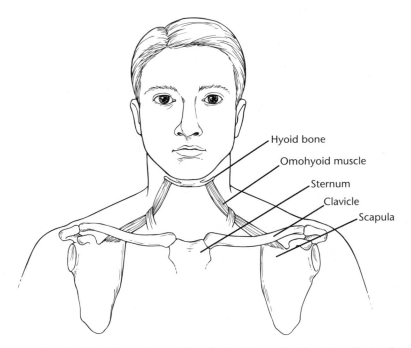

Hyoid bone
Omohyoid muscle
Sternum
Clavicle
Scapula

*Fig. 3-8*   Omohyoid muscle and its relationship to the hyoid and scapula.

Hence, deviations in shoulder girdle carriage may stress the function of the omohyoid muscle and contribute to the other factors underlying the TM disorder.

## ORGANS OF THE NECK AND THEIR SURROUNDING MUSCULATURE

J. PAUL ELLIS

It is difficult to memorize the muscles and organs of the neck region. Yet, it is imperative for the clinician to know the location of these structures in order to evaluate their involvement in disease. In each cervical spine case presented, the neck is carefully examined. Evaluation of this area consists of determining the motion characteristics of the cervical spine and palpating soft tissue structures to detect and ascertain organic disease that could be mimicking musculoskeletal problems. In each case certain organs of the neck area are palpated (for example, lymph nodes, thyroid, and carotid arteries) and the eyes, ears, nose and throat are examined. If palpable abnormalities are found on examination it is imperative that further evaluation, usually by referral, be considered. Any abnormalities in these organs can mimic or cause cervical spine pain and may be life threatening.

The organs mentioned are located in specific anatomic areas that are identified by their relationships to the muscles of the cervical spine. There are two major geometric regions of the cervical area: the anterior and the posterior cervical triangles. The contents of each of the triangles is presented in Table 3-6. The muscles that form the cervical triangles are landmarks used by the clinician to locate the organs. The sternocleidomastoid muscle (SCM) is a landmark for the chain of cervical nodes. The clinician can palpate the deep, superficial, and posterior chains that are located in their respective areas around the SCM. The thyroid gland is located behind the SCM and two fingers above the proximal end of the clavicle. By placing the fingers at this location, the clinician can palpate the gland when the patient is asked to swallow.

### Cervical triangles

The neck can be divided into two large triangles, the anterior and the posterior cervical triangles on each side. The *anterior triangle* is bounded by the anterior median line, the inferior border of the mandible, and the anterior border of the SCM (Table 3-7). The floor of the triangle is formed by the pharynx, the larynx, and the thyroid gland. The digastric and omohyoid muscles divide the anterior triangle into the *submandibular, submental, carotid,* and *muscular* triangles.[21]

The submandibular triangle lies between the inferior border of the mandible and the anterior and posterior bellies of the digastric muscle (digastric triangle). The floor of the triangle is formed by the mylohyoid muscle, the hyoglossus muscle, and the middle constrictor muscle of the pharynx. Its contents consist primarily of the submandibular gland and the hypoglossal nerve (CN XII). The submental triangle boundaries are the body of the hyoid bone, inferiorly, and the left and right anterior bellies of the digastric muscles. The two mylohyoid muscles make up its floor, and it contains the submental lymph nodes and small veins that unite to form the anterior jugular vein.[21,35] The submental lymph nodes receive lymph from the structures of the mouth and drain into the submandibular and deep cervical lymph nodes. The carotid triangle is bordered by the superior belly of the omohyoid, the posterior belly of the digastric muscle, and the anterior border of the SCM. It is considered a vascular triangle, with the common carotid artery and its branches ascending into it.[35] The *carotid sinus,* which is sensitive to changes in blood pressure, is located in the triangle and is innervated by CN IX, CN X, and sympathetic fibers. The *carotid sheath* is a tubular, thickly matted structure located next to the pretracheal fascia and in the carotid triangle. It contains

*Table 3-6*  Subdivisions of the anterior and posterior cervical triangles and their contents

| Triangle | Contents |
|---|---|
| **Anterior** | |
| Muscular | Infrahyoid muscles and thyroid and parathyroid glands |
| Carotid | Bifurcation of common carotid artery, superior thyroid artery, lingual artery, facial artery, occipital artery, ascending pharyngeal artery, internal jugular vein, ansa cervicalis, cervical sympathetic trunk, hypoglossal nerve, and superior laryngeal nerve |
| Submental | Lymph nodes and anterior jugular vein |
| Submandibular (digastric) | Facial artery, facial vein, submental artery, mylohyoid artery, external carotid artery, jugular vein, mylohyoid nerve, facial nerve, vagus nerve, submandibular gland, and part of the parotid gland |
| **Posterior** | |
| Supraclavicular (subclavian) | External jugular vein, suprascapular artery, and subclavian artery |
| Occipital | Occipital artery at the apex of the triangle and accessory nerve (CN XI) |

***Table 3-7*** Contents of the anterior cervical triangle

| | |
|---|---|
| Arteries: | Bifurcation of the common carotid artery and the superior thyroid, lingual, facial, occipital, ascending pharyngeal, submental, mylohyoid and external carotid arteries |
| Veins: | Internal jugular and facial veins |
| Nerves: | Ansa cervicalis, cervical sympathetic trunk, hypoglossal, superior laryngeal, mylohyoid, facial, and vagus nerves |
| Glands: | Part of the parotid gland and the submandibular and thyroid glands |
| Muscles: | Digastric, sternohyoid, sternothyroid, and omohyoid muscles |
| Other organs: | Larynx, trachea, and several lymph nodes |

the common carotid arteries, the internal jugular vein, the vagus nerve, and the ansa cervicalis. The *carotid body* is in proximity to the carotid triangle. It is a chemoreceptor that responds to changes in the chemical composition of blood.

The muscular triangle is bounded by the superior belly of the omohyoid muscle, the SCM, and the median plane of the neck. The triangle contains the infrahyoid muscles and the thyroid and parathyroid glands.

The posterior triangle contains nerves and vessels that supply the neck and upper limbs. The subclavian (third part), transverse cervical, suprascapular, and occipital arteries and the external jugular vein transverse through the posterior triangle. The subclavian artery supplies blood to the upper limb, the transverse cervical and suprascapular arteries branch from the thyrocervical trunk from the subclavian artery and supply the muscles of the scapular region. The occipital artery is a branch of the carotid artery and supplies the posterior half of the scalp. The external jugular vein drains most of the scalp and face and empties into the subclavian vein.

The nerves that pass through the posterior cervical triangle are the accessory part of the spinal accessory nerve (CN XI), nerves of the cervical plexus, and the upper part of the brachial plexus. The cervical plexus is made up of the ventral primary rami from the first four cervical levels. The lesser occipital nerve, the great auricular nerve and the transverse cervical nerve all originate from the ventral primary rami of C2 and C3. The lesser occipital nerve supplies the skin of the neck and scalp and the superior aspect of the ear. The greater auricular nerve supplies the skin of the neck, the inferior aspect of the auricle, and an area from the mandible to the mastoid process. The transverse cervical nerve innervates the skin over the anterior triangle of the neck; and the supraclavicular nerve supplies a small part

of the skin of the neck, the skin of the anterior aspect of the chest and shoulder and the acromioclavicular (AC) and sternoclavicular (SC) joints. The phrenic nerve arises from the ventral primary rami of C3 to C5 and is the motor nerve to the diaphragm.

The supraclavicular aspect of the brachial plexus (C5 to C7) passes through the lower aspect of the posterior triangle and innervates the upper extremity muscles. These muscles include the supraspinatus, infraspinatus, subscapularis, deltoid, and teres minor.

The posterior cervical triangle is divided by the inferior belly of the omohyoid muscle (Table 3-8). The triangle divides into a large superior occipital triangle and a small inferior supraclavicular triangle. At the superior aspect of the occipital triangle is the occipital artery. Also contained in this triangle is the accessory nerve as it innervates the trapezius and SCM. The supraclavicular (subclavian) triangle, located at the supraclavicular fossa of the neck, contains the external jugular vein and the subclavian artery.

### Suboccipital triangle

Located at the level of C1 to C2 deep in the posterior cervical musculature, the triangle contains the vertebral artery and the suboccipital nerve (dorsal ramus of C1). Passing just inferior to its lowest border (inferior oblique muscle) is the greater occipital nerve of C2. The suboccipital nerve innervates the muscles of the suboccipital triangle and the zygapophyseal joints of C1 and C2. The greater occipital nerve of C2 innervates the posterior aspects of the cranium. When this peripheral nerve is impinged upon or irritated it produces radicular pain along its route.

### Major arteries of the head and neck

This section will focus on the meningeal, the common carotid, and the vertebral arteries.

***Table 3-8*** Contents of the posterior cervical triangle

| | |
|---|---|
| Arteries: | Third part of the subclavian artery, transverse cervical, suprascapular, and occipital arteries |
| Veins: | External jugular and subclavian veins |
| Nerves: | Accessory (CN XI) and lessor occipital nerves, cervical plexus (ventral rami of C1 to C4; lesser occipital [C2], great auricular [C2, C3], transverse cervical [C2, C3], supraclavicular [C3, C4], and phrenic [C3 to C5] nerves), and supraclavicular part of the brachial plexus |

**Meningeal arteries.** The meningeal arteries supply both the bones of the calvaria and the meninges. The middle meningeal artery is the largest artery. It is a branch of the maxillary artery and is embedded in the external layer of the dura. It enters the skull through the foramen spinosum in the floor of the middle cranial fossa. As it passes the greater wing of the sphenoid bone it divides into the anterior (frontal) and the posterior (parietal) branches. A fracture in the temporal region of the skull may tear this artery leading to an epidural hematoma. The patient will experience headache that will lead to unconsciousness and possibly death in a very short period of time.

**Common carotid arteries.** The left common carotid artery arises from the aortic arch and ascends into the neck just posterior to the sternoclavicular joint. The right common carotid artery begins at the bifurcation of the brachiocephalic trunk behind the right sternoclavicular joint. Both ascend within the carotid sheath to the superior border of the thyroid cartilage where they divide into the internal and the external carotid arteries. The internal carotid artery continues into the skull without branching into the neck, enters the carotid canal in the petrous portion of the temporal bone, and enters the middle cranial fossa beside the dorsum sellae of the sphenoic bone. It then branches to supply the pituitary gland, the orbit, and most of the supratentorial portions of the brain.

The external carotid artery begins at the bifurcation of the common carotid artery (carotid sinus) and supplies the structures external to the skull.[35] The artery divides at the level of the carotid triangle into anterior, posterior, and medial branches. The anterior branch forms the superior thyroid, the lingual, and the facial arteries; the posterior branch forms the occipital and posterior auricular branches; and the medial branch forms the ascending pharyngeal artery. The facial artery is easily palpated because it supplies the submandibular gland.

**Vertebral artery.** The vertebral artery ascends from its origin, the subclavian artery, and enters the transverse foramen of the C6 cervical vertebra (the transverse foramen of C7 does not contain the vertebral artery). The vertebral artery then travels in the transverse foramen and wraps around the posterior aspect of the superior articular facet of C1 at the superior vertebral notch.[50] As presented in the cases, the anatomy of the vertebral artery is important to the clinician who applies a manual force to the cervical spine.

In all clinical presentations involving the cervical spine the patency of the carotid and vertebral arteries are evaluated by performing *George's test.* George's test consists of measuring the bilateral blood pressure and pulse rates, auscultation of the subclavian and carotid arteries, and three maneuvers—head rotation in a neutral position, Maigne's test, and de Kleijne's test. By specific positioning of the patient's head and neck and looking for neurologic signs, the patency of the carotid and vertebral arteries can be evaluated with 60% accuracy. The seated patient is asked to rotate the head to the right and the left, and then rotate, laterally bend, and extend in the seated (Maigne's) and supine (De Kleijn's) positions. Any signs of neurologic or vascular compromise (for example, nausea, tinnitus, vertigo, light headedness, slurring of speech, dizziness, or nystagmus) can indicate vascular compromise or stenosis of the carotid or vertebral arteries.

Controversy exists as to which vertebral artery is being evaluated by George's test. Taitz[49] states that contralateral vertebral artery blood flow is impaired when testing the patency of the ipsilateral artery. Selecki[45] found that the contralateral vertebral artery becomes kinked after 30 degrees of C1 to C2 rotation and that ipsilateral vertebral artery blood flow is impaired after 45 degrees. Vertebral artery compromise can cause clinical signs and symptoms.[50,53] The divisions of the vertebral artery help explain the stresses applied during cervical rotation. The vertebral artery is divided into four parts,[8a] with part 1 of the artery being from its origin at the subclavian artery to where it passes through the vertebral foramen of C6. Taitz and Arensburg[49] found that part 1 is commonly very tortuous. In part 1, the vertebral artery is joined by the vertebral vein and several branches from the inferior cervical ganglion; and when present, the cervicothoracic ganglion forms a plexus around the artery.

Part 2 of the vertebral artery is from C6 to C1. The vertebral veins and sympathetic nerve plexus accompany the artery in this area. As the artery enters the C1 vertebral foramen it makes an acute angle of 45 degrees to pass through the transvers foramen of the atlas.[50]

Part 3 begins as the vertebral artery travels from the vertebral foramen of C2. It is located posterior and medial to the rectus capitis lateralis. The vertebral artery, at this point, wraps around the superior articular pillar of the atlas to pass through the superior notch of the posterior arch (Fig. 3-9). The artery then passes under the posterior atlantooccipital membrane to begin the part 4, in which the artery runs medially and pierces the dura and arachnoid mater and travels through the foramen magnum. Once within the base of the skull it travels in the subarachnoid space along the clivus and joins with the opposite vertebral artery to form the basilar artery (Table 3-9).

There are three locations in which the patency of the vertebral arteries are tested during George's test: part

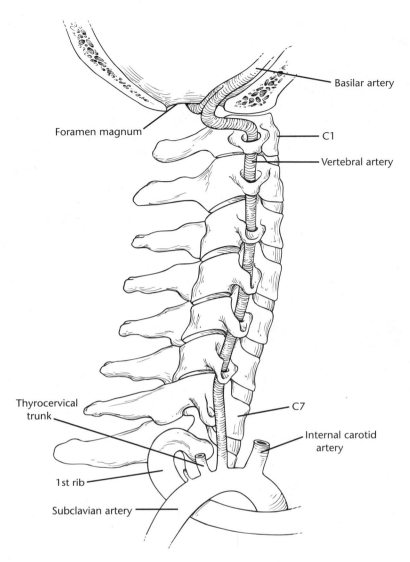

*Fig. 3-9* Projection of the vertebral artery through the transverse foramen to the foramen magnum of the cranium. The vertebral artery does not enter the vertebral foramen until C6 and has a tortuous path from C2 to the cranium.

1 is tested as it enters the C6 vertebral foramen, part 2 is tested between C2 and C1, and part 3 is tested when the artery wraps around the superior articular pillar of C1, possibly causing the artery to be kinked on opposite sides during the same maneuver. It is, therefore, impossible to say which vertebral artery is being evaluated when performing Maigne's and De Kleijne's tests. It is important for the clinician to be aware of the warning signs that indicate possible vertebral artery compromise, and if these signs are present, refers the patient for an angiogram to determine which artery truly lacks patency.

## Thoracocervical region of the neck (root of the neck)

The root of the neck, located between the thorax and the neck, contains the superior thoracic aperture through which all structures passing to and from the neck and thorax are located. The boundaries of the root of the neck are the first pair of ribs and their costal cartilage, laterally; the manubrium, anteriorly; and the body of the first thoracic vertebra, posteriorly. The arteries that pass through the thoracocervical region originate from the arch of the aorta and are the brachiocephalic trunk on the right side and the common carotid and the subcla-

*Table 3-9* The course of vertebal arteries in the foramen magnum

The vertebral artery unites with the contralateral vertebral artery to form the following:

- anterior spinal artery that travels along the length of the spinal cord
- two posterior spinal arteries
- two posterior inferior cerebellar arteries—supply inferior aspect of cerebellum and medulla
- basilar artery—from anastamosis of the right and left vertebral arteries
- posterior cerebral arteries that form the circle of Willis
- travels to occipital lobe and inferior portion of temporal lobe

vian arteries on the left side. The veins in the root of the neck are the anterior jugular, subclavian, and internal jugular veins. The nerves that pass through the root of the neck are the vagus (CN X) (parasympathetic to the

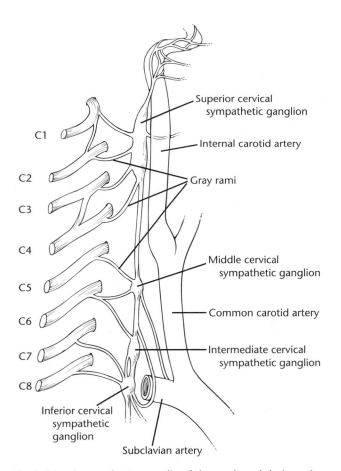

**Fig. 3-10** Sympathetic ganglia of the neck and their projection to the head. The cervical sympathetic ganglia receive innervation from the thoracic sympathetic chain ganglia and synapse with the cervical nerves (C1 to C8).

organs of the thorax and abdomen and motor to the larynx via the recurrent laryngeal nerve) and phrenic (sole motor nerve to the diaphragm) nerves and sympathetic trunks. The lymphatics and the thoracic duct also course through this area.

## AUTONOMIC NERVOUS SYSTEM OF THE HEAD AND NECK
### Sympathetic ganglia

Beginning at the first cervical vertebra, and anterolateral to the vertebral column, are three sympathetic ganglia (the superior, middle, and inferior or cervicothoracic [stellate] ganglia) (Fig. 3-10). These three ganglia receive their preganglionic fibers (white rami communicantes) from the upper levels of the thoracic vertebrae.[7] The postganglionic fibers leave the ganglia to travel along the arteries (most commonly the internal and external carotids), travel into the spinal nerves as gray rami (there are no white rami in the spinal nerves above T1), or travel by a direct route to the visceral branches (for example, the thyroid gland).

The superior cervical ganglion is the largest of the ganglia in the neck and is located at the level of C1 to C3. Postganglionic fibers from the superior cervical ganglion travel along the internal carotid artery and enter the cranial cavity to form the internal carotid plexus.[10] Other branches travel to the external carotid artery, C1 to C4 spinal nerves, and the cardiac plexus. The facial sweat glands are innervated by the sympathetic nerves traveling along the external carotid artery and the facial nerve (CN VII).

The middle sympathetic cervical ganglion is the smallest ganglion and may be absent. Lying adjacent to the C6 vertebra it has anterior and posterior branches that are continuous with the stellate ganglion.

The stellate ganglion is located between the base of the C7 transverse process and the neck of the first rib. The postganglionic gray rami may enter the C7 to T1 spinal nerves or make a cardiac branch or join the subclavian artery. Some of the rami that join the subclavian artery are large and split to ascend with the vertebral artery. They are collectively referred to as the vertebral nerve.

### Parasympathetic ganglia

The cranial portion of the parasympathetic division is located in the cranial nerves. The oculomotor (CN III), facial (CN VII), glossopharyngeal (CN IX), and vagus (CN X) nerves have parasympathetic ganglia that send preganglionic fibers to the effector organs (Fig. 3-11). The parasympathetic divisions of CN III, CN VII, and CN IX supply the head and neck whereas CN X supplies the organs in the thorax and viscera.

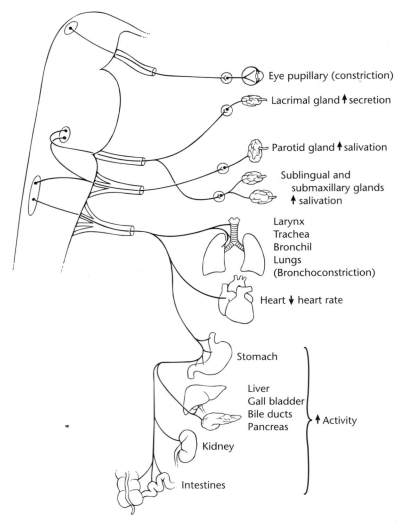

***Fig. 3-11***   Parasympathetic ganglia of the head originate from CN III, VII, IX, and X. The affects of these neurons' stimulation are presented in the illustration.

The oculomotor autonomic efferents are located in the Edinger-Westphal nucleus in the midbrain just ventral to the cerebral aqueduct of Sylvius. These fibers course in the oculomotor nerve to the ciliary ganglion where they synapse with postganglionic neurons. The postganglionic fibers of the ciliary ganglion travel to the eye and innervate the smooth muscle of the sphincter of the iris and the ciliary body. When stimulated, the pupil constricts and the lens thickens (see Fig. 2-11).

The cell bodies of the preganglionic fibers of the facial nerve are located in the superior salivatory nucleus (pons). Some of these nerves travel in the chorda typmani nerve that joins the mandibular division of the trigeminal nerve (CN V). These nerves continue to the submandibular ganglion and synapse with the postganglionic neurons that are secretomotor on the submandibular and sublingual salivary glands. Axons from the

pterygopalatine ganglion travel to the zygomatic nerve and terminate in the lacrimal gland, other glands, and mucous membranes of the palate and nasal mucosa.

The glossopharyngeal nerve preganglionic neurons originate in the inferior salivatory nucleus (medulla) and travel in the lesser petrosal nerve to the otic ganglion. In the otic ganglion they synapse with the postganglionic neurons that are secretomotor and travel in the auriculotemporal nerve (mandibular division of CN V) to the parotid gland.

The vagus nerve originates in proximity, both anatomically and functionally, to the glossopharyngeal nerve and it conveys 75% of the total parasympathetic efferent fibers.[10] The preganglionic fibers originate in the dorsal motor nucleus or the nucleus ambiguous in the medulla and travel in the vagus nerve to synapse in small ganglia located either in plexuses near the effector organs or in

**Table 3-10**    Common skull and sinus radiographic views

**Skull**

Anterior-posterior (A-P) view: petrous bone overlies orbits; good
    for evaluating frontal bone
Lateral view (right and left)
Caldwell's view: petrous bone lies below orbits; good for
    evaluating upper facial structures
Towne's view: (angled A-P view; good for evaluating occipital
    bone and petrous bone
Axial view: best view for evaluating skull base; TM joints and
    zygomatic arches are visible

**Sinuses**

Water's view: petrous bone not visualized; best for evaluating
    maxillary and frontal sinuses
Lateral view: spot view of sinuses
Axial view

the wall of the organ itself. The vagus nerve supplies parasympathetic fibers to the thorax, with cardiac, pulmonary, and esophageal branches and to the abdomen, with gastric and intestinal branches that join the celiac plexus en route to the stomach, small intestine, ascending colon, and most of the transverse colon, accessory glands, and kidneys.

## RADIOLOGY OF THE HEAD
JEFFREY COOLEY
GARY SCHULTZ

### Skull series

A variety of radiologic views can be taken for evaluating the skull and sinuses. The more common views include A-P, lateral, Caldwell, Towne's, and axia views (Table 3-10). Special views for evaluating the temporal, orbital, or mandibular regions can be found in most positioning texts.[1a,8b,42a] The value of plain film skull radiographs has diminished drastically with the advent of computed tomography (CT) and magnetic resonance imaging (MRI), although the high cost and limited availability of these advanced imaging procedures have allowed plain film skull radiography to retain its usefulness in some circumstances.

### Anatomy of the head

Although the clinician should have a basic knowledge of the anatomy of the head, evaluation of x-ray and other images in this region should be performed by individuals with extensive training in the nuances of head anatomy and pathology. Nevertheless, there are a few basic concepts to keep in mind.

When evaluating any bilateral structure, the symmetry should be examined. Also, the cortical margins should be checked closely to see if they are intact. This is especially important in the orbital regions, sinuses, and sella turcica. If the foramina are visible, they should be the correct size and symmetric. The sinuses should be looked at for proper pneumatization and the presence of fluid. The frontal sinuses may be absent or large, symmetric or asymmetric, all of which are normal, but the other sinuses should be well-formed and symmetric. Venous grooves may be seen in any location of the skull, although they predominate along the coronal suture and in the midparietal region. These should not be mistaken for fractures. Any visible cervical spine structures should also be evaluated.

### Lines of mensuration: skull[25a,55]

**Martin's basilar angle.** On a lateral view, one line is drawn from the nasion to the center of the sella tur-

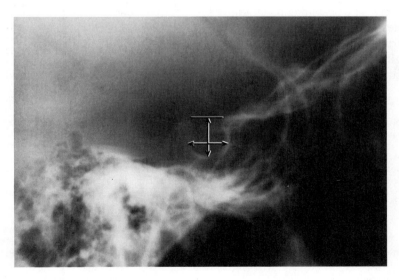

**Fig. 3-12**    Measurement of the sella turcica. The anterior-posterior and superior-inferior measurements on the lateral radiograph.

cica. A second line is drawn from the center of the sella to the anterior margin of the foramen magnum. The inferior angle formed by these two lines is measured. This angle should not exceed 152 degrees. An angle greater than 152 degrees may indicate platybasia, a dysplastic flattening of the skull base.

**Sella turcica measurements.** (Fig. 3-12) On a lateral view, two measurements are taken: anterior-posterior (A-P) depth and superior-inferior (S-I) depth. The A-P depth is measured from the widest distance between the anterior and posterior walls of the sella. The S-I depth is measured from a line drawn between the anterior and posterior clinoids, to the floor of the sella. The A-P measurement should not exceed 16 mm, and the S-I measurement should not exceed 12 mm. An increase in either of these measurements could indicate a space-occupying lesion within or near the pituitary fossa, or increased intracranial pressure. This measurement may also be made on a lateral cervical view, if visible; however, the sella will be less magnified on this view, and a measurement that is close to the above noted maximums may need to be evaluated with a lateral skull film or other imaging.

## Temporomandibular joint

Plain film evaluation of the temporomandibular joint is rapidly becoming outdated. Several views can be used to evaluate the TMJ, including the lateral, the off-lateral, and the axial orientations.[1a] The position of the condylar heads within the joints can be evaluated, and position and motion can be assessed by obtaining open- and closed-mouth projections. The overlying anatomy makes evaluation for early osseous pathology difficult. Plain film tomography can resolve this problem but provides little information on the soft tissue changes, such as disc location and integrity. The best imaging modality to evaluate the soft tissues of the TM joint is MRI, and for evaluation of the cortical and soft tissue structures, CT arthrography. Imaging for purely muscular complaints (trigger points, strain) is unwarranted.

## REFERENCES

1. Axelsson S, et al: Arthrotic changes and deviation in form of the temporomandibular joint- and autopsy study, *Swed Dent J* 11:195, 1987.
1a. Ballinger PW, editor: *Merrill's atlas of roentgenographic positions and standard radiologic positions,* St. Louis, 1990, Mosby.
2. Basmajian J, Slonecker C: *Grant's method of anatomy: A clinical problem-solving approach,* ed 11, Baltimore, 1989, Williams & Wilkins.
3. Bell WE: *Temporomandibular disorders,* ed 2, Chicago, 1986, Yearbook Medical Publishers.
4. Belser UC, Hannam AG: The influence of altered working-side occlusal guidance on masticatory muscles and related jaw movement, *J Prosthet Dent* 53:406, 1985.
5. Belser UC, Hannam, AG: The contribution of the deep fibers of the masseter muscle to selected tooth-clenching and chewing tasks, *J Prosthet Dent* 56:629, 1986.
6. Bourbon B: Anatomy and biomechanics of the TMJ. In Kraus S, editor: *TMJ disorders: Management of the craniomandibular complex,* New York, 1988, Churchill Livingstone.
7. Chusid J: *Correlative neuroanatomy and functional neurology,* ed 17, Los Altos, 1979, Lange.
8. Clemente C: *Gray's anatomy,* Philadelphia, 1985, Lea & Febiger.
8a. Cramer G: The cervical region. In Cramer G, Darby S, editors: *Basic and clinical anatomy of the spine, spinal cord, and ANS,* St. Louis, 1995, Mosby.
8b. Cullinan AM: *Optimizing radiographic positioning,* Philadelphia, 1992, Lippincott.
9. Curl DD, Stanwood G: Chiropractic management of capsulitis and synovitis of the temporomandibular joint, *J Orofacial Pain* 7:283, 1993.
10. Darby S: Neuroanatomy of the autonomic nervous system. In Cramer G, Darby S, editors: *Basic and clinical anatomy of the spine, spinal cord, and ANS,* St. Louis, 1995, Mosby.
11. Dikmen S, McLean A, Temkin N: Neuropsychological and psychosocial consequences of minor head injury, *J Neurol Neurosurg Psych* 49:1227, 1986.
12. Dwyer A, Aprill C, Bogduk N: Cervical zygapophyseal joint pain patterns. I. A study in normal volunteers, *Spine* 15:453, 1990.
13. Eriksson PO, et al: Symptoms and signs of mandibular dysfunction in primary fibromyalgia syndrome (PSF) patients, *Swed Dent J* 12:141, 1988.
14. Gelb H: The optimum temporomandibular joint condyle position in clinical practice, *Int J Periodontics Restorative Dent* 5:34, 1985.
15. Graber T, Swain B: *Current orthodontic concepts and techniques,* ed 2, Philadelphia, 1975, Saunders.
16. Gronwall D, Wrightson P: Delayed recovery of intellectual function after minor head injury, *Lancet* 2:606, 1974.
17. Hannam AG, et al: The relationship between dental occlusion, muscle activity and associated jaw movement in man, *Arch Oral Biol* 22:25, 1977.
18. Hartmann F, et al: The lateral pterygoid muscle: Anatomic dissection and medical imaging. Perspectives in the treatment of M.P.D.S. *Actual Odontostomatol (Paris)* 163:545, 1988.
19. Heffex L, Jordan S, Going R Jr: Determination of the radiographic position of the temporomandibular joint disk, *Oral Surg Oral Med Oral Pathol* 65:272, 1988.
20. Hellsing G: Human jaw muscle motor behavior. II. Reflex and receptor mechanisms, *Swed Dent J* 12:47, 1988.
21. Hollinshead WH: *Textbook of anatomy,* ed 3, Maryland, 1974, Harper & Row.
22. Hubbard D, Barker D, Banks R: The muscle spindle. In Engel A, Banker B, editors: *Myology,* New York, 1986, McGraw-Hill.
23. Hubbard D, Berkoff G: Myofasical trigger points show spontaneous needle EMG activity, *Spine* 18:1803, 1993.
24. Jackson MK, et al: Statistical analysis of clinical, radiographic, and histologic features of temporomandibular arthropathy, *Oral Surg Oral Med Oral Pathol* 63:162, 1987.
25. Jamsa T, Kirveskari P, Alanen P: Malocclusion and its association with clinical signs of craniomandibular disorder in 5-, 10- and 15-year old children in Finland, *Proc Finn Dent Soc* 84:235, 1988.
25a. Keats TE, Lusted LB: *Atlas of roentgenographic measurements,* St. Louis, 1990, Mosby.
26. Kessler RM, Hertling D: *Management of common musculoskeletal disorders,* Philadelphia, 1983, Harper & Row.
27. Kirveskari P, et al: Effect of elimination of occlusal interferences on signs and symptoms of craniomandibular disorder in young adults, *J Oral Rehabil* 16:21, 1989.
28. Levin HS, et al: Neurobehavioral outcome following minor head injury: A three-center study, *J Neurosurg* 66:234, 1987.
29. Levy PH: A form and function concept of occlusion and the maxillomandibular relationship, *J Prosthet Dent* 33:149, 1975.
30. Liedberg J, Westesson PL: Sideways position of the temporomandibular joint disk: Coronal cryosectioning of fresh autopsy specimens, *Oral Surg Oral Med Oral Pathol* 66:644, 1988.
31. Liu ZJ, Wang HY, Pu WY: A comparative electromyographic study of the lateral pterygoid muscle and arthrography in patients with temporomandibular joint disturbance syndrome sounds, *J Prosthet Dent* 62:229, 1989.

32. Lundh H, Westesson PL: Long-term follow-up after occlusal treatment to correct abnormal temporomandibular joint disk position, *Oral Surg Oral Med Oral Pathol* 67:2, 1989.

33. MacDonald JW, Hannam AG: Relationship between occlusal contacts and jaw-closing muscle activity during tooth clenching, Part I, *J Prosthet Dent* 52:718, 1984.

34. Meyers LJ: Possible inflammatory pathways relating temporomandibular joint dysfunction to otic symptoms, *Cranio* 6:64, 1988.

35. Moore, K: *Clinically oriented anatomy,* ed 3, Baltimore, 1992, Williams & Wilkins.

36. Myers J: Newly described muscle attachments to the anterior band of the articular disk of the temporomandibular joint, *JADA* 117:437, 1988.

37. Okeson JP: *Management of temporomandibular disorders and occlusion,* St. Louis, 1989, Mosby.

38. Okey, C: The cervical spine hyperflexion-extension (whiplash) injuries, Los Angeles College of Chiropractic's Eighth Annual Interdisciplinary Symposium, 1995.

39. Pinto O: A new structure related to the temporomandibular joint and the middle ear, *J Prosthet Dent* 12:95, 1962.

40. Pullinger AG, Seligman DA, Solberg WK: Temporomandibular disorders. Part II. Occlusal factors associated with temporomandibular joint tenderness and dysfunction, *J Prosthet Dent* 59:363, 1988.

41. Rimel RW, et al: Disability caused by minor head injury, *Neurosurgery* 9:221, 1981.

42. Riolo ML, Brandt D, TenHave TR: Associations between occlusal characteristics and signs and symptoms of TMJ dysfunction in children and young adults, *Am J Orthod Dentofacial Orthop* 92:467, 1987.

43. Rutherford, WH: Sequelae of concussion caused by minor head injuries, *Lancet* 1:1, 1977.

43a. Rowe LJ, Yochum TR: Radiographic positioning and normal anatomy. In Yochum TR, Rowe LJ, editors: *Essentials of skeletal radiology.* Baltimore, 1987, Williams & Wilkins.

44. Schneider MJ: Tender points/fibromyalgia vs. trigger points/myofascial pain syndrome: A need for clarity in terminology and differential diagnosis, *J Manipulative Physiol There* 18:398, 1995.

45. Selecki BR: The effects of rotation of the atlas on the axis: Experimental work, *Med J Aust* 1:1012, 1969.

46. Solberg WK, et al: Malocclusion associated with temporomandibular joint changes in young adults at autopsy, *Am J Orthod* 89:326, 1986.

47. Stegnenga B, de Bont LG, Boering G: Osteoarthrosis as the cause of craniomandibular pain and dysfunction: A unifying concept, *J Oral Maxillofac Surg* 47:249, 1989.

48. Stuss DT, et al: Reaction time after head injury: fatigue, divided and focused attention, and consistency of performance, *J Neurol Neurosurg Psych* 52:742, 1989.

49. Taitz C, Arensburg B: Erosion of the foramen transversarium of the axis, *Acta Anat* 134:12, 1989.

50. Thiel, HW: Gross morphology and pathoanatomy of the vertebral arteries, *JMPT* 14:133, 1991.

51. Travell J, Rinzler S, Herman M: Pain and disability of the shoulder and arm, treatment by intramuscular infiltration with procain hydrochloride, *JAMA* 120:417, 1942.

52. Weiss HD, Stern BJ, Goldberg J: Post-traumatic migraine: chronic migraine precipitated by minor head or neck trauma, *Headache* 31:451, 1991.

53. White AA, Panjabi MM: *Clinical biomechanics of the spine,* ed 2, Philadelphia, 1990, Lippincott.

54. Wood WW, Takada K, Hannam AG: The electromyographic activity of the inferior part of the human lateral pterygoid muscle during clenching and chewing, *Arch Oral Biol* 31:245, 1986.

55. Yochum TR, Rowe LJ: Measurements in skeletal radiology. In Yochum TR, Rowe LJ, editors: *Essentials of skeletal radiology,* vol 1, Baltimore, 1987, Williams & Wilkins.

## SUGGESTED READINGS

Cramer GD, Darby SA: *Basic and clinical anatomy of the spine, spinal cord and ANS,* St. Louis, 1995, Mosby.

Curl DD, editor: *Chiropractic approach to head pain,* Baltimore, 1994, Williams & Wilkins.

Moore KL: *Clinically oriented anatomy,* ed 3, Baltimore, 1992, Williams & Wilkins.

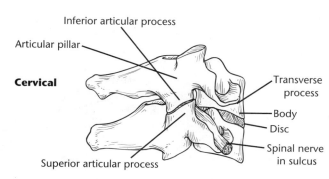

***Fig. 4-1*** Typical cervical vertebra and its exiting spinal nerve.

### KEY TERMS

*Typical and atypical
  vertebral bodies*
*Intervertebral foramin*
*Spinal curvature*
*Bone density*
*Sacroiliac joints*
*Nerve roots*
*Sympathetic nervous system*
*Cauda equina*
*Lumbar intervertebral disc
  biomechanics and
  nutrition*

*Spinal motion (kinetics and
  kinematics)*
*Coupled motions of the
  vertebrae*
*Lumbo-pelvic rhythm
  (flexion-relaxation
  phenomenon)*
*Orthopedic provocative tests*
*Radiology of the spine*

## FUNCTIONAL ANATOMY OF THE CERVICAL SPINE

J. PAUL ELLIS

There are seven cervical vertebrae: four typical (C3 to C6) and three atypical (C1, C2, and C7). This section will focus on the cervical vertebrae, the muscles of this area, and the correlation of this area to Cases 8 and 9.

### Typical cervical vertebrae

All typical cervical vertebrae have a body, two pedicles, two transverse processes, two laminae, and one spinous process. The spinal canal in the cervical spine is triangular and the transverse processes are trough-shaped with anterior and posterior tubercles located at its lateral borders. The spinal nerve exits the intervertebral foramen (IVF) at its inferior aspect and traverses along the trough of the transverse process. The transverse foramen, located anterior to the spinal nerve, houses the vertebral artery as it travels to the brain (Fig. 4-1).

**Uncinate processes of the cervical spine.** Uncinate processes, located at the superior lateral borders of the vertebral bodies, unite with the anterior inferior lip of the vertebral body above to form the *uncovertebral joints.* Present only in the cervical spine (C3 to C7), the uncovertebral joints (the joints of Von Luschka) are synovial-diarthrodial joints that consist of the uncinate

processes and the anterior inferior lip of the vertebral body above. The joint assists in controlling lateral bending and flexion in the cervical spine. Uncinate hypertrophy is a common cause of IVF compromise (Fig. 4-2). As presented in Case 9, patients with this problem show signs of a nerve root radiculopathy during certain spinal motions.

**Articular processes of the typical cervical spine (facet joints).** There are four articular processes (facets) located at the pedicle-laminar junction. The superior articulating facets of the typical cervical vertebra face the posterior at a 45-degree angle to the horizontal plane. The inferior articular facet of the vertebra above join with the superior articular facet of the vertebra below to form the *zygapophyseal joint* (Z joint; a synovial-diarthrodial joint). Along with the intervertebral disc, the shape, size, and direction of the joint surface determines the direction and the amount of intersegmental motion that occurs between the vertebrae.[37,125]

**Cervical zygapophyseal joint.** Anatomically, the Z joints of the spine consist of bony articular facets whose articular surfaces are covered with hyaline cartilage. Periosteum found on the diaphysis is not present on the bone in synovial joints. A space exists between the ending of the periosteum and the beginning of the hyaline cartilage, and osteophytic formation occurs in this area.[137] Between the facets and their hyaline cartilage cover is synovial fluid that nourishes the hyaline cartilage. The synovium is an extension of the capsule, which produces the synovial fluid, and is located on the joint capsule as a fold or tab that may cover part of the hyaline cartilage. The impingement of the synovial tabs between the joint surfaces is thought to be one of the causes of spinal pain and a cause of joint restriction.[41,103]

Encircling the joint is the capsule. The fibrous joint capsule consists of two layers. The deepest layer is perpendicular to the facet plane and attaches from the

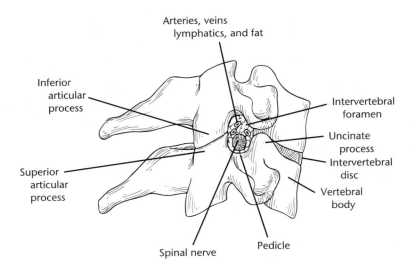

***Fig. 4-2*** Cervical intervertebral foramen borders and contents. The uncinate process sits at the anterior aspect of the intervertebral foramin (IVF). Uncinate hypertrophy is a common cause of IVF impingement. It can decrease IVF area and impinge on the dura, nerve root, or spinal nerve, producing radicular signs and symptoms.

superior facet to the inferior facet. The more superficial layer attaches to the ligamentum flavum on both sides.[37]

The sensory nerve supply to the Z joint is from the medial branch of the dorsal ramus (posterior primary rami) from the spinal nerves above, below, and at the same level.[66,79] Three of the four types of sensory receptors are located in the capsule: types I, II, and IV. Type I consists of sensitive static and dynamic mechanoreceptors that are continually supplying proprioceptive feedback. Type II receptors are less sensitive mechanoreceptors that are dynamic, and type IV receptors are slow-conducting (unmyelinated) nociceptive mechanoreceptors.[132] Because the joint capsule has a rich supply of nociceptive fibers any motion that causes an excessive mechanical stretch or a chemical irritant will cause the patient to perceive pain.

### Atypical cervical vertebrae

The atlas (C1) is a unique vertebra in appearance and function. It does not have the same anatomic structures as do the other vertebrae and is a transitional vertebra from the skull (occiput) and the cervical vertebra of C2 (Fig. 4-3). The first 25 degrees of flexion/extension occur between occiput and C1, where at C1-C2, the zygapophyseal joints are arranged in such a manner that greater than 50% of cervical spine rotation occurs at this joint. Rotation can easily occur at this articulation without neural compromise because its joint contains a large vertebral arch and lacks a vertebral body. The shape of the facets also assists in this rotational component and limits flexion/extension and lateral bending. The axis (C2), as its name implies, is an axis of rotation for C1 during cervical spine rotation. Again, being a transi-

tional vertebra, C2 is more like the typical cervical vertebrae at its inferior articular facets, with the intersegmental motion between C2-C3 being similar to the typical cervical vertebrae (Fig. 4-4).

### Muscles of the cervical spine

There is controversy in the literature regarding muscle activity during spinal motion. Clinically, muscles work in groups, and the majority of muscle activity occurs by eccentric action. The juxtapositional muscles of the spine are small, have a short moment arm, and help stabilize the spine during motion. The larger muscles produce spinal motion because they are farther from the axis of rotation, have longer moment arms, and can produce more force. Table 4-1 presents the major muscles involved in cervical spine motion. These muscles work in synchrony to produce motions of the cervical spine.

Generally speaking, during cervical spine flexion, most of the movement results from the eccentric activity of the posterior cervical musculature. During extension, the anterior cervical musculature is eccentrically contracting, and lateral bending is produced by eccentric activity on the contralateral side and rotation is produced by concentric activity of the contralateral sternocleidomastoid muscle (SCM). Other muscles also participate in these motions and assist in spinal stability. The muscles that assist the contralateral SCM during cervical rotation are described in Table 4-1.

### Ligaments of the cervical spine

Many ligamentous structures support the axis-atlas articulation. The transverse ligament holds the dens in

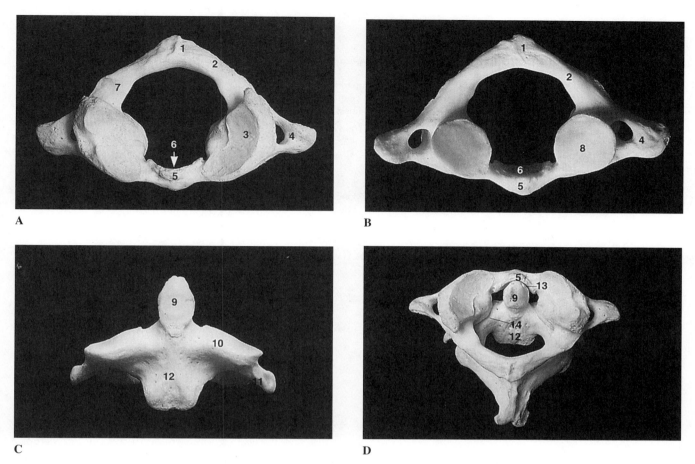

*Fig. 4-3* Occiput-C1 articulation. **A,** Atlas, from above. **B,** Atlas, from below. **C,** Atlas, from the front. **D,** Atlas and axis articulated, from above and behind. 1, Posterior tubercle of atlas, replacing the usual vetebral spine; 2, posterior arch, much longer than the anterior arch (5); 3, lateral mass with superior articular facet, concave and kidney-shaped, to articulate with the occipital condyle of the skull as the atlantooccipital joint, for flexion and extension movements between the skull and the atlas; 4, transverse process with foramen for the vertebral artery; 5, anterior arch; 6, facet on its posterior surface (arrow), to articulate with the dens of the axis (9, 13); 7, groove for vertebral artery, which leaves the foramen in the transverse process and lies here before turning up to enter the skull through the foramen magnum; 8, facet on lower surface of lateral mass, flat and round (compare with the upper surface, 3) to articulate with the superior articular facet of the axis (10) as the lateral atlantoaxial joint (14); 9, dens (odontoid process) of axis, continuous with the body (12); 10, superior articular facet, for articulation with the lateral mass of the atlas (8, 14); 11, transverse process (foramen not seen in this front view); 12, body of axis; 13, for rotation movements between atlas and axis, median atlantoaxial joint; 14, lateral atlantoaxial joint for rotation movements between atlas and axis. (From: McMinn RM, Gaddum-Rosse P, Hutchings RT, Logan BM: *McMinn's functional and clinical anatomy,* St. Louis, 1995, Mosby, with permission.)

place against the anterior arch of C1, the alar ligaments extend from the sides of the dens to the lateral margins of the foramen magnum and control rotation and side-to-side movements of the head.[90] The tectorial membrane is the superior continuation of the posterior longitudinal ligament and covers the alar and transverse ligaments. The posterior and anterior longitudinal ligaments are broad and thick in the cervical spine and traverse the entire length of the spine. The ligamentum flavum is a highly elastic ligament that attaches from lamina to lamina and is located on the anterior aspect of the zygapophyseal joint where the capsular ligaments attach from the superior to the inferior facet and are perpendicular to the zygapophyseal joint surfaces. The purpose of the ligaments is to control movements so that joint integrity is not breached.

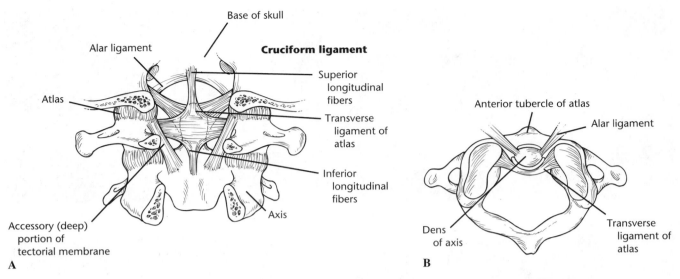

*Fig. 4-4*   The C1-C2 (Atlanto-dens) articulation and its supporting structures. **A,** Posterior view. **B,** Superior view.

## FUNCTIONAL ANATOMY OF THE THORACIC SPINE AND RIBS

GARY M. GREENSTEIN

The thoracic spine (dorsal spine) is made up of 12 true (movable) vertebrae consisting of seven typical and five atypical segments. The thoracic vertebrae have distinct features that distinguish them from the cervical or lumbar vertebrae. Each thoracic vertebra consists of one body, two pedicles, two transverse processes, four articulating facets, two laminae, and one spinous process (Fig. 4-5). The vertebral body is heart shaped and consists of *costovertebral facets* located at the superior and the inferior-anterior aspects. The head of the rib is attached to these facets. The *costovertebral joints* of the typical thoracic vertebrae connect the ribs to the vertebral bodies. They consist of the demifacet located at the posterior-inferior portion of the vertebral body described above, the intervertebral disc, the posterior-superior demifacet of the vertebral body below, and the head of the rib. The T6 rib, for instance, is joined to the T6 and T7 bodies and the T7 costotransverse joint. The *costotransverse joint* is the articulation of the costotransverse facet on the transverse process of the thoracic vertebra and the tubercle on the neck of the rib. The costotransverse facets are present on all thoracic vertebrae except T11 and T12 (the atypical vertebrae). In total there are 12 articulations on the typical thoracic vertebra. The articulations consist of (1) four articular facets on the articular processes, (2) four demifacets at the costovertebral joint, (3) two costotransverse facets, and (4) two intervertebral disc (IVD) articulations at the intervertebral joints.

Case 11 discusses a young woman who has scoliosis (lateral curvature) in the thoracic area. The average presentation of the thoracic spine is a 5-degree, right-sided apex curve located between T6 and T8. Any measurement greater than 5 degrees is considered indicative of scoliosis. The size and shape of a scoliotic vertebra is presented in Figure 4-6. The biomechanics of such a vertebra is different from that of a normal vertebra. Coupled motions in a scoliotic spine reverse from normal thoracic motion. The scoliotic spine is similar to the lumbar vertebrae, in which on rotation, the coupled motion of lateral bending is in the opposite direction. Muscle origins and insertions remain constant but the actions of these muscles change the overall spinal response. Table 4-2 presents the muscles that are involved in normal thoracic spine motion.

### Zygapophyseal joints of the thoracic spine

The superior articular processes (facets) of the thoracic vertebrae are flat on their articulating surface, are at a 60-degree angle to the horizontal plane, and are externally rotated to approximately 20 degrees.[125] As in other areas of the spine, the facet direction determines the motion that is present in the area. The major movement that occurs in the thoracic vertebrae is trunk rotation. Rotation is coupled, as in the cervical region, with lateral bending to the same side.

### Ribs

There are 12 pairs of ribs located in the thoracic area of the spine. The upper seven ribs connect directly to the sternum (true or vertebral sternal ribs) via the costal cartilage. The lower five are classified as false ribs. Ribs 8, 9, and 10 connect indirectly to the sternum through

**Table 4-1** Muscles, motions, and innervations in the cervical spine

| Muscle Action | Innervation |
| --- | --- |
| **Muscles involved in cervical spine flexion** | |
| *Eccentric action* | |
| Trapezius | CN XI |
| Splenius cervicis | Dorsal primary rami |
| Iliocostalis cervicis | Dorsal primary rami |
| Longissimus cervicis | Dorsal primary rami |
| Spinalis cervicis | Dorsal primary rami |
| *Concentric action* | |
| Longus colli | Ventral primary rami |
| Scalene musculature | Anterior primary rami |
| Sternocleidomastoideus | CN XI |
| **Muscles involved in cervical spine extension** | |
| *Eccentric action* | |
| Longus capitis | Ventral primary rami |
| Rectus capitis anterior | Ventral primary rami |
| Sternocleidomastoideus | CN XI |
| *Concentric action* | |
| Rectus capitis posterior major and minor | Ventral primary rami |
| Obliquus capitis superior | Ventral primary rami |
| Semispinalis capitis | Dorsal primary rami |
| Splenius capitis | Dorsal primary rami |
| Longissimus capitis | Dorsal primary rami |
| Trapezius | CN XI |
| **Muscles involved in cervical spine lateral bending** | |
| *Eccentric and concentric action** | |
| Splenius capitis | Dorsal primary rami |
| Splenius cervicis | Dorsal primary rami |
| Longissimus capitis | Dorsal primary rami |
| Longissimus cervicis | Dorsal primary rami |
| Iliocostalis cervicis | Dorsal primary rami |
| Scalene musculature | Ventral primary rami |
| **Muscles involved in cervical spine rotation** | |
| *Ipsilateral* | |
| Splenius capitis | Dorsal primary rami |
| Longissimus capitis | Dorsal primary rami |
| Obliquus capitis inferior | Ventral primary rami |
| Major and minor rectus capitis posterior | Ventral primary rami |
| *Contralateral* | |
| Sternocleidomastoideus | CN XI |

*Eccentric muscle activity during lateral bending produces contralateral motion. Concentric action produces ipsilateral cervical spine lateral bending motion.*

the costal margin of the seventh costal cartilage (vertebrochondral ribs). Ribs 11 and 12 are floating, or vertebral ribs, that have a cartilaginous tip at their anterior aspect but end in the investment of the muscles of the anterior abdominal wall.[6]

Ribs are curvilinear flattened structures surrounded with a thin outer cortex of bone. They possess a large medullary cavity that has an abundant blood supply. The endosteum and periosteum of the ribs are well developed, providing the ribs with many free nerve end-

ings that elicit a deep, dull ache when fracture occurs (sclerotogenous pain pattern). Rib fractures can usually be palpated by the clinician because they are superficial structures and have a rich nerve supply.

## Sympathetic nervous system

The sympathetic nervous system is located in the thoracolumbar area of the spine. It extends from the first thoracic spinal segment to lumbar segment L3. The cell bodies of the neurons are located in the mediolateral gray matter of the spinal cord. The axons (preganglionic fibers) of these cell bodies exit the cord with the ventral root, enter the spinal nerve, and separate from the motor axons to form the white *rami communicantes* (myelinated) of the paravertebral chain ganglia (Fig. 4-7). These axons may innervate the chain at that level or may ascend or descend along the ganglionic trunk. Each preganglionic fiber synapses with many postganglionic neurons that are distributed among many different paravertebral ganglia.[34] The multitude of synapses permits coordinated activation of sympathetic neurons at several spinal levels.

The postganglionic neurons exit from the trunk by way of the gray *rami comuunicantes* (unmyelinated). The first four preganglionic fibers (T1 to T4) synapse in the paravertebral chain ganglia and travel along those ganglia in a superior direction to the stellate and superior cervical ganglion. The postganglionic fibers then synapse at the eye and the lacrimal and salivary glands. From approximately T5 to T12, the preganglionic fibers travel from the spinal cord through the paravertebral chain ganglia and synapse at the celiac ganglion and the *superior mesenteric ganglion*. The postganglionic fibers of the celiac ganglion innervate the liver, stomach, small intestine, pancreas, kidneys, large intestine, and rectum. The postganglionic fibers from the superior mesenteric ganglion follow the thoracic splanchnic nerve and innervate the adrenal medulla. The most caudal part of the sympathetic chain (L1 to L3) bypasses the paravertebral chain ganglia and synapses in the *inferior mesenteric ganglion*. The post ganglionic fibers innervate the large intestine, rectum, bladder, and reproductive organs.

Many organic maladies resemble neuromusculoskeletal problems in the thoracic spine and surrounding areas. Table 4-3 presents some of the more common afflicted organs and their usual pain referral patterns.

## CLINICAL ANATOMY OF THE LUMBAR REGION AND THE SACROILIAC JOINTS
GREGORY CRAMER

The lumbar portion of the vertebral column is very sturdy and is designed to carry the weight of the head, neck, trunk, and upper extremities. However, the lumbar region is also a frequent source of pain of spinal origin, making a thorough knowledge of this region es-

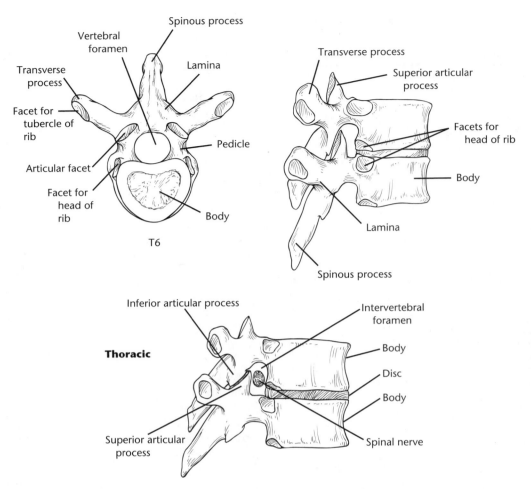

*Fig. 4-5* Typical thoracic vertebra and its exiting spinal nerve.

sential to understanding the various causes of low back pain (Cases 13 and 14). In addition, a thorough understanding of the anatomy of the lumbar region helps clinicians design the best possible treatment program for their patients.

The extent to which low back pain can be attributed to pathology or to dysfunction of the sacroiliac joint (SIJ) has been a matter of discussion for many decades. Currently attention is being focused on the SIJ as a primary source of low back pain.[24] One reason for this is that herniation of the intervertebral disc is now known to be a rather infrequent cause of low back pain, accounting for less than 10% of the cases of pain in this region.[24] On the other hand, pain arising from the SIJ is reported to account for more than 20% of low back pain complaints[74] and is implicated to some extent in more than 50% of the cases of low back pain.[24] This makes the SIJ a clinically important area. An understanding of the unique and interesting anatomy of this joint is essential for the proper diagnosis and treatment of pain arising from this articulation.

## Lumbar region*

This section will present the typical characteristics of lumbar vertebrae, the ligamentous structures unique to the lumbar region, the lumbar vertebral canal, and the intervertebral foramina. A brief description of the unique characteristics of L5 and the lumbosacral articulation will follow. The section will conclude with a brief discussion of the nerves, vessels, and related viscera of the lumbar region. This will be followed by a separate section discussing the sacroiliac joint.

**Lumbar lordosis and characteristics of typical lumbar vertebrae.** Under normal conditions, the lumbar lordosis is more prominent than is the cervical lordosis. It extends from T12 to the L5 intervertebral disc and the greatest portion of the curve occurs between the L3 and L5. The lumbar lordosis is created by the increased height of the anterior aspect of both the lumbar verte-

---

*Adapted from Cramer, G: The lumbar region. In Cramer G, Darby S. *Basic and clinical anatomy of the spine, spinal cord, and ANS*, St. Louis, 1995, Mosby.

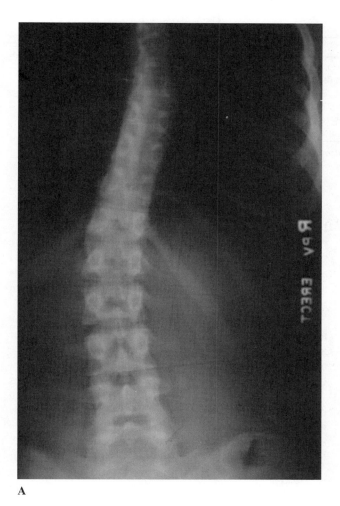

**A**

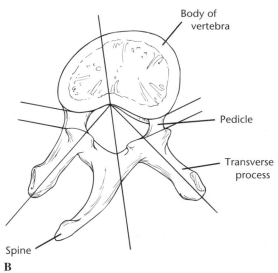

**B**

*Fig. 4-6* Presentation of a scoliotic vertebra. **A,** Radiograph depicts scoliotic spine. **B,** Illustration of thoracic spine vertebra at apex of scoliotic curve from radiograph.

**Body of vertebra**

**Pedicle**

**Transverse process**

**Spine**

bral bodies and the lumbar intervertebral discs, with the discs contributing more to the lordosis than the increased height of the vertebral bodies. An increase or a decrease of the lumbar lordosis may contribute to low back pain.[91]

**Lumbar vertebral structures.** When viewed from above, the vertebral bodies of the lumbar spine are large and kidney shaped with the concavity facing posteriorly. The vertebral bodies are wider from side to side (lateral width) than from front to back and are taller in front (anteriorly) than behind. Therefore, as mentioned above, the vertebral bodies are partially responsible for the creation and maintenance of the lumbar lordosis (Fig. 4-8).

The lateral width of the lumbar vertebrae increases from L1 to L3. The L4 and L5 are somewhat variable in width.[129]

The blood supply to the vertebral bodies is quite extensive and complex, consisting of periosteal arteries, nutrient arteries, and equatorial arteries.[14,28]

The pedicles of the lumbar spine are short but very strong. They attach lower on the vertebral bodies than do the pedicles of the thoracic region but higher than those of the cervical region. Therefore, each lumbar vertebra has a superior vertebral notch that is less distinct than that of the cervical region. On the other hand, the inferior vertebral notch of lumbar vertebrae is very prominent.

Each transverse process of a typical lumbar vertebra projects posterolaterally from the junction of the pedicle and the lamina of the same side. It lies anterior to the articular process and posterior to the lumbar intervertebral foramen.

The lumbar transverse processes are long with the transverse processes of L3 being the longest. These processes are flat and thin from front to back. They are also narrower, from the superior to the inferior aspect, than their thoracic counterparts.

Unique to the lumbar spine are the accessory processes. Each accessory process projects posteriorly from the junction of the posterior and inferior aspect of the transverse process with the corresponding lamina. These processes serve as attachment sites for the longissimus thoracis muscles (lumbar fibers) and the medial intertransversarii lumborum muscles.[129]

**Articulating processes.** Each superior articular process possesses a hyaline cartilage–lined superior articular facet that is oriented in the vertical plane. The articular surface of a typical superior articular facet can be gently curved with the concavity facing medially, or the articular surface can be angled abruptly (Fig. 4-9). When the articular surface is angled abruptly, two rather distinct articulating surfaces are formed.[113] One surface faces posteriorly and forms an almost 90-degree angle with the second surface, which faces medially. As with the curved facet, this concavity also faces posteriorly

*Table 4-2*   Muscles of the thoracic spine*

| Thoracic spine motion | Muscles |
| --- | --- |
| Right rotation | Left external oblique (c), right internal oblique (c) |
| Left rotation | Right external oblique (c), left internal oblique (c) |
| Flexion | Erector spinae: iliocostalis (e), longissimus (e), spinalis (e) |
| Extension | Rectus abdominous (e); bilateral external, internal, and transverse obliques (e) |
| Right lateral bending | Left quadratus lumborum (e), left erector spinae (e), deep thoracic musculature (e) |
| Left lateral bending | Right quadratus lumborum (e), right erector spinae (e), deep thoracic musculature (e) |

*Muscles work in groups and the majority of their activity is eccentric. The actions performed do not involve application of an external force to resist the motion occurring.*
*e, Eccentric muscle activity; c, concentric muscle activity.*

and medially. In either case (curved or angled articular surfaces) the shape will conform almost perfectly with the inferior articular facet of the vertebra above.

The orientation of the superior articular facets varies from one vertebral level to another. A line passed across each superior articular facet, on transverse computerized tomography scans, shows that the L4 superior facets (and therefore the L3-L4 Z joints) are more sagitally oriented than are the L5 facets. Also, the S1 superior facets (and therefore the L5-S1 Z joints) are more coronally oriented than are the L4 and L5 facets.[121] The next section on zygapophyseal joints discusses the orientation of the superior and inferior articular facets in greater detail.

Unique to the lumbar spine are the mammillary processes that project posteriorly from the superior articular processes of lumbar vertebrae. Each mammillary process is a small rounded mound of variable size. Some processes are almost indistinguishable whereas others are relatively prominent. The mammillary processes serve as attachment sites for the multifidi lumborum muscles.

The inferior articular processes of lumbar vertebrae are convex anteriorly and laterally. They possess inferior articular facets that cover their anterolateral surface, and similarly to the superior articular facets, the inferior ones also vary in shape. Even though articular processes vary from one vertebral level to another, and even from one side to another, the superior and inferior articulating processes of a Z joint conform to each other in shape. This conformation is such that each inferior articular facet usually fits remarkably well into the posterior

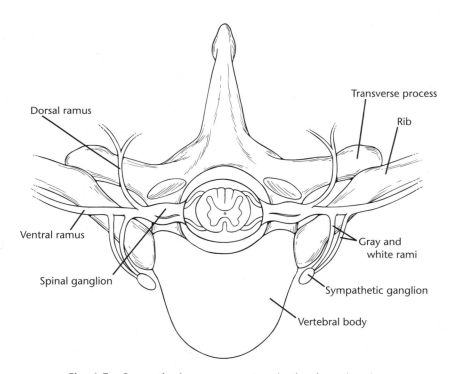

*Fig. 4-7*   Sympathetic nervous system in the thoracic spine.

*Table 4-3* Organic pain that can mimic musculoskeletal problems in the upper trunk, neck, and head regions

| Pain origin | Pain location |
|---|---|
| Heart | Left or right cervical carotid area, into the left upper extremity to the fifth digit and across the chest |
| Lungs | Cervical spine |
| Liver and gall bladder | Right midscapular region and scapular spine |
| Diaphragm | Midscapular region |
| Stomach, pancreas, duodenum | Epigastric area and midback |

and medial concavity of the adjoining superior articular facet.

**Zygapophyseal joints: general considerations.** The lumbar zygapophyseal joints (Z joints) are clinically sig-

nificant (Case 13). This section will focus on the clinically significant and unique aspects of the lumbar Z joints.

The lumbar Z joints are considered to be complex synovial joints that are oriented in the vertical plane.[129]

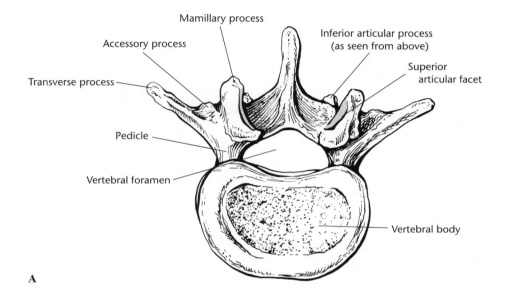

A

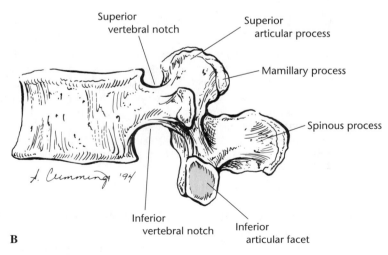

B

*Fig. 4-8* Typical lumbar vertebra and its exiting spinal nerve. (From: Cramer G, Darby S: *Basic and clinical anatomy of the spine, spinal cord, and ANS.* St. Louis, 1995, Mosby, p. 441, with permission.)

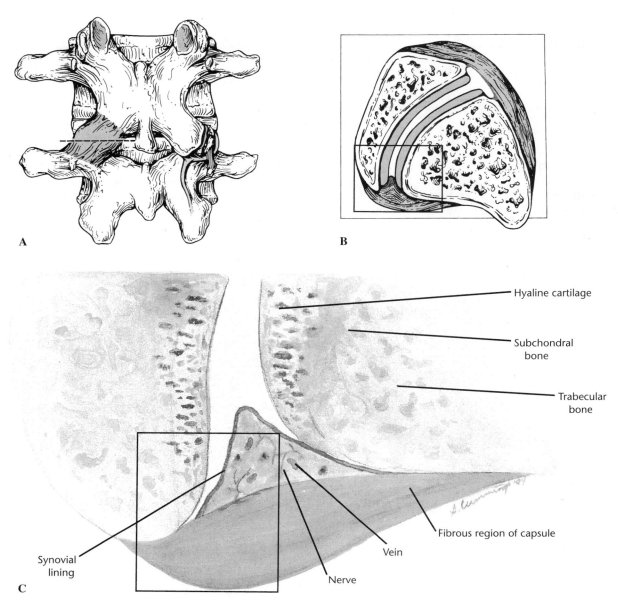

**A**

**B**

Hyaline cartilage

Subchondral bone

Trabecular bone

Fibrous region of capsule

Vein

Nerve

Synovial lining

**C**

***Fig. 4-9*** The zygapophyseal joint (Z joint). Illustrations **A** and **B** demonstrate the Z joint from a posterior view and a horizontal section respectively. Illustration **C** represents the Z joint after magnification (~×10). The articular cartilage, subchondral bone, and articular capsule are prominently displayed. In addition, a Z joint synovial fold is also very prominent. Notice that the articular capsule has an outer tough fibrous region. The center of the synovial fold is more vascular and contains adipose tissue. A nerve can be seen passing through this region. A synovial lining can be seen on the deep surface of the articular capsule and the synovial fold. (From: Cramer G, Darby S: *Basic and clinical anatomy of the spine, spinal cord, and ANS.* St. Louis, 1995, Mosby, p. 441, with permission.)

Their shape varies with the shape of the superior and inferior articular facets (see previous section). Therefore, the lumbar Z joints are concave posteriorly and, in fact, have been described as being biplanar in orientation.[116] This means that they have a coronally oriented, posterior-facing, anteromedial component and a large sagitally oriented, medial-facing, posterolateral component. Taylor and Twomey[116] state that the lumbar Z joints are coronally oriented in children and the large sagittal component develops as the individual matures. The sagittal component limits rotation, whereas the coronal component limits flexion. More specifically, the shape of the lumbar Z joints allows for considerable flexion in the lumbar region, but the size of the joints is what eventually limits flexion at the end of the normal range of motion. Therefore, the long contact surfaces between the coronal component of the superior articular processes and the adjacent inferior articular processes limit flexion by "restraining the forward translational component of flexion."[116]

Even though the size of the Z joints eventually limits flexion, approximately 60 degrees of flexion can occur before the bony restraints of the lumbar articular processes prevent further movement. However, the size and shape of the Z joints greatly limit rotation. During rotation of the lumbar region, distraction, or gapping, occurs between adjacent lumbar articular facets (the superior facet of the vertebra below and the inferior facet of the vertebra above) on the side of rotation. For example, right rotation results in gapping of the facets on the right side. Also during rotation, the two opposing facets of the opposite side are pressed together. This causes them to act as a fulcrum for the distracting facets on the side of rotation.[100]

Extension of the lumbar region is limited by the inferior articular process on each side of a lumbar vertebra contacting the junction between the lamina and the superior articular process of the vertebra below. This junction between the lamina and the superior articular process is known as the pars interarticularis.

**Variation in size and shape of the zygapophyseal joint.** Considerable variation exists between individual Z joints at different lumbar levels and also between the left and right Z joints at the same vertebral level. The shapes range from a slight, gentle curve that is concave posteriorly, to a pronounced, dramatic, posteriorly concave curve and, in some cases, to a joint in which the posterior and medial components face one another at an angle of nearly 90 degrees. Generally, the Z joints of the upper lumbar levels are more sagittally oriented than are those of the lower lumbar levels. This makes the lower lumbar joints more susceptible to recurrent rotational strain.[73]

**Articular capsules.** An articular capsule covers the posterior aspect of each lumbar Z joint. The ligamentum flavum covers the anterior and medial aspect of the Z joint. The articular capsule is quite tough, possesses a rich sensory innervation, and is well vascularized.[55] The outer fibers of the articular capsule are horizontally directed, coursing from the posterolateral to the anteromedial direction.[100] These fibers extend a considerable distance medially and become continuous with the lateral fibers of the interspinous ligament. These characteristics of the capsule help limit forward flexion.[100] Laterally, each articular capsule is frequently continuous with the articular cartilage lining the superior articular facet. There is a gradual transition from the fibrous

tissue of the capsule to fibrocartilage and finally to the hyaline cartilage of the superior articular facet.[116] Each capsule has a rather large superior and inferior recess that extends away from the joint. The capsular fibers surrounding these recesses are very thin and loose, and there may be openings where neurovascular bundles enter the recesses.[116] Paris[100] states that effusion within the Z joint may enter the superior recess and as little as 0.5 ml of effusion may cause the superior recess of the capsule to enter the anteriorly located IVF. Once in the IVF, the capsule may compress the exiting spinal nerve. Such a protrusion of the Z joint is known as a *synovial cyst.*[133]

The superior and inferior recesses are filled with *fibro-fatty pads.* These pads are well vascularized and are lined with a synovial membrane. They also protrude a significant distance into the superior and inferior aspect of the Z joint.[41] Engle and Bogduk[41] report that adipose tissue pads probably develop from undifferentiated mesenchyme of the embryologic Z joint. Furthermore, they indicate that in certain instances mechanical stress to the joint may cause an adipose tissue pad to undergo fibrous metaplasia that results in the formation of a *fibroadipose meniscoid* (an adipose tissue pad with a fibrous tip of dense connective tissue). They felt that both the adipose tissue pads and the meniscoids "play some form of normal functional role."[41]

In addition, "fringes" of synovium extend from the capsule to the region between the articular facets. These fringes fill the small region where the facets do not completely approximate one another.

As mentioned previously, fatty synovial folds may sometimes develop a fibrous tip that extends between the joint surfaces leading to compression of the folds between the articular surfaces.[28,116] These protruding synovial folds have been associated with the early stages of degeneration.[104] Other types of projections (meniscoids) into the joint space are entirely fibrous in nature.[116] Rauschning[104] frequently found hemarthrosis and effusion in the Z joints, which was associated with tearing of the meniscal folds or "nipping" of these folds between the joint surfaces.

Certain Z joint folds possess nociceptive fibers.[54,55] Entrapment within a Z joint of these innervated folds could be a primary source of back pain and muscle tightness (spasm) even without traction of the capsule (Case 13).

Degenerative changes of the Z joints frequently accompany aging. Kirkaldy-Willis et al[73] stated that such changes include an inflammatory reaction at the synovial lining of the Z joint, changes of the articular cartilage, loose bodies in the Z joint, and laxity of the joint capsule. All these events result in joint instability.[73] Alterations of the Z joints (left and right) at any given vertebral level are frequently accompanied by degenerative changes in the intervertebral disc at the same level

Degeneration of the disc leads to increased rotational instability of the Z joints, resulting in further degeneration of these structures. Such degenerative changes in the Z joints usually result in increased bone formation (leading to arthrosis or spur formation), which can compress the exiting spinal nerve.[104] Less frequently do degenerative changes take the form of erosion of the superior articular process.[73] This can lead to degenerative spondylolisthesis.

Osteophytes (or bony spurs) often develop with age on the superior and inferior articular processes. Frequently, this occurs along the periphery of the Z joint along the attachment sites of the ligamentum flavum or the articular capsule.

**Laminae of the lumbar spine.** The laminae in the lumbar region are broad and thick but do not overlap one another completely. Therefore, in contrast to the thoracic region, a distinct space exists between the laminae of adjacent lumbar vertebrae. This space allows for relatively easy access to the spinal subarachnoid space and is used in many diagnostic and therapeutic procedures.

The region of the lumbar lamina located between the superior and inferior articular processes is known as the *pars interarticularis*. This section fractures easily, resulting in a condition known as *spondylolysis* (see Cases 6, 11, and 15). As a result of spondylolysis, the vertebral body, pedicles, and superior articular processes can displace anteriorly. This anterior displacement is known as *spondylolisthesis* (see Cases 6, 11, and 15). Spondylolysis and spondylolisthesis are most common at L5. However, they may occur at any lumbar level.

**Spinous process.** The spinous processes of the lumbar vertebrae are broad from the superior portion to the inferior portion, narrow from side to side, and project directly posteriorly. They are, more or less, flat and rectangular in shape. Their posterior and inferior ridge is thickened for the attachment of ligaments and muscles.

## Lumbar vertebral foramen and lumbar vertebral canal

**General considerations.** The vertebral foramina in the lumbar region are generally triangular, although they are somewhat more rounded in the upper lumbar vertebrae and more triangular or trefoil shaped in the lower lumbar vertebrae. The triangular shape of the vertebral foramina of the middle and lower lumbar vertebrae is reminiscent of the shape of these openings in the cervical region; however, the lumbar foramina are smaller than those of the cervical region but are larger and more triangular than the rounded foramina of the thoracic region.

The size of the vertebral canal ranges from 12 to 20 mm in its anterior to posterior dimension at the midsagittal plane and 18 to 27 mm in its transverse diameter. Stenosis is defined as a narrowing beyond the lowest value of the normal range.[35]

Adipose tissue, nerves, and vessels are located within the epidural space of the vertebral canal. The internal vertebral venous plexus is particularly important clinically in the epidural space of the lumbar vertebral canal.

**Internal vertebral venous plexus.** The internal vertebral venous plexus is located deep to the bony elements of the vertebral foramina (the laminae, spinous processes, pedicles, and vertebral body). This plexus is embedded in a layer of loose areolar tissue known as the epidural (extradural) adipose tissue. The internal vertebral venous plexus has been given many additional names partly because of its clinical importance to the epidural venous plexus, the extradural venous plexus, and Batson's channels (see Case 18).

The internal vertebral venous plexus consists of many interconnected longitudinal channels. Several run along the posterior aspect of the vertebral canal and several others run along the anterior aspect of the canal. The anterior channels drain the vertebral bodies via large basivertebral veins. The basivertebral veins pierce the center of each vertebral body and communicate with the internal plexus posteriorly and the external vertebral venous plexus anteriorly. The posterior communication of the basivertebral veins with the anterior internal vertebral venous plexus occurs by means of small veins that run from the basivertebral veins, around the posterior longitudinal ligament, to reach the anterior internal vertebral venous plexus.

The veins of the internal vertebral venous plexus contain no valves and, therefore, the direction of drainage is posture and respiration dependent. Inferiorly, this plexus is continuous with the prostatic venous plexus in men, and, superiorly (in both men and women), it is continuous with the occipital dura mater venous sinus of the posterior cranial fossa. Therefore, prostatic carcinoma may metastasize via this route to all regions of the spine and to the meninges and the brain (see Case 18).

**Neural elements within the lumbar subarachnoid cistern.** The vertebral foramen of L1 contains the conus medullaris. The conus medullaris ends at the level of the L1 intervertebral disc. The remainder of the lumbar portion of the vertebral canal contains the cauda equina (Fig. 4-10). The cauda equina is bathed in the cerebrospinal fluid of the subarachnoid space. The subarachnoid space in the lumbar vertebral canal is quite large when compared with the cervical and thoracic regions. Because of its size, the subarachnoid space below the level of the L1 vertebral foramen is known as the lumbar cistern. Also within the lumbar vertebral canal are the meninges (pia mater, attached to rootlets; arachnoid;

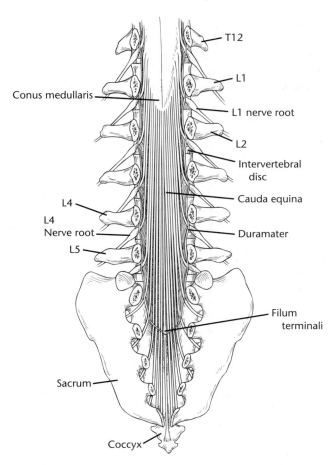

**Fig. 4-10** The lumbar vertebral canal and cauda equina. The posterior arches of the lumbar vertebrae have been removed to reveal the lumbar vertebral canal and the cauda equina.

and dura mater, which surrounds the arachnoid and to which the arachnoid is closely applied).

**Dural attachments within the vertebral canal.** The dura mater of the lumbar spine has a series of attachments to neighboring vertebrae and ligaments. These attachments are found at each segmental level and are usually found in the region of the intervertebral disc.[104] They have been referred to as the "dural attachment complex"[36] or "Hoffman ligaments."[36,104] A thorough description of these structures is beyond the scope of this section and can be found in Cramer.[28]

Stimulation of the anterior aspect of the lumbar spinal dura mater has resulted in pain felt in the midline, radiating into the low back and superior aspect of the buttock.[40] This pattern of pain referral is also seen in irritation of the posterior longitudinal ligament.

**Lumbar intervertebral foramina and nerve root canals.** Many of the features that make the region of the lumbar IVF different from those of the rest of the spine result from the unique characteristics of the lum-

bar and sacral spinal nerves. Because the spinal cord ends at approximately the first lumbar intervertebral disc, the lumbar and sacral dorsal and ventral roots must descend, sometimes for a considerable distance, within the subarachnoid space of the lumbar vertebral canal. This region of subarachnoid space is known as the *lumbar cistern.* The exiting nerves (dorsal and ventral rootlets or roots) leave the lumbar cistern by entering a sleeve of dura mater. This usually occurs slightly inferior to the level of the intervertebral disc at the level *above* the IVF that the roots will eventually occupy. For example, the L4 roots enter their dural sleeve just beneath the L3-L4 disc and then course inferiorly and laterally to exit the L4-L5 IVF. The fact that the neural elements pass over an intervertebral disc before exiting through an IVF is of clinical significance (see Case 14) (Fig. 4-11).

More specifically, upon leaving the subarachnoid space of the lumbar cistern, the exiting dorsal and ventral roots pass at an oblique inferior and lateral angle and retain a rather substantial and very distinct covering of dura mater. This covering, known as the *dural root sleeve,* will surround the neural elements and their accompanying radicular arteries and veins until they leave the confines of the IVF. Frequently the dorsal and ventral rootlets that arise from the spinal cord do not all

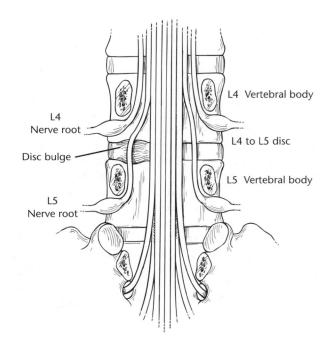

**Fig. 4-11** Diagram simplifying the relationship between the lumbar intervertebral discs and the exiting nerve roots. Notice that a bulge of the L4-L5 intervertebral disc affects the L5 nerve roots. The S1 roots have not yet entered their dural root sleeve and remain in the subarachnoid space of the lumbar cistern. Their location in the subarachnoid space allows the S1 roots to "float away" from the bulging disc.

unite to form dorsal and ventral roots until they are well within the dural root sleeve.[36,104] In addition, the dorsal and ventral roots combine to form the mixed spinal nerve while they are within the distal aspect of the funnel-shaped dural root sleeve. This latter union occurs at the level of the IVF. The exiting mixed spinal nerve has been found to be larger than the combined size of the individual dorsal and ventral roots.[33] Upon reaching the lateral edge of the IVF, the dural root sleeve becomes continuous with the epineurium of the mixed spinal nerve. Many authors[18,80,104,123] consider the region beginning at the exit of the neural elements from the lumbar cistern and continuing to the lateral edge of the IVF, as being of significant clinical importance. Possibly because of the clinical significance of this region several terms, such as lumbar radicular canal,[123] nerve root canal, or simply, root canal have been used to describe it.[104] A full discussion of the subtle differences between the regions described by these terms can be found elsewhere.[28] The term nerve root canal (NRC) will be used in the following paragraphs when discussing the course of the dural root sleeve and its contents and the term intervertebral foramen will be used to describe the terminal part of the NRC that lies between the pedicles of two adjacent vertebrae.

**Entrapment of the neural elements.** Compression, or entrapment, of neural elements as they pass through the NRC or the IVF can occur.[78] Causes of such compression include degenerative changes of the superior articular facets and posterior vertebral bodies, intervertebral disc protrusion, and pressure from the superior pedicle of the IVF.[62,87,123]

*Anatomy of the nerve root canals.* The size of the NRCs varies considerably from the upper to the lower lumbar segments. They are smaller at the level of L1 and L2 because, after exiting the lumbar cistern, the L1 and L2 nerves course almost directly laterally to reach the IVF. This led Crock[30] to state that the concept of a NRC at L1 and L2 is useless, because the beginning of the dural root sleeve lies against the inferior and medial aspect of the upper pedicle of the IVF. Therefore, there is no true dural "canal" for these nerve roots.

The NRCs become progressively longer from L1 to S1 as the dural root sleeves exit at a more oblique inferior angle. Therefore, the NRCs of L5 and S1 are the longest and the most susceptible to damage from pathology of surrounding structures.[30]

All of the exiting rootlets or roots course over an intervertebral disc either just before entering their dural root sleeve (L1 and L2) or, in the case of L3 to S1, directly in the region where they enter the dural root sleeve. However, only the S1 dural root sleeve (and contents) passes completely over an intervertebral disc (the L5 disc). The S1 NRC passes through a movable and narrow opening between the L5 disc anteriorly and

the L5 to S1 ligamentum flavum posteriorly. Therefore, the S1 nerve is exposed to possible compression both anteriorly (disc protrusion) and posteriorly (ligamentum flavum bulging or buckling or hypertrophy of the superior articular process of the sacrum) in this region.[104]

*Clinical conditions related to the nerve root canals.* Resorption of the intervertebral disc (particularly at the L5 to S1 level) causes narrowing of the IVF at the same level (the L5 to S1 IVF in this instance), and also narrowing of the NRC of the nerve exiting at the IVF below (the S1 NRC in this instance). Crock[30] states that the remaining annulus fibrosis of the disc may bulge posteriorly, bringing the posterior longitudinal ligament along with it. The superior articular facet of the segment below (S1) moves superiorly and anteriorly, again compressing the NRC (S1). The combination of posterior annulus bulge and anterior displacement of the superior articular facet of the vertebra below can result in dramatic narrowing of the NRC that runs between these two structures.[2,104] Osteophyte (bony spur) formation is fairly common, both from the vertebral body along the attachment of the annulus fibrosis and from the superior articular process along the attachment of the ligamentum flavum. These spurs can further compress the neural and vascular elements of the NRC.[2,104]

*Intervertebral foramina proper.* When viewed from the side of the lumbar region, the lumbar IVFs face laterally. A typical lumbar IVF (Fig. 4-12) is sometimes described as being shaped like an inverted teardrop or an inverted pear.

The spinal nerve is formed in the superior one third of the IVF by the union of the dorsal and ventral roots. This union occurs in the lateral aspect of the IVF. At the medial aspect of the IVF, the dorsal and ventral roots are very close to the medial and inferior aspects of the superior pedicle that forms the upper boundary of the IVF.[30] The neural elements in the upper region of the IVF are accompanied by a branch (or sometimes branches) of the lumbar segmental artery, the *superior segmental (pedicle)* veins connecting the external and internal vertebral venous plexuses and the sinuvertebral nerve.[104] The spinal nerve occupies approximately one third of the IVF in the lumbar region. This allows for crowding by the articular facets during extension.[18,104] The inferior aspect of the IVF is usually narrowed to a slit by the annulus fibrosis, which normally bulges slightly posteriorly. The inferior aspect of the IVF is also narrowed by the posteriorly located ligamentum flavum. The *inferior segmental (discal)* veins usually lie in this narrow space. Similarly to the superior segmental (pedicle) veins, these segmental veins also unite the internal vertebral venous plexus with the external vertebral venous plexus. Branches of the segmental veins unite with the ascending lumbar vein.

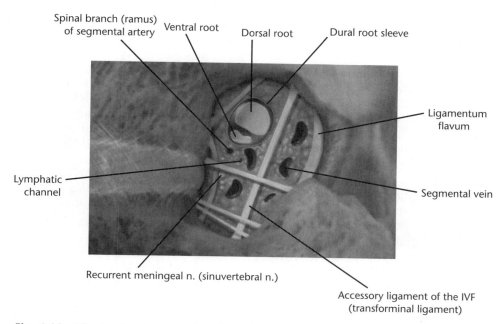

Spinal branch (ramus) of segmental artery — Ventral root — Dorsal root — Dural root sleeve — Ligamentum flavum — Lymphatic channel — Segmental vein — Recurrent meningeal n. (sinuvertebral n.) — Accessory ligament of the IVF (transforminal ligament)

***Fig. 4-12***   The lumbar intervertebral foramen (IVF). Notice the borders of the IVF. Also notice the structures which normally traverse the IVF. The most common locations of the transforaminal ligaments are also shown on this illustration. (Illustration by Dino Juarez, The National College of Chiropractic.)

## Unique aspects of the lumbar vertebrae, ligaments, and range of motion of the lumbar region

**Fifth lumbar vertebra.** The vertebral body of the fifth lumbar vertebra is the largest of the entire spine. It is taller anteriorly than posteriorly and this contributes to the increase in the lower lumbar lordosis (the lower lumbar lordosis is frequently called the lumbosacral angle). The spinous process of L5 is the smallest of those of the lumbar vertebrae. It projects inferiorly and its posterior aspect is more rounded than the rest of the lumbar spinous processes. The transverse processes of this vertebra are much wider than those of the rest of the lumbar spine. In fact, they originate from the entire lateral aspect of the pedicles and their origin continues posteriorly to the adjacent lamina. However, they do not extend as far laterally as do other lumbar transverse processes. The lateral aspect of the transverse processes of L5 also angles slightly superiorly, with the angulation beginning at about the midpoint of each of the two (left and right) processes.

**Lumbosacral articulation** The lumbosacral articulation actually consists of several articulations between L5 and the sacrum. It has two components: (1) the joining, via the fifth intervertebral disc, of the inferior aspect of the body of L5 with the body of the first sacral segment and (2) the joints between the left and right inferior articular processes of L5 and the superior articular processes of the sacrum. The curvature of these latter joints is not as great as that of the Z joints of the rest of the lumbar spine. The plane of articulation of the lumbosacral zygapophyseal joint is subject to much variation, ranging between 20 and 90 degrees from the sagittal plane (the average range is 40 to 60 degrees). Frequently asymmetry, known as *tropism,* exists between the left and right L5-S1 Z joints. Lippitt[82] reported that tropism may be a cause of premature degeneration and pain, but the clinical significance of tropism remains a matter of controversy.

The L5-S1 intervertebral disc is typically narrower than the intervertebral discs of the rest of the lumbar spine.[94] This may contribute to the IVF at this level being smaller than the IVFs of the rest of the lumbar spine. Recall that the spinal nerve at this level is the largest. Therefore, more than one third of the L5-S1 IVF is occupied by the mixed spinal nerve. Even though the intervertebral disc and IVF are smaller in this region, the L5-S1 articulation is, by far, the most movable of all of the lumbar joints (5 degrees of unilateral rotation, 3 degrees of lateral bending, 10 degrees of flexion, and 10 degrees of extension). These factors, along with others,[28] make the L5 roots and mixed spinal nerve vulnerable to compression as they traverse the L5 NRC.

The intra-articular space of the left and right lumbosacral Z joints is usually wider than the spaces in the remainder of the lumbar spine. A recess normally exists along the inferomedial edge of the lumbosacral Z joints. This recess is filled with a very large intra-articular synovial fold that is composed primarily of adipose tissue. Another intra-articular synovial protrusion usually projects into the superior and medial aspect of the L5-S1 Z joint.[55] These synovial folds are susceptible to entrapment between the opposing L5-S1 articular facets and are a likely source of low back pain and subsequent muscle tightness. Gentle, well-controlled spinal manipulation to open the facets to allow an entrapped synovial fold to be pulled out of the joint by its attachment to the joint capsule has been suggested as the treatment of choice for this condition.[55]

Five percent of the population have a transitional segment between the lumbar spine and the sacrum.[94] This takes the form of either a "lumbarization" of S1 or, more frequently, a "sacralization" of L5. *Sacralization* refers to elongation of the transverse processes of L5 with varying degrees of fusion or articulation with either the sacral ala or the iliac crest. The union between L5 and the sacrum may be bilateral, but it is usually only unilateral. The L5 to S1 intervertebral disc in cases of sacralization is normally significantly thinner than that of typical L5 to S1 segments.[94] Also, because it is usually devoid of nuclear material, this disc will rarely undergo pathologic change or degeneration to the degree seen in discs above the sacralized segment.[94]

**Ligaments of the lumbar region.** The ligaments of the lumbar region include the following: the articular capsules of the zygapophyseal joints, ligamenta flava, supraspinous ligament, interspinous ligaments, intertransverse ligaments, and anterior and posterior longitudinal ligaments (Fig. 4-13). The iliolumbar ligaments (left and right), which are found only in the lower lumbar region, will also be covered in this section.

A unique characteristic of the anterior longitudinal ligament (ALL) in the lumbar region is that it is wider from side to side than in the thoracic region. It is also thicker than the posterior longitudinal ligament.[59] It extends across the anterior aspect of the vertebral bodies and intervertebral discs to attach inferiorly to the sacrum. The ALL functions to limit extension, and it may be torn during extension injuries of the back and spine. It receives sensory (nociceptive and proprioceptive) innervation from branches of the gray communicating rami of the lumbar sympathetic trunk. Therefore, damage to this ligament during extension injuries can be a direct source of pain.

The anterior and the posterior longitudinal ligaments (PLLs), collectively, have been termed the intercentral ligaments because they connect the anterior and posterior surfaces of adjacent vertebral bodies (centra), respectively.[59] They also attach the vertebral bodies to the intervertebral discs and are important in *stabilizing* the spine during flexion (PLL) and extension (ALL). They also function to *limit* flexion (PLL) and extension (ALL) of the spine.

The PLL in the lumbar region appears denticulated, that is, it is narrow over the posterior aspect of the vertebral bodies and flares laterally at each intervertebral disc, where it attaches to the posterior aspect of the annulus fibrosis.

The PLL receives sensory innervation from the recurrent meningeal nerve (sinuvertebral nerve). Recent

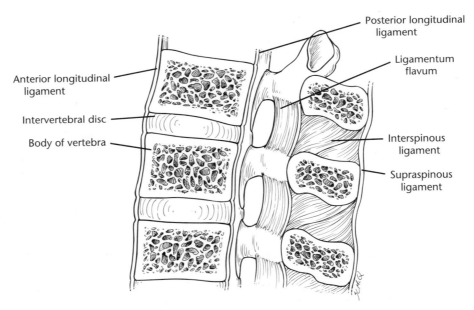

Anterior longitudinal ligament

Intervertebral disc

Body of vertebra

Posterior longitudinal ligament

Ligamentum flavum

Interspinous ligament

Supraspinous ligament

*Fig. 4-13*   A midsagittal section demonstrating the ligaments of the lumbar region.

studies[75] substantiate previous assumptions that the PLL is pain sensitive and indicate that the PLL (at least in the lumbar region) is *highly* sensitive to pain.

The paired (left and right) ligamenta flava of the lumbar region are the thickest of the entire spine. They extend between the laminae of adjacent vertebrae throughout the lumbar region, including the junction between the laminae of L5 and those of the S1 segment. Each ligamentum flavum is thickest medially and passes laterally to form the anterior joint capsule of the Z joint. The most laterally situated fibers attach to the pedicle of the vertebra below.

A typical lumbar interspinous ligament consists of three sections: the anterior, the middle, and the posterior.[7,14] These three parts run between adjacent spinous processes, filling the gap along the length of these processes. A full description of the three portions of this ligament can be found elsewhere.[28]

The interspinous ligaments can be torn, and in one study, the fibers were found to be ruptured in up to 21% of cadavers examined.[7]

The interspinous ligaments and the supraspinous ligament limit the end range of lumbar flexion and are the first to sprain during hyperflexion of the lumbar region.[64]

The supraspinous ligament is strongest in the lumbar region. Classically, it has been described as extending to the sacrum.[129] However, others[7] believe that the supraspinous ligament ends at L5 and does not extend to the sacrum; Paris[100] states that it usually ends at L4 and, rarely at L5, never extending to the sacrum. The strong fibers of origin of the lumbar erector spinae muscles (thoracolumbar fascia) take the place of this ligament inferior to the spinous process of L4.[100] This fascia continues inferiorly to the median sacral crest. Bogduk and Twomey[14] do not consider the supraspinous ligament to be a true ligament in the lumbar region because it is primarily made up of very strong tendinous fibers of the longissimus thoracis and multifidus muscles and crisscrossing fibers of the thoracolumbar fascia. In addition, a condensation of the membranous (deep) layer of the superficial fascia forms the superficial layer of the "supraspinous ligament."[14]

The term "supraspinous ligament" continues to be used quite frequently by clinicians and researchers alike. In such instances reference is being made to the tough combination of midline tendons of the longissimus thoracis muscle, the intersecting fibers of the thoracolumbar fascia, and the membranous layer of superficial fascia. The term "lumbar supraspinous restraints" would seem to more accurately reflect the true nature of the fibrous band of tissue found along the posterior aspect of the lumbar spinous processes and interspinous spaces.

Currently, the intertransverse ligaments are thought to be composed of two lamellae.[7] The posterior lamella of the intertransverse ligaments passes medially to the posterior aspect of the zygapophyseal joint. It is pierced by the posterior primary division and continues medially to help reinforce the Z joint capsule from behind.

The anterior lamella of the intertransverse ligaments passes medially to form a layer of fascia over the intervertebral foramen. Here it is pierced by the anterior primary division and the spinal branches of lumbar segmental arteries and veins. The anterior lamella then continues anteriorly and medially, to become continuous with the anterior longitudinal ligament. The accessory (transforaminal) ligaments that span the IVF are probably condensations of the anterior lamella of the intertransverse ligament.[14]

The left and right iliolumbar ligaments pass from the left and right transverse processes of L5 (and occasionally L4) to the sacrum and iliac crest of the same side. These ligaments probably function to stabilize the L5 to S1 junction, helping to maintain the proper relationship of L5 on S1, a function that is enhanced after degeneration of the L5 intervertebral disc.[96] In addition, the ligaments probably limit axial rotation of L5 on S1. Because the iliolumbar ligament is innervated by posterior primary divisions of the neighboring spinal nerves, it may possibly be a primary source of back pain.

**Lumbar intervertebral discs.** In general, the intervertebral discs of the lumbar region are the thickest of the spine. They are similar in composition to the discs in the other regions and consist of a central nucleus pulposus, an outer annulus fibrosis, composed of 15 to 25 lamellae,[119] and the cartilaginous (vertebral) end plates that form the superior and inferior surfaces of the IVDs (Fig. 4-14).

The function of the lumbar IVDs is similar to that of the IVDs throughout the spine. That is, they absorb loads placed on the spine from above (axial loading) and allow for some motion to occur.[64] The lumbar discs become shorter during the day because they carry the load of the torso. They usually regain their shape within 5 hours of sleep (creep). During the active hours the discs require movement to maintain proper hydration. In fact, decreased movement and decreased axial loading have been strongly associated with disc degeneration.[119]

The lumbar IVDs are thicker anteriorly than posteriorly. This helps in the formation of the lumbar lordosis. Liyang et al[83] found that the shape of the lumbar IVDs changes significantly during flexion and extension of the lumbar region. Flexion narrowed the anterior aspect of the disc by approximately 1 to 5 mm and increased the height of the posterior aspect of the disc by approximately 1.5 to 3 mm.

Because each lumbar disc is in contact with two or three pairs of dorsal roots,[115] bulging, or protrusion, of

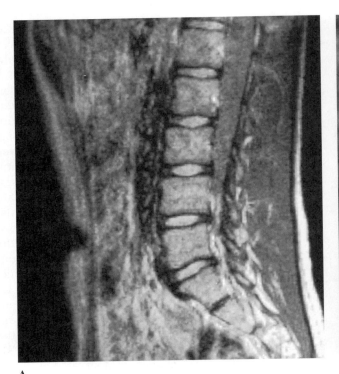

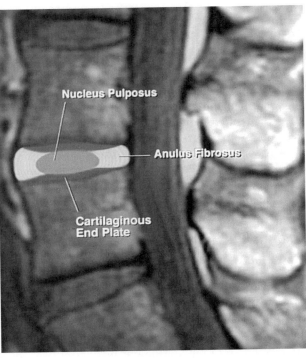

A                              B

*Fig. 4-14*   **A,** Midsagittal magnetic resonance imaging scan of the lumbar region, showing the intervertebral discs and the adjacent vertebral bodies. **B,** Same scan as in **A** with the parts of the intervertebral disc labeled. (Photographs by Ron Mensching and illustration by Dino Juarez, The National College of Chiropractic. From: Cramer G, Darby S: *Basic and clinical anatomy of the spine, spinal cord, and ANS.* St. Louis, 1995, Mosby, p. 441, with permission.)

the IVD is a major cause of radicular pain (Case 14). However, it should be kept in mind that each IVD is innervated by sensory nerve endings and, as a result, can be a primary source of back pain.[113] The IVD receives both nociceptive and proprioceptive fibers. The posterior aspect of the disc receives innervation from the recurrent meningeal nerve (sinuvertebral nerve) and the lateral and anterior aspects of the disc are supplied by branches of the gray communicating rami of the lumbar sympathetic trunk.[15,40]

Bogduk and Twomey[14] have described a series of events that explains the mechanism by which the IVD can be a primary source of pain in the absence of IVD herniation. They describe two mechanisms by which the IVD may cause pain without herniation. The first is by means of torsional injuries to the disc and the second is by compression of the IVD. In addition, internal disc disruption can directly affect the IVD.

The ranges of motion between individual lumbar vertebrae and various combinations of adjacent vertebrae[28] are beyond the scope of this chapter. The most clinically useful ranges of motion are those of the entire lumbar region and those of the lumbosacral (L5-S1) articulation (see Cases 13 and 14). These are listed in Table 4-4.

## Soft tissues of the lumbar region: nerves and vessels

The muscles associated with the lumbar region are listed in Table 4-5. This section on soft tissue structures of the lumbar region will focus on vessels and nerves related to the lumbar spine. Many of these structures are located on the internal surface of the posterior abdominal wall and are associated with the anterior and lateral aspects of the lumbar vertebral column.

*Table 4-4*   Total ranges of motion for the lumbar and lumbosacral regions

| **Lumbar Region** |
| --- |
| Flexion: 60 degrees |
| Extension: 20 degrees |
| Unilateral lateral flexion: 25 to 30 degrees |
| Unilateral axial rotation: 10 to 15 degrees |
| **Lumbosacral (L5-S1) motion segment** |
| Combined flexion and extension: 20 degrees |
| Unilateral lateral flexion: 3 degrees |
| Unilateral axial rotation: 5 degrees |

*Table 4-5*   The layers of the muscles of the back including the lumbar area

Layer 1. Extrinsic muscles: These muscles attach the thoracic spine to the upper limb and consist of the trapezius and latissimus dorsimuscle (cervical and thoracic spine).
Layer 2. Intermediate extrinsic muscles: These consist of the serratus posterior inferior muscle (thoracic and lumbar spine).
Layer 3. Superficial layer of deep back muscles: splenius muscles (cervical spine).
Layer 4. Intermediate layer of deep back muscles: These consist of the erector spinae, iliocostalis, longissimus, and spinalis (cervical, thoracic, and lumbar spine).
Layer 5. Deep layer of deep back muscles: These muscles lie below the erector spinae muscles (especially the spinalis) and sit in the groove between the spinous process and the transverse process of the vertebrae. This layer is collectively known as the transversospinalis group and consists of the following muscles: (1) the multifidus—poorly developed in the thoracic region, (2) the rotatores—best developed in the thoracic region, (3) the intertransversarii, and (4) the levator costorum (cervical, thoracic, and lumbar spine).
Posterior abdominal wall: (1) PSOAS, (2) iliacus, and (3) quadratus lumborum (lumbar spine).

*Modified from Moore KL:* Clinically oriented anatomy, *ed 3, Baltimore, 1992, Williams & Wilkins.*

## Nerves of the lumbar region: dorsal and ventral roots, mixed spinal nerves, posterior and anterior primary divisions, and sinuvertebral nerves.

The innervation of the lumbar portion of the vertebral column and the soft tissue structures of the lumbar region is a topic of extreme clinical importance. A knowledge of the innervation of the spine gives the clinician a better understanding of what could be causing a patient's pain. Because the basic neural elements associated with the spine have been covered in previous chapters, this section will concentrate on those aspects of innervation unique to the lumbar region.

The cauda equina and exiting roots and spinal nerves have been discussed previously, under "Neural elements within the lumbar subarachnoid cistern" and "Lumbar intervertebral foramina and nerve root canals," respectively. This section will cover the dorsal and ventral roots and the mixed spinal nerve briefly will concentrate on aspects of the neural elements after they have left the confines of the IVF. Since the majority of spinal structures are innervated by either the recurrent meningeal nerves or the posterior primary divisions, these nerves and the structures they innervate will be covered in more detail below. This will be followed by a discussion of the anterior primary divisions and the lumbar plexus. It should be remembered that the lateral and anterior aspects of the IVDs and the ALL are innervated by branches of the lumbar sympathetic trunk and the lumbar gray rami communicantes.

### General considerations.

Three types of nerve endings have been found in almost all of the structures in the lumbar vertebral column that receive a nerve supply. These include free nerve endings, nonencapsulated endings, and encapsulated endings.[13] This would indicate that most innervated structures of the spine are sensitive to pain, pressure, and proprioception.[65,127]

Of particular interest and, on occasion, of particular frustration to clinicians and researchers alike is that there is an overlap of innervation throughout the spine, and this has been particularly well documented in the lumbar region.[48] Most spinal structures seem to be innervated by nerves from at least two adjacent vertebral levels. This led Edgar and Ghadially[40] to state, "The poor localization of much low back pain and its tendency to radiate may be related to this neurological pattern." This can make the task of identifying the cause of low back pain particularly challenging at times.

### Dorsal and ventral roots and mixed spinal nerves.

The dorsal and ventral roots of the lumbar spine travel inferiorly as the cauda equina. They then course through the nerve root canal before exiting the IVF. The nerve roots can be irritated by many structures and pathologic processes. These include disc protrusion or other space occupying lesions, structural lesions of the vertebral canal, chemical irritation, and intrinsic radiculitis.[12] Before exiting the IVF the dorsal and ventral roots unite to form a mixed spinal nerve. Each lumbar mixed spinal nerve emerges from a lumbar intervertebral foramen and immediately divides into an anterior primary division (ventral ramus) and a posterior primary division (dorsal ramus).

### Recurrent meningeal (sinuvertebral) nerves.

The recurrent meningeal nerves (RMNs) at each level innervate many structures located within the IVF and the vertebral canal. Because they have been found to carry fibers that conduct nociception (pain), structures innervated by these nerves are considered to be capable of producing back pain[53]; however, in addition to nociceptive input, the RMNs also probably carry fibers for thermal sensation and proprioception.[40]

The RMNs are found at each IVF of the vertebral column. Each RMN originates from the most proximal portion of the anterior primary division just distal to the IVF that it will eventually reenter. The RMN receives a branch from the closest gray communicating ramus and then enters the anterior aspect of the IVF close to the pedicle that forms the roof of this opening. Usually more than one RMN enters each IVF, and up to six have been found at one level.[40] Consequently, compression of the RMNs within the confines of the IVF may be a cause of back pain.[40]

Upon entering the IVF, the RMNs ramify extensively. There is a great deal of variation associated with their distribution within the vertebral canal.[60] Usually each gives off a large ascending branch and smaller descending and transverse branches, although the transverse branch is not always present. The ascending branch usually extends superiorly for at least one vertebral level above its level of entrance. The branches of the RMNs anastomose with those of adjacent vertebral segments including those of the opposite side of the spine.[12,40,60] They innervate the posterior aspect of the IVD, the PLL, the periosteum of the posterior aspect of the vertebral bodies, the epidural venous plexus, and the anterior aspect of the spinal dura mater. Therefore, all of these structures have been implicated as possible sources of back pain. In addition, compression of the RMNs in the vertebral canal may be a cause of spinal stenosis.[40] However, because of the great variability in the distribution of the RMNs, the pattern of pain referral as a result of nociceptive input received from them may also be quite inconsistent.

**Posterior primary divisions.** Whereas the recurrent meningeal nerves innervate the structures located on the anterior aspect of the vertebral canal, the posterior primary rami innervate those structures of the posterior aspect of the vertebral canal (the vertebral arch structures). This difference in innervation may be of significance; the recurrent meningeal nerves may be responsible for relaying information related to potential or real harm, to the neural elements of the vertebral canal, and the posterior primary divisions may be responsible for relaying information related to the structural integrity of the spine.[40,53]

Each posterior primary division (PPD) of the lumbar region leaves the mixed spinal nerve at the lateral border of the IVF and passes over the transverse process of the lower vertebra participating in the formation of the IVF (for example, the L3 nerve passes over the L4 transverse process). The nerve passes posteriorly and sends a twig to the intertransversarius medialis muscle and continues posteriorly where it divides into a medial and a lateral branch. The medial branch passes deep to the mamillo-accessory ligament and supplies sensory innervation to the Z joint and then motor innervation to the multifidi. This innervation to the multifidi has been found to be very specific.[16] The medial branch of the PPD innervates those fibers that insert onto the spinous process "of the same segmental number as the nerve."[16] The medial branch then continues further medially to innervate the rotatores and interspinous muscles. It also provides sensory innervation to the interspinous ligament, the supraspinous "ligament," possibly the ligamentum flavum, and the periosteum of the posterior arch, including the spinous process. Along its course, the medial branch anastomoses with medial branches of adjacent levels and also sends an inferior branch to the Z joint of the level below.[12,40,53] Therefore, each Z joint is innervated by medial branches of at least two PPDs.[12]

The lateral branch of the PPD supplies motor innervation to the erector spinae muscles. Bogduk[13] found that the lateral branch supplies the iliocostalis lumborum muscle, whereas an intermediate branch stems from the lumbar PPDs to supply the longissimus thoracis muscle. After innervating the longissimus thoracis muscle, the intermediate branches form an anastomosis with the intermediate branches of adjacent levels. The PPD of L5 has only two branches, a medial branch with a typical distribution and a more lateral branch that corresponds with the intermediate branches of higher levels because it innervates the longissimus thoracis muscle. The L1, L2, and L3 lateral branches are sometimes known as the superior *cluneal nerves* (e.g., Maigne's Syndrome). They supply sensory innervation to the skin over the upper buttocks. Neither the medial branches of the PPDs nor any branches of the L4 and L5 posterior primary divisions supply the skin of the back.[53]

### Anterior primary divisions and lumbar plexus

The anterior primary divisions (APDs), or ventral rami, branch from the mixed spinal nerves at the lateral border of the IVF and immediately enter the psoas major muscle. The ventral rami of the first four lumbar nerves then branch within the substance of the psoas major muscle to form the lumbar plexus. The psoas major muscle may provide some protection for the dorsal and ventral roots from traction forces placed on the peripheral nerves of the lumbar plexus.[33]

Note that the lumbar plexus is derived from the ventral primary rami of only the first four lumbar nerves. The vertral ramus of L5 unites with a branch of the ventral ramus of L4 to form the lumbosacral trunk. The lumbosacral trunk then enters the pelvis to unite with the APDs of the sacral mixed spinal nerves and, in doing so, helps to form the sacral plexus. Frequently the twelfth thoracic (subcostal) nerve also participates in the lumbar plexus. Table 4-6 lists the branches of the lumbar plexus along with the closely related subcostal nerve and lumbosacral trunk.

### Autonomic nerves of the lumbar region

The abdominal and pelvic viscera receive their motor innervation from autonomic nerves derived from both the sympathetic and parasympathetic nervous systems. Sensory nerves originating from the same visceral structures also travel along the sympathetic and parasympathetic nerve fibers. The diffuse nature of the sympathetic and parasympathetic systems is responsible for the equally diffuse nature of the sensory innervation that travels along with them. This is one reason pain from an abdominal or pelvic viscus may "refer" to a region some distance from the affected organ.[53]

*Table 4-6*    The branches of the lumbar plexus

| Nerve | Motor and sensory innervation |
| --- | --- |
| Subcostal nerve (T12) | Sensory—region under the umbilicus |
| Iliohypogastric nerve (L1) | Motor—pyramidalis and quadratus lumborum muscles<br>Sensory—gluteal, inguinal, and suprapubic region |
| Ilioinguinal nerve (L1) | Motor—anterior abdominal wall |
| Genitofemoral nerve (L1 and L2) | Motor—anterior abdominal wall<br>Femoral branch: sensory—femoral triangle<br>Genital branch: motor—dartos and cremaster muscles |
| Lateral femoral cutaneous nerve (L2 and L3) | Sensory—lateral aspect of the thigh |
| Femoral nerve (L2, L3, and L4) | Sensory—anterior thigh<br>Motor—psoas and iliacus muscles (before leaving the abdominopelvic cavity posterior to the inguinal ligament)<br>Motor—quadratus femoris and pectineus muscles (distal to the inguinal ligament) |
| Obturator nerve (L2, L3, and L4) | Sensory—medial aspect of the thigh<br>Motor—adductor muscles of the thigh |
| Lumbosacral trunk (L4 and L5) | The lumbosacral trunk is not officially a part of the lumbar plexus. This nerve passes inferiorly to participate in the sacral plexus. It therefore serves as a connection between the lumbar and sacral plexuses. |

Sympathetic innervation of the abdominal viscera is derived from two sources, the thoracic and the lumbar splanchnic nerves. The parasympathetic innervation is by either the left and right vagus nerves or the pelvic splanchnic nerves. A discussion of specific nerves that make up both the sympathetic and parasympathetic divisions of the autonomic nervous system and their clinical relevance is beyond the scope of this section and can be found elsewhere.[32]

## CLINICAL ANATOMY OF THE SACROILIAC JOINT*
CHAE-SONG RO
GREGORY D. CRAMER

The sacroiliac joint (SIJ) is an articulation between the auricular surface of the lateral aspect of the sacrum and the auricular surface of the medial aspect of the ilium (Figs. 4-15 and 4-16) (see Case 15). Previously, this joint was classified as an amphiarthrosis. However, it is now classified as an *atypical synovial joint* with a well-defined joint space and two opposing articular surfaces.[24] The auricular surface is shaped like an inverted "L."[129] Other authors have described it as being "C"-shaped.[24] The superior limb of this surface is oriented anteriorly and superiorly, and the inferior limb is oriented posteriorly and inferiorly. An articular capsule lines the anterior aspect of the joint, whereas the posterior aspect of the joint is covered by the interosseous sacroiliac (SI) ligament. No articular capsule has been found along the posterior joint surface.

The sacral auricular surface has a longitudinal groove, known as the *sacral groove,* along its center, which extends from the upper end to the lower end. The posterior

rim of this groove is very thick and is known as the *sacral tuberosity.* The iliac auricular surface has a longitudinal ridge, known as the *iliac ridge,* which corresponds to the sacral groove. The inferior end of this iliac ridge ends as the *posterior inferior iliac spine* (PIIS). The sacral groove and the iliac ridge interlock for stability and help to guide movement of the SIJ.

The region within the posterior concavity of the SIJ is covered by the interosseous ligament and consists of three *fossae.* The *middle* fossa is the approximate location of the axis of SIJ rotation. It is approximately around this fossa that the iliac ridge moves circularly in the sacral groove. Posterior to the auricular surface of the ilium is the *iliac tuberosity.* The anterior aspect of the iliac tuberosity inserts into the middle sacral fossa, creating a pivot around which the iliac ridge turns within the sacral groove.[4] Between the iliac tuberosity and the iliac ridge there is a *sulcus.* The sulcus promotes stability by interlocking with the sacral tuberosity. Finally, anterior and superior to the iliac tuberosity there is a depression that interlocks with an additional elevation on the posterior and superior surface of the sacral ala (alar tuberosity). Therefore, stability of the SIJ is promoted by a series of "tongues and grooves."[106] Figure 4-15 shows this series of interlocking elevations and depressions that aid the stability of the SIJ. This series of interlocking prominences and depressions become more enhanced and irregular with age.

### Ligaments of the sacroiliac joint

The fibrous articular capsule of the SIJ is only located along the anterior surface of the joint. It is lined internally with a synovial membrane, and is innervated with nociceptive and proprioceptive nerve endings. There is no articular capsule along the posterior border of the SIJ.

* Adapted from Ro CS, Cramer G: The sacrum, sacroiliac joint, and coccyx. In Cramer G, Darby S: *Basic and clinical anatomy of the spine, spinal cord, and ANS.* St. Louis, 1995, Mosby.

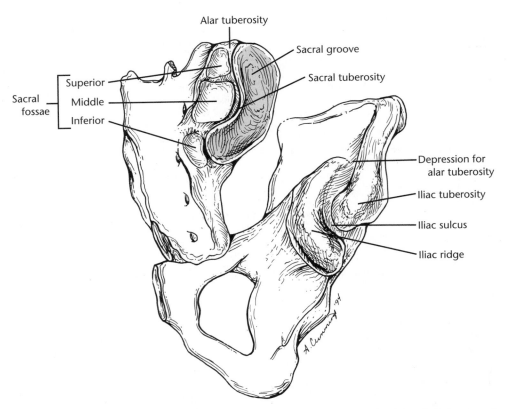

Sacral fossae — Superior / Middle / Inferior

Alar tuberosity

Sacral groove

Sacral tuberosity

Depression for alar tuberosity

Iliac tuberosity

Iliac sulcus

Iliac ridge

***Fig. 4-15*** Medial surfaces of the right sacrum and ilium. The series of elevations and depressions associated with the sacroiliac joint are accentuated in this illustration. These elevations and depressions are thought to help increase stability of the sacroiliac joint. (From: Cramer G, Darby S: *Basic and clinical anatomy of the spine, spinal cord, and ANS.* St. Louis, 1995, Mosby, p. 235, with permission.)

The interosseous ligament of each SIJ connects the three sacral fossae (see above) to the area around the iliac tuberosity. The interosseous ligament consists of superficial and deep layers.

The pelvic surface of each SIJ is covered by the anterior, or ventral, SI ligament. The ventral SI ligament passes across the anterior aspect of the SIJ in the horizontal plane. It does not support the joint as strongly as do either the interosseous or the posterior SI ligaments.[47] The ventral SI ligament fuses with the articular capsule of the pelvic side of the SIJ and is thicker inferiorly, near the region of the posterior inferior iliac spine.[124]

The posterior (dorsal) SI ligament is made up of two rather distinct parts. The long posterior SI ligament originates from the posterior superior iliac spine and the sacral tubercles of S3 and S4. It runs vertically along the posterior aspect of the SIJ and ends by blending inferiorly with the sacrotuberous ligament. The short posterior SI ligament originates from the sacral tubercles of S1 and S2. It runs in the horizontal plane and covers the SIJ posteriorly.

There are two accessory SI ligaments that are important for maintaining the stability of the SIJ. A third ligament, the iliolumbar ligament, provides additional stability to the region. The sacrotuberous ligament runs inferiorly and laterally from the posterior and inferior aspect of the sacrum to the ischial tuberosity. The lesser sciatic foramen is formed between this ligament and the sacrospinous ligament (discussed next). The sacrospinous ligament runs from the anterior surface of the sacrum (fused second, third, and fourth segments) to the spine of the ischium. The greater sciatic foramen is located superior to this ligament.

The sacrotuberous and sacrospinous ligaments limit anterior and inferior nodding (nutational) motion of the sacrum at the SIJ. This is accomplished by restricting the extent that the sacral apex can move posteriorly and superiorly when the promontory of the sacrum nods anteriorly and inferiorly.

The iliolumbar ligament connects the iliac crest with the adjacent transverse process of the L5 vertebra. Part of the iliolumbar ligament also attaches to the anterior and superior part of the sacrum. The iliolumbar ligament

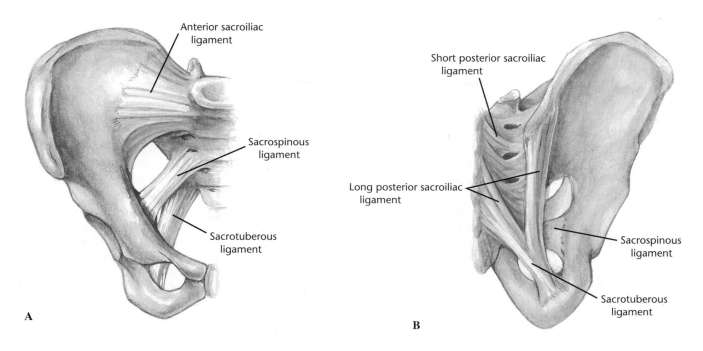

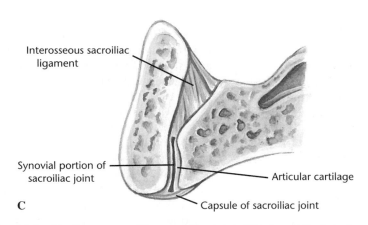

***Fig. 4-16***   The ligaments of the sacroiliac joint (SIJ). **A** and **B,** Anterior and posterior views of the SIJ respectively. **C,** SIJ in horizontal section. Notice the capsule of the SIJ is only present anteriorly. (From: Cramer G, Darby S: *Basic and clinical anatomy of the spine, spinal cord, and ANS.* St. Louis, 1995, Mosby, p. 237, with permission.)

helps to limit lateral tilting of the pelvis and gapping of the SIJ.

### Innervation of the sacroiliac joint

The SIJ is richly innervated, and the joint capsule has both nociceptors (pain receptors) and proprioceptors (joint position sensation receptors). This would indicate that the sensory receptors of the SIJ relay information related to movement and joint position and in doing so may help to keep the body upright and balanced. The most pain sensitive structures in this region are the posterior inferior iliac spine and the superior portion of the

sacroiliac fissure.[95,102] The specific innervation of the SIJ is quite variable, even between the left and right sides of the same individual.

The anterior (pelvic) part of the SIJ is innervated by the APDs of L2 through S2[9] with L4 and L5 being the most frequent source of innervation.[24] The posterior part of the SIJ, according to most authors, is innervated by PPDs of S1 and S2. However, the innervation of this part of the joint is probably more extensive than being limited to just the upper sacral segments. Bernard and Cassidy[9] state that the posterior part of the SIJ is innervated by the lateral branches of the PPDs of L4 to

S3. Ro[105] found that the lateral branch of the L5 PPD extended inferiorly and passed between the superficial layer of interosseous SI ligament and the posterior SI ligament.

The variability of SIJ innervation from person to person and even from the left to the right side of the same person, may be one reason for the wide range of pain referral patterns described by patients experiencing discomfort of SIJ origin (see Case 15).[9] Furthermore, the wide variation of referral patterns may help to explain the difficulty researchers and clinicians have in identifying the incidence of SIJ dysfunction.

The microscopic anatomy of the zygapophyseal joints, intervertebral discs, and the sacroiliac joints is beyond the scope of this section. These topics are covered rather extensively in Stathopoulos P, Cramer G: The microscopic anatomy of the zygapophyseal joints and intervertebral discs and Ro CS, Cramer G: The sacrum, sacroiliac joint, and coccyx. In Cramer G, Darby S: *Basic and clinical anatomy of the spine, spinal cord, and ANS.* St. Louis, 1995, Mosby.

## BIOMECHANICS OF THE SPINE
### The cervical spine
RAYMOND BRODEUR

As presented in the anatomy section, the neck and cervical spine are very complicated and anatomically compact spaces with many vital organs. Thorough evaluation of the musculoskeletal aspects of the cervical spine requires a familiarity with the biomechanics of the region. This section will focus on the normal biomechanics of this region.

**Kinematics of the cervical spine.** In cervical spine evaluation patients are asked to voluntarily move their neck in a predetermined direction (active range of motion). The clinician evaluates the total range of motion that occurs in each direction by palpating and observing patients while they move their neck. There are two areas of concern to the clinician when evaluating the kinematics of the cervical spine: (1) global kinemat-

ics of the head as it moves relative to the thorax and (2) intervertebral (intersegmental) kinematics.

The most important factor in the evaluation of global kinematics of the cervical spine is total range of motion (ROM).[114,131] There are many clinical measuring devices that are used to assess cervical spine range of motion. The clinical tool most commonly used by clinicians, physical therapists, and occupational therapists is the hand-held goniometer. This instrument is only as accurate as the proficiency of the examiner. The measuring device quantifies total ROM in one plane. Other research goniometers have been developed that attempt to quantify cervical spine ROM more accurately. Using these other devices, Dvorak et al[38,39] found that the ROM decreases with age and that the active ROM is usually smaller than passive ROM (5%–10%) (Table 4-7). Further statistical evaluation of these findings indicated that the variabilities of the measurements on repeated examinations are larger in active range measurements than in passive measurements (variability of 12 to 17 degrees in active ROM measurements versus variability of 8.1 to 14.1 degrees in passive ROM measurements). This indicates that passive ROM measurements may be a more reliable tool for measuring total motion.

Lind et al[81] used radiographs to evaluate flexion/extension and lateral bending of the cervical spine from the occiput to C7. Motion radiography is considered the gold standard for measuring spinal motion. They found that for flexion/extension, the mean ROM was 93 degrees and for total left-to-right lateral flexion, the mean range was 90 degrees. This suggests that some of the motion reported by Dvorak is occurring in the thoracic spine and also provides evidence that when examining a patient for total active ROM of the cervical spine, it is necessary to assess the thoracic spine (T3 to T4). The thoracic spine may contribute 16 to 63 degrees of total cervical spine motion.

Rotation of the cervical spine occurs primarily at C1 to C2.[125] Clinically, this motion can be isolated from the rest of the cervical spine by fully flexing the neck. This

*Table 4-7* Electronic goniometric measurements of the cervical spine during passive range of motion evaluation

| | | Range of motion (degrees) | | | | | |
| | | Full flexion/extension | | Left/right lateral bending | | Left/right axial rotation | |
| Author | Age (years) | Male | Female | Male | Female | Male | Female |
| --- | --- | --- | --- | --- | --- | --- | --- |
| Post (1987) | All ages | 120 | | 90 | | 130 | |
| Magee (1987) | All ages | 150–160 | | 40–90 | | 140–180 | |
| Dvorak (1992) | 20–29 | 153 | 149 | 101 | 100 | 184 | 182 |
| | 30–39 | 141 | 156 | 95 | 106 | 175 | 186 |
| | 40–49 | 131 | 140 | 84 | 88 | 157 | 168 |
| | 50–59 | 136 | 127 | 88 | 76 | 166 | 152 |
| | 60+ | 116 | 133 | 74 | 80 | 146 | 154 |

motion locks the facet joint and prevents rotation at the lower cervical spine.[130] Dvorak and coworkers[38,39] measured the passive ROM of the head during maximum cervical spine flexion. They found the average rotation to be between 66 degrees and 75 degrees. Interestingly, the ROM for this joint increased with age to range between 77 and 85 degrees. It is likely that this increase with age is a compensation of the atlas-axis joint for the loss of rotation at other intervertebral joints.

**Axis of rotation and cervical kinematics.** The location of the axis of rotation changes according to how motion is performed. For example, in flexion of the cervical spine with the chin tucked in, the axis of rotation will be in the upper cervical spine, whereas the same motion without the chin tucked in has a different axis of rotation. Measurement of spinal motion needs to be clinically standardized. If injury is present in the cervical spine the axis of rotation moves accordingly. Work by Osterbauer et al[98] and Winters et al[130] have shown that the helical (three-dimensional) axes of rotation in flexion/extension is different in patients who have whiplash injuries to their cervical spine. They found that the axis translates upward in the whiplash patients indicating that less motion occurs in the lower cervical spine after a whiplash injury.

### Cervical whiplash

Scientific evaluation of whiplash injuries to the cervical spine have focused on the biomechanics of the rear-end collision, with the driver wearing a lap and harness belt (see Case 8). Anatomic considerations consist of the driver's head, neck (cervical spine and all involved structures), and trunk (thorax and thoracic spine). Whether a vehicle is stationary or traveling, the inertia and momentum of the driver's head, neck, and trunk are equal to those of the vehicle. When a collision occurs between two vehicles, the inertia and momentum of the vehicle and the driver's trunk are proportionately changed. Since the head and the neck are not directly harnessed to the automobile their momentum and inertia are not changed. The head is "left behind" causing the neck and cervical spine to move (accelerate) into extension. When the anterior cervical muscles (the spindle) senses the sudden (impulsive) change in their length caused by neck extension, they concentrically contract to prevent injury. Their contraction causes the whipping action of neck flexion (deceleration).[46,117]

**Intervertebral kinematics of the cervical spine.** Most of the in-vivo kinematic studies of the cervical spine have concentrated on flexion and extension. These motions are considered to be strictly planar motions and are easier to evaluate scientifically than are rotation and lateral bending, which are multiplanar motions. Therefore, plain film x-ray examination is well suited to study flexion and extension kinematics in the spine.

The segmental flexion and extension ROMs between the vertebrae is presented in Table 4-8. Of interest is the variability of intersegmental motion between authors. Penning[101] presented a range of 25 to 45 degrees of flexion extension between occiput and C1, whereas Dvorak[39] found an average of 14.1 degrees in the same area. This difference is caused primarily by the research techniques used by the authors. Penning did not have the sophisticated computer equipment and precision that were used in Dvorak's study. From Table 4-9 it is observed that the major motion of the occiput (CO)- and C1 joint is flexion and extension (that is, nodding). Kraemer and Patris[76] also measured the motion of the intervertebral joints in flexion and extension from the neutral position. Of interest is that 52% of the subjects displayed slight extension intersegmental motion between occiput-C1 when they were asked to flex their cervical spine. This phenomenon is described as *paradoxical motion* (Fig. 4-17). At full cervical spine flexion the occiput-C1 motion ranges from −26 degrees (− indicates extension) to 13 degrees of flexion. In addition, they found the extension of this joint during cervical spine flexion decreased with age. For subjects less than 20 years of age, the average C0-C1 angle on cervical spine flexion was −9 degrees, with the extension angle decreasing to near zero for ages 40 to 69. The C0-C1 angle becomes a flexion angle only for subjects over the age of 70 years.

The cervical spine has the greatest ROM of the total spine.[8] The type of motion that occurs in the cervical spine is the result of the shape and direction of the articulating facets, the shape of the cervical disc, and the surrounding ligamentous structures.[125] The major determinant of intersegmental motion is facetal shape and the direction in which the facet surfaces are oriented in the zygapophyseal joint. Panjabi et al.[99] using functional spinal units, quantified intersegmental spinal motion. They found that intersegmental motion was governed by the zygapophyseal facetal plain direction. The facets in the cervical spine are flat-surfaced structures that are directed 45 degrees off the horizontal plane (see Fig. 4-1).

*Table 4-8* Motion of the intervertebral joints in flexion and extension measured from the neutral position

| Level | Flexion (degrees) | Extension (degrees) |
| --- | --- | --- |
| C0-C1 | −0.82 ± 4.63 | 13.97 ± 6.51 |
| C1-C2 | 5.76 ± 4.44 | 5.56 ± 4.38 |
| C2-C3 | 5.10 ± 2.81 | 3.86 ± 3.20 |
| C3-C4 | 7.20 ± 3.46 | 6.10 ± 4.13 |
| C4-C5 | 7.39 ± 3.65 | 8.08 ± 4.60 |
| C5-C6 | 7.49 ± 3.96 | 7.25 ± 4.74 |
| C6-C7 | 8.46 ± 4.03 | 4.32 ± 3.73 |

*Table 4-9*    Total intervertebral flexion and extension range of motions for the cervical spine*

| Vertebral joint | Penning (1978) | Kraemer and Patris (1989) | Lind (1989) | Dvorak (1993) |
|---|---|---|---|---|
| C0-C1 | 30 [25-45]† | 13.1 | 14 (15)‡ | 14.1 (4.9) |
| C1-C2 | 30 [25-45] | 11.3 | 13 (5) | 12.0 (3.0) |
| C2-C3 | 12 [5-16] | 9.0 | 10 (4) | 17.2 (3.9) |
| C3-C4 | 18 [13-26] | 12.3 | 14 (6) | 17.2 (3.9) |
| C4-C5 | 20 [15-29] | 15.5 | 16 (6) | 21.1 (3.5) |
| C5-C6 | 20 [16-29] | 14.7 | 15 (8) | 22.6 (4.2) |
| C6-C7 | 15 [6-25] | 12.7 | 11 (7) | 21.4 (3.7) |

*All values are in degrees
†Ranges reported by the authors
‡Standard deviation

**Coupling motion in the cervical spine.** Kinematic evaluation of intersegmental motion of the typical cervical vertebrae shows that the major motions in this area are flexion/extension and rotation. Lateral bending also occurs with little hindrance. The uncovertebral joints do, however, limit excessive lateral bending, which helps prevent kinking of the vertebral artery as it traverses through the transverse foramen.[17] Each motion of the spine has another motion that is coupled to it (all intersegmental motion may have five coupled motions). Primary intersegmental motion of the typical cervical vertebrae is coupled with secondary motions. The secondary motion for typical cervical vertebral rotation is lateral bending; flexion and extension are coupled with anterior and posterior translation, respectively; and lateral bending is coupled with rotation. The motions that coupled with rotation and flexion and extension form a strong couple, meaning that the respective lateral bending and translation is significant and should be palpated by the clinician. Lateral bending is coupled with

rotation. It is a minor couple and cannot be palpated by a clinician. The secondary (coupled) motions in the cervical spine are presented in Table 4-10. All couples presented in Table 4-10 occur with the normal lordotic curve of the cervical spine. If the lordotic curve is reversed (kyphosis) by flexing the cervical spine, the secondary couple reverses.[125] This is a valuable technique for the examining clinician who, at times, cannot find a problem in spinal motion in a patient who still has pain. Coupled motion can be changed in any area of the spine by changing the curve in the sagittal plane. If the lordotic curve in the cervical or lumbar spine or the kyphotic curve in the thoracic spine are reversed by flexion or extension, the couple is reversed and the restriction may be found.

Motion palpation is an attempt by the clinician to evaluate intersegmental spinal motion. During motion palpation, the clinician evaluates spinal motion by placing his/her hands on the moving vertebra and the verte-

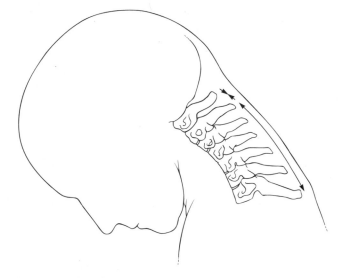

*Fig. 4-17*    Paradoxical motion of occiput-C1 and C1-C2 during cervical spine flexion.

*Table 4-10*    Primary and secondary motions of typical vertebra in the cervical, thoracic, and lumbar spine*

| Primary motion | Secondary (coupled) motion |
|---|---|
| **Cervical and thoracic spine** | |
| Flexion | Anterior translation |
| Extension | Posterior translation |
| Right rotation | Right lateral bending |
| Left rotation | Left lateral bending |
| Right lateral bending | Right rotation (C3-T4) |
| | Left or right rotation (T4-L1) |
| Left lateral bending | Left rotation (C3-T4) |
| | Left or right rotation (T4-L1) |
| **Lumbar spine** | |
| Flexion | Anterior translation |
| Extension | Posterior translation |
| Right rotation | Left lateral bending |
| Left rotation | Right lateral bending |
| Right lateral bending | Left rotation |
| Left lateral bending | Right rotation |

*Coupled motion during lateral bending is a weaker couple than during spinal rotation.

bra below. This procedure is performed by passively moving the vertebra through its joint play and into its end-range. Greenman[57] elaborated on these concepts and developed the concept of the physiologic barrier (Fig. 7-1). Joint play is the motion that occurs between two vertebrae to reach the end of motion (active motion). End-feel determines the motion of the joint when it is at the end of its normal range (passive motion). At the end-range the joint is displaced by the clinician pushing on the spinous process or articular process.

**Coordinate system.** In research, a coordinate system is developed to define spinal motion. Most commonly used is the right-handed cartesian coordinate system.[125] In our example above of cervical spine flexion, the primary motion is forward rotation about the X-axis and its secondary coupled motion is forward translation along the Z-axis. The right-handed cartesian coordinate system describes these motions as +RX for forward rotation about the X-axis and +TZ as forward translation along the Z-axis.

**Spinal motion of the atypical cervical vertebrae.** Spinal motion of the atypical cervical vertebrae demonstrates a different couple. The atypical vertebrae in the cervical spine are C1, C2, and C7. This section will pay particular attention to C1 and C2 motions. C7 has the same general primary and coupled motion as the typical vertebrae but has slightly more rotation that makes its motion similar to thoracic spine motion.

The shape and direction of the facets determine the motion that occurs between these vertebrae.[109a,125] The first joint that will be discussed is the occiput-C1 joint articulation. Two occipital condyles are located at the most inferior aspect of the occiput. The condyles are cup shaped and converge anteriorly. The superior articular processes of the atlas are saucer shaped and converge anteriorly. Because of this unique shape, the occiput-C1 joint's major motion is described as *nodding*. Twenty-five degrees of flexion and extension in the cervical spine is produced by this joint.[125] Other intersegmental motions at this level are very limited. Only 5 degrees of lateral bending and rotation occur between the occiput and C1.[125] Coupled motion during rotation is in the contralateral direction (that is, right rotation produces left lateral bending).

The superior articular processes of the axis (C2) sit along the horizontal plane, are convex in the sagittal plane, and meet with the convex inferior articular processes of C1. The dens of C2 meets with the anterior tubercle of C1 and forms the atlanto-dens interspace. The atlas and dens are supported by the transverse ligament that is attached to the medial tubercle of the lateral masses of the atlas. The major motion that occurs between the atlas and the axis is rotation. The first 40 degrees (greater than 50% of total cervical spine rotation) in either direction occurs predominantly at this joint and should be palpated by the clinician.[8] The coupled motion between C1 and C2 during rotation is upward vertical translation (+TY). As the head is returned to the neutral position C1-C2 translates downward (−TY) (Fig. 4-18).[125] The tertiary couple at C1-C2 during rotation is lateral bending and is in the same direction as occiput-C1 (it is in the opposite direction of the typical cervical vertebrae during rotation). The purpose of opposite lateral bending at occiput-C1 and C1-C2 compared to the typical cervical vertebrae during rotation is to keep the head erect during this motion.

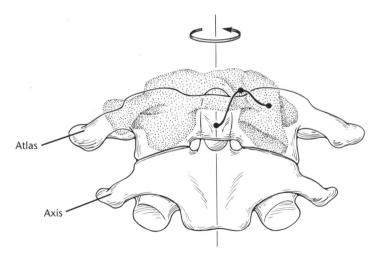

Atlas

Axis

*Fig. 4-18*  The coupled motion of the atlas during cervical spine rotation. Note that the center of mass of the atlas translates superior and slightly inferior while rotating (solid line). Illustration depicts left cervical rotation. (Adapted from: White AA, Panjabi MM: *Clinical biomechanics of the spine*, ed 2, Philadelphia, 1990, Lippincott.)

If the coupled motions of the vertebrae were in the same direction the head would be laterally flexed during rotation. Other motions at C1-C2 are limited because of the facet's surface structure and its direction.

## BIOMECHANICS OF THE THORACIC SPINE

The superior articular facet of the thoracic vertebra is 60 degrees off the horizontal plane and 20 degrees rotated from the sagittal plane. The inferior articular facet joins to form the Z joint. The Z joint's orientation allows trunk rotation and limits lateral bending and flexion.[8] The ribs also limit thoracic spine lateral bending. The major motion, therefore, in the thoracic area is rotation of the trunk. Rotation is generally considered to be 90 degrees in either direction. On rotation of the thoracic spine, the secondary coupled motion is lateral bending to the same side.[125] The lateral curvature presented on rotation is caused by the secondary coupled motion of lateral bending. The spinous direction corresponds with the direction of the spinous processes of the lower cervical spine. As long as the kyphotic curve (lordotic curve in the cervical spine area) is present the coupled motion of rotation will be lateral bending to the same side.[84,125] As is presented in Case 11, this coupled motion does not exist.

In structural scoliosis there is no change of the curve on flexion (Adam's test) or lateral bending. Rotation, in a scoliotic spine, is usually limited because of the shape of the vertebra and the tropism present in the facets. It has been noted on an A-P radiograph that the spinous process is facing the concavity in scoliosis.[125] Other coupled motion of the thoracic spine is presented in Table 4-10.

Rib motion has been described as being similar to a bucket handle. On inspiration ribs move up and out, and in the opposite direction on exhalation. These motions are caused by synchronous action of the diaphragm, the intercostal muscles, and inflation and deflation of the lungs.

Kinetically, the ipsilateral internal oblique and contralateral external oblique muscles concentrically contract to cause trunk rotation. Lateral bending of the trunk is caused by contralateral eccentric action of the erector spine, quadratus lumborum, and the deep lumbar musculature.

## BIOMECHANICS OF THE LUMBAR SPINE

Low back pain is the most frequent complaint of patients visiting the clinician's office,[93] with pain of mechanical origin being the most frequently observed subtype.[29] Proper diagnosis of maladies of the low back is extremely difficult. The anatomic structures that could be contributing to the patient's pain are endless. To obtain a working diagnosis, the clinician needs to be familiar with the biomechanics of the area involved. This section will discuss the biomechanics of lumbopelvic rhythm and the IVD and their relevance to Cases 13 to 17.

### Lumbopelvic rhythm: flexion-relaxation phenomenon

Lumbopelvic rhythm is derived from motion of the skeletal system (kinematics) and muscle activity (kinetics). Flexion at the waist totals 90 degrees. Kinematically, starting from anatomic position of 0 degrees the lumbar spine flexes the first 45 to 60 degrees, followed by rotation of the pelvis within the hip joints to 90 degrees. Kinetically, the first muscle action to occur anteriorly offsets the center of gravity. This begins the process of forward bending. A 3 to 5 millisecond concentric action of the rectus abdominis muscle anteriorly displaces the center of gravity. The erector spine muscles (iliocostalis, longissimus, and spinalis) eccentrically contract and allow lumbar flexion to approximately 60 degrees. During this time the gluteus maximus and hamstring muscles statically act to prevent tilting of the pelvis. At 60 degrees, the sequence reverses. The erector spine statically contract and the gluteus maximus and hamstrings eccentrically contract allowing further flexion. At 90 degrees, all muscles are quiescent and the patient is hanging by the ligaments.[45,58] The total range of motion of the lumbar spine in flexion is 60 degrees, with the final 30 degrees of flexion being accomplished by pelvic anterior rotation.

Examination of patients with pain in the lumbar spine includes active range of motion that involves lumbar flexion. Of interest is the fact that the initiation of the patient's pain complaints at different phases of lumbar flexion informs the clinician about which anatomic structures could be causing the problems.[58] In Case 15 (SI joint pathology) the patient describes pain that occurs at 90 degrees. In patients with IVD disease (see Case 14) or lumbar sprain or strain, pain will most likely be initiated almost immediately upon flexion. The injury to the surrounding spinal musculature, including the erector spinae muscles, initiates pain when these tissues are active. In Case 14 the patient's pain develops when compression and shear stresses increase in the IVD, at the beginning of lumbar flexion. In Case 13 (facet syndrome) pain is not elicited on flexion but only on lumbar extension. This is not always true in facet injuries. The capsular ligaments are stressed during both lumbar flexion and extension,[125] and because of the rich nociceptive supply, injury to these ligaments can produce pain perception during either motion.

### Biomechanics of the lumbar intervertebral disc (IVD)

The IVD is an anterior vertebral structure that is located between adjacent vertebral bodies. It is a ligamentous structure in that it attaches bone to bone. Securely attached to the bony structures of the end plates by Sharpey's fibers, the IVDs have a layer of hyaline cartilage between their collagenous structures and the vertebral bodies (Fig. 4-19). Considered an amphiarthrodial joint, the IVD allows limited motion between the adjacent vertebral bodies. They stabilize the spine and at the same time allow movement between adjacent vertebrae giving the spine its flexibility and its ability to absorb and distribute loads.[19]

The IVD has three components: the annulus fibrosis, nucleus pulposus, and hyaline cartilage. Like other connective tissues the disc consists of a small number of cells embedded in an abundant extracellular matrix with an elaborate framework of macromolecules filled with water.[19] The annulus fibrosis consists of 12 to 20 concentric collagenous rings that surround the water-abundant nucleus.[125] Because the adult disc does not contain a direct blood supply, the cells within its structure depend on the transport of molecules through the matrix.[63,109] The framework and matrix water content depend upon the proteoglycan concentration.[120]

The human IVD consists of four concentrically arranged components: (1) the nucleus pulposus located in the center, (2) a transition zone between the inner annulus fibrosus and the nucleus with cells that resemble chondrocytes, (3) a fibrocartilaginous inner annulus fibrosis with similar chondrocytic cells as the transition zone, and (4) the outer annulus ring of densely packed collagen fibril lamellae with fibroblast-like or fibrocyte-like cells. In the young disc the vertebral end plates initially consist of hyaline cartilage, and the nucleus contains notochordal cells.[109] With age, the end plates contain calcified cartilage and bone and the nucleus contains chondrocyte-like cells.[20,135]

The tensile strength of the IVD results from its collagenous fibers, where its stiffness and resilience to compression (damping properties) are derived from the interaction of proteoglycans and water.[110] Located at the outer aspect of the annulus, collagen accounts for as much as 70% of the dry weight of the annulus but comprises less than 20% of the central nucleus of a young person. By contrast, proteoglycans will account for 50% of the nucleus in a young person and will be present in low quantities in the outer annular fibers.

A major cause of disc degeneration is inadequate disc nutrition.[42] Disc cells rely on diffusion of nutrients from the blood vessels at the periphery of the annulus and within the vertebral bodies. The age-related decline in arteries supplying the annulus and the calcification of the cartilage end plates impair nutrient delivery and waste removal.[19] However, when disc prolapse occurs, an increase in vascularity occurs around the protruded nucleus.[136]

During flexion the "healthy" annulus bulges anteriorly approximately 1.75 mm and tensile forces occur in the posterior annular fibers. Nucleus pulposus motion is controversial.[125] In the healthy disc the nucleus moves posteriorly on flexion and anteriorly on extension. However, it does not move as a solid but acts as a viscoelastic material and diffuses according to the loads applied to the IVD.[77,125] The pathologic characteristics of the IVD change in that the biomechanics are not well understood. What is known is that the nucleus responds to external pressure and will flow to an area of least resistance. When annular fibers "break down" the nuclear material will flow to the area of least resistance.[125]

Vibration and resonance are two factors that affect the integrity of the IVD (see Case 14). All objects have an inherent vibration. The inherent vibration of the human body is approximately 4.5 Hz. Resonance occurs when two objects vibrate at the same frequency. When this happens a summation of vibration occurs and possible changes in the structures can be facilitated. Resonance seems to have a direct affect on the IVD. It

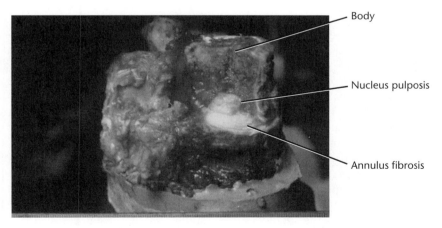

*Fig. 4-19*   Typical lumbar "healthy" intervertebral disc in a functional spinal unit (FSU) from a cadavaric spine.

increases the internal pressure of the disc and its shear flexibility that, in turn, decreases its resistance to buckling, thereby causing stress at the posterior region of the disc leading to possible protrusion.[128]

## BIOCHEMISTRY OF THE INTERVERTEBRAL DISC
JEDDEO PAUL

Each IVD is composed of proteoglycans and cartilage. The proteoglycans are proteins conjugated to linear heteroglycan polysaccharides, whereas cartilage is a dense form of connective tissue consisting of cells (extracellular matrix or ground substance) and insoluble collagen fibers embedded in a matrix of ground substance.[20] The cells within the matrix include chondrocytes, fibroblasts, macrophages, and mast cells, all of which are responsible for the synthesis of the matrix components and collagen.

The normal disc consists of a soft, spongy, gel-like central portion, the nucleus pulposus, and surrounding it is a tough fibrous ring, the annulus fibrosus, organized into lamellae of coarse collagen fibers. The nucleus pulposus is highly hydrated, especially in young discs, accounting for 80% to 88% of the disc volume.[25] Generally, the annulus fibrosus is less hydrated than the nucleus pulposus.

The three components present in the IVD are collagen, proteoglycans, and water, with water accounting for 90% of the volume of the normal disc. The collagen types of the annulus fibrosus are types I and II with type I constituting 40% of the total collagen and type II, 60%. The collagen of the nucleus pulposus is exclusively of the type II fibrils and is lower in collagen content than is the annulus fibrosus. In general, type II collagen fibers deform and absorb compressive forces better than the other types of collagen.[134] Whereas the collagen fibers exist as a network providing intervertebral connections, the proteoglycans, which are highly anionic, allow hydration of the disc tissues. This swelling tendency of the normal disc is due to the high osmotic pressure exerted by the highly charged glycosaminoglycans of the proteoglycans.[1,10,25]

The proteoglycans making up the disc material are conjugated proteins of glycosaminoglycans (GAGs)[86], a class of linear heteropolysaccharides. The GAGs of the disc proteoglycans include chondroitin sulfate A, B, and C, hyaluronic acid, and keratan sulfate.[1,10,89] Chondroitin sulfate, also a polysaccharide of the disc cartilage, has the repeating disaccharide unit consisting of glucuronic acid and $N$-acetylgalactosaminosulfate, with each unit alternating via $\beta(1-3)$ and $\beta(1-4)$ glycosidic linkages, with the linkages themselves also appropriately alternating. The molecule entraps water, forming gels.[1,10,52] It is linear, has no branches, and has molecular mass of 50,000 to 100,000 daltons and is the smallest of the glycosaminoglycans.

There are three kinds of chondroitin sulfates: chondroitin A or chondroitin-4-sulfate, chondroitin B or

dermatan sulfate, and chondroitin C or chondroitin-6-sulfate.[67] Chondroitin-4-sulfate and chondroitin 6-sulfate are composed of repeating units of glucuronic and acid $N$-acetylgalactosamine-4-sulfate or $N$-acetylgalactosamine-6-sulfate, respectively. Chondroitin B, another 4-sulfated species, consists of the repeating disaccharide unit L-iduronic acid-$N$-acetylgalactosamine-4-sulfate with each unit linked via $\beta(1-3)$ and $\beta(1-4)$ glycosidic linkages, with alternation of both the monosaccharide residues and the glycosidic linkages.[1,10]

Hyaluronic acid is a heteroglycan of glucuronic acid and $N$-acetyl that are linked through glucosamine $\beta(1-3)$ and $\beta(1-4)$ glycosidic linkages, with both the monosaccharide residues and the linkages alternating. Thus, the molecule is linear, has no branching, and consists of the repeating disaccharide unit. The molecular mass of hyaluronic acid is variable, ranging from several hundred thousand to several million daltons. It is polyanionic, viscous, gelatinous, and sticky.

Keratan-6-sulfate is a linear heteroglycan with the repeating disaccharide unit $\beta$-D-galactose-$N$-acetylglucosamine-6-sulfate linked via $\beta(1-4)$ and $\beta(1-3)$ glycosidic linkages with both the monosaccharide residues and the $\beta$ linkages alternating in the molecule.[112]

There are two types of keratan sulfate having the same chemical constitution but differing in distribution: type II keratan sulfate is found in connective tissue and type I is more abundant in the cornea of the eye. Another difference is that when the keratan sulfates bind to proteins to form proteoglycans, keratan sulfate I binds covalently to L-asparagine residues on the protein whereas type II binds covalently to threonine or serine residues on the protein. Keratin sulfate II is attached to the same polypeptide backbone as is chondroitin sulfate, forming aggregates with the extracellular matrix of cartilage.

### Structure and biosynthesis of proteoglycans

Hyaluronic acid combines only loosely with proteins but the chondroitin sulfates combine covalently with a single core protein rich in serine and threonine to form a large aggregate of 3 to $6 \times 10^6$ daltons. These glycosaminoglycan-protein complexes are called *proteoglycans,* which are 90% carbohydrate and about 10% protein in composition.

The globular ends of the core proteins associate noncovalently with a long filament of hyaluronic acid running through and constituting the backbone of the aggregate.[10] This association is stabilized by small link proteins. On the core protein are chains of keratan sulfate, five to six disaccharide units long, and chondroitin sulfate 40 to 50 disaccharide units long. The keratan sulfate chain is 6 nm long and the chondroitin sulfate chain, 20 to 30 nm long.

The chondroitin sulfates are linked to the core protein through an oligosaccharide sequence of two galactose units followed by one xylose unit that forms a β-glycosidic linkage to serine or threonine side chains on the core protein. The keratan sulfates, on the other hand, are linked through the oligosaccharide to asparagine side chains on the core protein and thus involve different covalent bonds. After every 25 repeating units of hyaluronic acid there is one proteoglycan subunit attached. The hyaluronic acid backbone is 450 to 4200 nm long and has 140 subunits of proteoglycans attached laterally. The molecule has an extended structure (bottle-brush structure) (Fig. 4-20) resulting from electrostatic repulsion of numerous negative charges present.

With increasing age the proportion of nonaggregated proteoglycans increases and the size of the proteoglycan molecule decreases, especially in the nucleus. These changes begin early in life and may be one of the events that lead to disc degeneration.[21,22,63,71,97]

## PROVOCATIVE TESTING OF THE SPINE
DORRIE TALMAGE

### Provocative maneuvers of the cervical spine

An orthopedic examination includes a thorough history, vital signs, inspection, superficial, deep, and joint play palpation, percussion, other instrumentation, range of motion evaluation, orthopedic provocative maneuvers, neurologic examination, radiologic examination (and other studies if needed), and laboratory evaluation (H.v.I.P.P.I.R.O.N.E.L.). Each component of the examination provides a piece of the diagnostic puzzle, and when put together, can give a profile of the patient's problem leading to a more accurate working diagnosis.[44]

Provocative maneuvers are designed to provoke the patient's symptoms, and they therefore test the integrity of different anatomic structures within a given region. In this text, cases are presented that utilize commonly encountered provocative maneuvers. In the cervical spine common provocative tests are the axial compression test (Jackson's test), Spurling's test, distraction test, maximal foraminal compression test, shoulder depression test, and Valsalva's maneuver.

Which provocative test to chose is determined by the history and previous physical examination findings. The provocative test sequence is from the least invasive to the most invasive test. Test invasiveness is determined by the amount of stress being applied to the anatomic structures being provoked. The discussion of these tests will center around the following: (1) the anatomic structures being assessed, (2) positive findings, (3) the interpretation of the findings, and (4) their relationship to the cases.

There are many provocative tests for the cervical spine. The anatomic structures commonly tested are

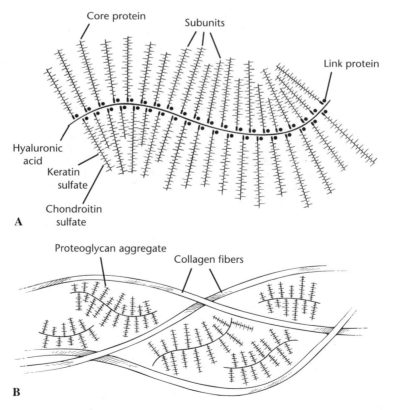

**Fig. 4-20**   **A, B,** Illustration of a proteoglycan and its biochemical components.

dural tension, foraminal and vertebral canal patency, and muscle, tendon, or ligamentous injuries.[122] Table 4-11 presents the more common tests of the cervical spine and the anatomic structures they are testing. Some of the more common tests will be discussed here.

In the cervical spine, axial compression (Jackson's test) is one of the least invasive cervical tests. It is recommended that this test be performed first on the neck with acute pain, and if positive, it would be unnecessary to perform additional compression tests (such as Spurling's or maximal foraminal compression tests). If the clinician feels that a false negative result has been obtained, then one of the more invasive compression tests can be performed. Invasive maneuvers are indicated if the patients has chronic pain, low intensity pain, or if a screening examination is desired. A positive compression test is the reproduction of radicular pain caused by a space-occupying lesion in the vertebral canal. The lesion either decreases available space within the canal to cause impingement or prevents the involved structures from moving properly within the canal.

Three anatomic structures within the vertebral canal and IVF cause radicular pain. They are the dural sheath, nerve roots, and spinal nerves.[23] Compression alone of these anatomic structures results in numbness or tingling, or as a pins-and needle sensation into a dermatome. If these structures are stretched or irritated (for example, from inflammation or impingement) they will produce radicular pain. Even though a positive test (radicular pain) may not be elicited, it is important to remember that localized or sclerotogenous or myoto-genous pain (nonradicular, dull, and achy in character) may be provoked. If this occurs it should be recorded as a negative test, but that pain is produced.[11,27,85]

If there is irritation of the apophyseal joints (as in a facet syndrome) compression will lead to approximation of the facets creating a response of the pain stretch receptors of the joint capsule or nociceptive mediators in the subchondral bone.[107] Facet involvement does not result in radicular pain and will produce a negative test result.

When a compression test is performed on the cervical spine the facet joints approximate, causing stretch of the surrounding capsule. If the capsule has been injured or becomes fibrotic, the pain receptors are far more responsive to motion, thereby eliciting pain. In IVD disease, compression will increase the intradiscal pressure, potentially leading to further protrusion or further release of inflammatory chemical mediators (such as prostaglandins, bradykinins, and others).[51] In the presence of osteophytes that protrude into the IVFs or the central canal, specifically from the uncinate processes, compression can cause further penetration or entrapment of the involved spinal root, thus leading to radicular pain (see Case 9).

The distraction maneuver in the cervical spine tests the following anatomic structures: the apophyseal joints, joints of Von Luschka (uncovertebral joints), spinal nerve roots, spinal ligaments, intervertebral foramina, intervertebral discs, and surrounding musculature.[11,27]

A positive test is a relief of symptoms. Relief of symptoms indicates decompression of the nerve root (in the

*Table 4-11*  Some common provocative tests used to evaluate the spine

| Provocative test | Anatomic structures being tested | Positive finding(s) |
|---|---|---|
| **Cervical spine** | | |
| Jackson's compression test | Dural sheath, nerve root, spinal nerve | Radicular pain |
| Spurling's compression test | Dural sheath, nerve root, spinal nerve | Radicular pain |
| Maximal foraminal compression test | Dural sheath, nerve root, spinal nerve | Radicular pain |
| Distraction test | Dural sheath, nerve root, spinal nerve | Relief of radicular pain |
| Shoulder depression test | Dural sheath, nerve root, spinal nerve brachial plexus | Radicular pain to one or more dermatomes |
| E.A.S.T. test | Subclavian artery | Vascular compromise |
| Eden's test | Scalene musculature | Radiculopathy to multiple dermatomes or vascular compromise |
| **Thoracic spine** | | |
| Wright's hyperabduction test | Pectoralis minor | Vascular compromise, subclavian artery TOS |
| Tests for anterior thoracic wall | Peripheral nerve, muscles | Radicular pain, dull ache |
| **Lumbar spine** | | |
| Straight leg raise (SLR) | Dural sheath, nerve root, spinal nerve | Radiculopathy to one dermatome usually |
| Braggard's test | Dural sheath, nerve root, spinal nerve | Radiculopathy to one dermatome usually |
| Bekhterev's test | Dural sheath, nerve root, spinal nerve | Radiculopathy to one dermatome usually |
| Neri's bow string test | Dural sheath, nerve root, spinal nerve | Radiculopathy to one dermatome usually |

E.A.S.T., *Elevated arm stress test;* TOS, *thoracic outlet syndrome.*

IVF) by a space-occupying lesion (for example, disc protrusion and osteophytes), and in this case the patient would describe a lessening of radicular symptoms (see Case 6).[27,51,85] An exacerbation of the patient's pain (sclerotogenous or myotogenous) usually indicates a probable soft tissue injury in the apophyseal joints, uncovertebral joints, muscles, ligaments, or any combination of the above. During distraction of the cervical spine, the ligaments, muscles, and joint capsule are being stretched. If these structures are compromised by either a muscular strain or a ligamentous sprain then symptoms are produced.

The anatomic structures that are being assessed by the shoulder depression test are the spinal nerve roots, cervical and brachial plexi, and the IVD. A positive test is radicular pain on the side of shoulder depression (see Case 10). The test may also provoke nonradicular pain (a negative test result) by stretching the surrounding soft tissues (such as ligaments and muscles).[85] In this test, considerable tension is placed on the nerve roots or plexi. If adhesions, disc herniations, or osteophytes have developed, this tension may be sufficient to provoke a positive response.

Valsalva's maneuver tests for a space-occupying lesion within the central or lateral vertebral canals. The structures that are being tested are the spinal cord, nerve roots, and the surrounding dura.

The test is performed by asking the patient to "take a deep breath, hold it, and bear down as though they are having a bowel movement." The patient is asked if this maneuver increases their presenting complaints or creates pain of a radicular nature. This maneuver, in the presence of a space-occupying lesion, creates an increase in intrathecal pressure causing an exacerbation of pain. A space-occupying lesion may take the form of a tumor, disc herniation or an osteophyte.[27,51,85]

### Provocative maneuvers of the thoracic spine

Few provocative maneuvers have been developed for the evaluation of the thoracic spine. Some of the maneuvers that are utilized on the thoracic spine are from lumbar spine provocative tests. The more common tests used to evaluate the thoracic spine are presented in Table 4-11. These tests are designed to reproduce the patient's chief complaint, usually sclerotogenous, myotogenous pain. One exception is Shepelmann's test that reproduces a radicular pain indicative of an intercostal neuritis. Tests designed to diagnose rib fracture or compression fracture (Case 12) will reproduce sclerotogenous localized pain. Again, the tests are performed in the order of the least provocative to the most provocative.

### Provocative maneuvers of the lumbar spine

There are a multitude of provocative maneuvers related to the low back. The majority of tests used to evaluate

the lumbar spine are designed to determine dural compromise and nerve root motion within the IVF. The more common provocative tests to evaluate the lumbar spine are presented in Table 4-11. These tests are positive when radicular pain is reproduced.[56] They are testing the ability of the dural sheath, nerve root, or spinal nerve to move properly during tension.[43] These tests are considered positive only when the lumbar spine is moving, in the first 60-70 degrees of spinal flexion (lumbo-pelvic rhythm). In these tests, either the involved lower extremity is raised (that is, SLR) or the patient is asked to bend at the waist in the seated (sciatic tension test and Bechterew's test) or the standing position (Neri's bowstring test and Lewin's test). The tests are positive only when radicular pain is present before 60-70 degrees of flexion.[49,50,85]

Anatomic structures that can result in a space-occupying lesion within the spinal canal and produce radiculopathy are the IVDs, tumors, ligaments (hypertrophy), facets (hypertrophy), or osteophytes.

Muscle evaluation is also an important aspect of provocative testing. Length-tension tests evaluate the flexibility of muscles and determine whether a joint can move through its range of motion without hindrance from the involved muscles. Muscle testing also provocatively evaluates muscle strength. Muscle testing "rules" and the muscle grading system are presented in Table 4-12. Other provocative procedures consist of deep tendon reflex, sensory, and pain evaluations.

## RADIOLOGY OF THE SPINE

JEFFREY COOLEY
GARY SCHULTZ

The type of radiographic series ordered depends on several factors, including additional patient information required, patient data (age, sex), and the likelihood of the findings affecting treatment. Two views taken at 90 degrees are considered the legal minimum in most instances.[5,31] This section will present the standard views taken for each spinal area and the common line markings used to evaluate these areas.

### Radiography of the cervical spine

The typical series consists of the anterior-posterior open mouth (APOM) view, anterior-posterior lower cervical (APLC) view, lateral cervical view, and, when necessary, the oblique views (Fig. 4-21). Specific views are used to evaluate complex regions of anatomy, or spinal placement at extremes of motion (Table 4-13). The Davis series consists of seven views including the five views presented and flexion and extension views (see Case 9).[88,108]

### Lines of mensuration of the cervical spine[69,137]

The following measurements are meant to be utilized as approximations of alignment and should not be con-

*Table 4-12*  Rules of muscle testing and the muscle grading system

The muscle being tested is isolated by positioning of the limb as best as possible to isolate the muscle.
The muscle and joint are positioned at one half of the distance of total motion.
The patient is asked to contract the muscle against resistance by applying a concentric action against a static position, that is, the patient is asked to hold a position and not let the clinician move the joint.
Resistance is applied by the clinician for a minimum of 6 seconds.
Resistance is applied by the clinician in a crescendo-decrescendo manner.
The muscle being tested is not overpowered. Enough resistance is applied by the clinician to determine whether the muscle is able to resist a load with gravity.

Muscle grading system:
0   no muscle action, a flaccid muscle
1   slight muscle action, not enough to cause limb motion and barely felt by the examiner
2   muscle action but patient has problems resisting gravity
3   functional muscle, resistance against gravity, but patient is not able to resist an applied load
4   muscle resistance against gravity with mild resistance
5   muscle resistance against gravity with resistance

sidered exact measurements. Minor variations in positioning and mensuration techniques could alter the results of these measurements significantly (for example, placing the patient's neck in too much extension for the lateral view may increase the cervical lordosis). Additionally, a measurement that is outside of the normal range may still be normal for that individual.[69] As such, clinical application of radiography is often tenuous, and the radiographic findings should not overshadow the clinical findings without sufficient reason.

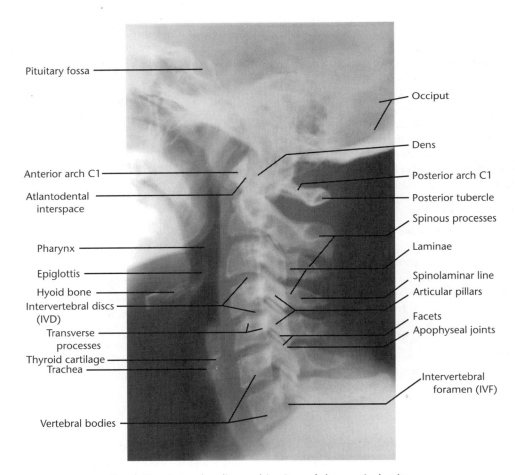

*Fig. 4-21*  Lateral radiographic view of the cervical spine.

*Table 4-13*   Common cervical spine views

| | |
|---|---|
| Anterior-posterior lower cervical view (APLC) | Lower cervical spine in the frontal plane |
| Anterior-posterior open mouth view (APOM) | Upper cervical spine in the frontal plane |
| Lateral view | Entire cervical spine in the sagittal plane; C1 and C7 must be visible to avoid missing abnormalities |
| Anterior oblique views (right and left) | Best for evaluating the cervical IVFs |
| Additional views | |
| Flexion and extension lateral view | Mechanical instability and end-range of motion |
| Fuch's view | Upper cervical spine in patients who cannot open their mouths |
| Pillar or Boyleston view | Articular pillars, views may be bilateral for comparison |

**McGregor's line.** This line is used to evaluate for basilar invagination. The only drawback to this line is that it can be affected by changes in the shape of the occiput unrelated to basilar invagination.[126] On a lateral view, a line is drawn from the posterior aspect of the hard palate to the most inferior surface of the occiput. The tip of the odontoid process should not project above this line more than 8 mm in men or 10 mm in women.

**Atlantodental interspace.** On a lateral view, the distance between the posterior surface of the anterior arch of C1 and the anterior surface of the dens is measured. This can also be measured on flexion and extension lateral views. During flexion, the measurement should be taken at the midaspect of the joint, since the superior aspect may widen more than the inferior aspect. The maximum measurement (in any position) in adults is 3 mm and in children, 5 mm. An increase in this measurement indicates loss of integrity of the transverse ligament, which is seen in such conditions as rheumatoid arthritis and pharyngeal infections, as well as in traumatic rupture of the ligament.

**George's line.** On a lateral view, a line is drawn along the posterior aspects of all the vertebral bodies. These lines should be in relatively good alignment, thus forming a smooth, continuous line. The line can also be drawn on flexion and extension lateral views. A break in the continuity of this line suggests listhesis of a vertebra on the one below. The amount of slippage should be measured. Two millimeters or less of displacement or translation is considered to be within physiologic limits.[31]

**Posterior cervical line.** On a lateral view, a line is drawn connecting the spinolaminar (posterior cervical) lines from C1 to T1 (if visible). Like George's line, this should form a relatively smooth, continuous line, and it should be drawn in conjunction with George's line. When using this line, it should be borne in mind that the spinolaminar lines are not always vertically oriented. In this instance, the superior aspects of the spinolaminar lines should be lined up. This will allow for a smoother line. It should be recalled that the C1 posterior arch is often short, which will disrupt this line.[61, 68] In this instance, the atlantodeutal interspace (ADI) and George's line should still be normal.

**Sagittal diameter of the spinal canal.** On a lateral view, the shortest distance from the posterior aspect of the vertebral body to the spinolaminar line is measured. The distance between the posterior aspect of the dens and the posterior cervical line is measured at C1. The ranges for diameter by level are listed in Table 4-14. However, these ranges do not consider the physical characteristics of individual patients. An alternative method to evaluate the canal diameter from C2 to C7 is based on the fact that generally, this diameter should be no less than 82% of the vertebral body width at that same level. For example, if the C4 vertebral body measures 20 mm, then the canal diameter at that level should measure no less than 16 mm. A smaller measurement could indicate canal stenosis and may predispose the patient to developing symptoms of stenosis from less significant pathology.[70,88] Measurements that are higher than normal could indicate a space-occupying lesion such as a tumor or neural anomaly.

**Cervical gravity line.** On a neutral lateral view, a vertical line is drawn down from the apex of the odontoid process. This line should intersect the C7 vertebral body. If the line falls anterior to C7, it indicates anterior carriage of the head. This is commonly seen in whiplash patients (Case 8) in association with loss of the lordosis. If the line falls posterior to C7, it indicates posterior carriage of the head (an uncommon finding).

**Cervical lordosis.** There are several ways to measure the cervical lordosis. A popular method is to measure the lordotic angle. A line is drawn through the anterior

*Table 4-14*   Measurements of sagittal canal diameter in the cervical spine

| Level | Diameter (mm) | |
|---|---|---|
| | Minimum | Maximum |
| C1 | 16 | 31 |
| C2 | 14 | 27 |
| C3 | 13 | 23 |
| C4 to C7 | 12 | 22 |

and posterior tubercles of C1. Another line is drawn along the inferior end plate of C7. Perpendicular lines are constructed from these lines. At the point of intersection of these lines, the superior angle is measured. The normal range is 35 to 45 degrees. An angle smaller than 35 degrees indicates hypolordosis and greater than 45 degrees indicates hyperlordosis.

The problem with this line is that the patient can have an alordotic cervical spine below C1, but have significant extension of C1 on C2 and a normal angle overall. With this in mind, other methods have been developed, such as the cervical depth measurement. With this measurement, a line is drawn on a lateral view from the most superior posterior point of the dens to the posterior inferior corner of the C7 body. The greatest distance from this line to the posterior aspect of the vertebral bodies is measured. The range is 7 to 17 mm, with the smaller measurement indicating hypolordosis.

The positioning of the patient is important, as this will affect these measurements. The significance of an abnormal lordotic measurement is questioned, since many individuals with altered lordoses have no apparent clinical findings. It can, however, suggest alteration of muscular balance or ligamentous integrity.

**Retropharyngeal and retrotracheal spaces.** Two measurements are made on a neutral lateral view: the distance from the anteroinferior corner of the C2 vertebral body to the posterior border of the pharyngeal air shadow (retropharyngeal) and the distance from the anteroinferior corner of the C6 vertebral body to the posterior border of the tracheal air shadow (retrotracheal). The maximum measurement for the retropharyngeal space is 7 mm and for the retrotracheal space, 20 to 21 mm. An increase in either of these measurements indicates the presence of a space-occupying lesion, including hematoma, infection, and tumor.

### Thoracic spine and rib series

A number of radiographic views have been described to evaluate the osseous and soft tissue anatomy of the thoracic spine. Frontal (A-P) and lateral (left) views are the standard evaluation projections (Fig. 4-22). Additional views often supplement the frontal and lateral views.[5,31,108] Views of the ribs are commonly acquired

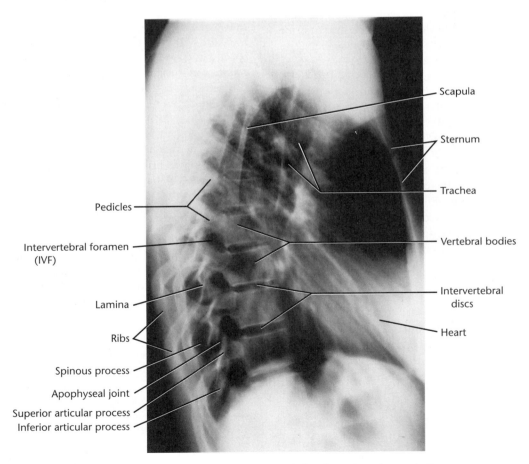

*Fig. 4-22*   Lateral radiographic view of the thoracic spine and ribs.

with the patient in three different positions, allowing optimum evaluation of these complex bones.

## Lines of mensuration of the thoracic spine[69,137]

**Scoliosis: Cobb's method.** Cobb's method, overall, is considered the most accepted method of measuring the degree of curvature of a scoliosis (Case 11).[56a] Other methods are used, but these are not presented. On a frontal radiograph, the top and bottom of the convexity are determined. This is achieved by identifying the points at each end of the convexity where the end plates are parallel. When the discs appear open-wedged on the opposite side of the convexity, this is too far, and the angle will start to decrease. This is often the most difficult part of measuring the scoliosis, because the end plates are not always easily identified. Sometimes one can only "eyeball" the end of the curve, making sure the same segments are used in any later evaluations. Once the top and bottom of the curve have been determined, lines are drawn along the top end plate of the superior segment and the bottom end plate of the inferior segment (this can be modified to use the top and bottom of the pedicles, respectively, if the end plates are not visible). Perpendicular lines are drawn from both of these lines, and the superior angle formed is measured at their intersection.

A measurement of 10 degrees or greater should be termed a scoliosis. Also, a minimal change of ± 5 degrees between any additional measurements must be found before a change in the curvature can be considered significant.

**Risser's sign.** Risser's sign relates to the appearance of the iliac crest apophyses, and is used as an estimator of skeletal maturity in scoliosis patients (see Case 11). It can be seen on any frontal film that demonstrates the iliac crests. The normal apophysis appears at the lateral aspect of the iliac crest (near the anterior superior iliac spine [ASIS]). As the patient ages, the medial edge of this apophysis progresses towards the medial end of the crest. Once it reaches the medial end of the crest, it is seen as a long, linear opacity above the iliac crest, separated by a thin, lucent band that represents the physis. When the apophysis first appears, the patient is at Risser stage 1. When the apophysis reaches the posterior superior iliac spine (PSIS) region, they are at Risser stage 4, and when the apophysis fuses to the crest, the patient is at Risser stage 5.

Originally, it was felt that once a patient reached Risser 4, they were skeletally mature and that little, if any, progression would occur within an existing scoliosis.[104a] Further studies[69,93a] into this phenomenon have shown that a considerable amount of skeletal growth can still occur at Risser stage 4, and even small amounts at Risser 5. However, once Risser stage 5 is reached, most patients are skeletally mature, and there is a sig-

nificant reduction in the likelihood of a patient's scoliosis progressing more than a few degrees.

Even though Risser's sign is considered one of the most accurate plain film estimates of skeletal maturity in the adolescent age group, its limitations suggest that it should only be used in combination with other factors when evaluating for the likelihood of progression of a scoliosis.

### Osteoporosis

Although plain x-ray films are generally unreliable in the early detection and assessment of osteoporosis, plain-film findings of osteoporosis can be a helpful adjunct to the diagnosis. The trabecular bone becomes sparse, resulting in overall reduction in bone density. In the vertebral bodies, the primary stress-bearing trabeculae are vertically oriented, and they will appear accentuated because of resorption of the secondary stress-bearing horizontal trabeculae. This accentuation of vertical trabeculae is usually seen at multiple, contiguous levels.

Thinning of the cortices is also visible on plain films and results in "pencil-thin" cortices of the segments. This means that the end-plate margins will demonstrate thinned subchondral cortex, and the pedicles will appear to have less cortical thickness.

As is presented in Case 12, nontraumatic compression deformities are a sure sign that bone density is compromised. These compression deformities may take several shapes. First, an isolated central end-plate impression may be present. This bowing of the end plate into the vertebral body suggests inability of the trabeculae to withstand the weight-bearing stresses placed upon them.[125] Secondly, biconcave end-plate deformities may be present. This is nothing more than impressions of both superior and inferior end plates. This pattern of compression has been termed the "fish vertebrae" appearance. Thirdly, the segment may lose anterior vertebral body height with maintenance of the end-plate integrity. Historical correlation is necessary to distinguish this pattern of collapse from traumatic collapse. Lastly, the segment may demonstrate loss of anterior and posterior vertebral body height. This pattern of compression is impossible to distinguish from collapse of the vertebral segment from neoplastic infiltration and frequently demands further evaluation using laboratory tests, advanced imaging techniques, and even biopsy. Additionally, fractures of the ribs are quite common, and can result from a wide range of insults, including "bear hugs," coughing spasms, and chiropractice adjustments.

Case 12 demonstrates the typical spontaneous nature of vertebral fractures, although trivial trauma such as jarring the heel after stepping off a curb, or forceful muscular contraction of the paraspinal or abdominal muscles can cause collapse as well. As with any fracture, edema and hemorrhage will result, and this may be seen as deviation of the paraspinal pleural reflections in the thoracic spine. Normally, the paraspinal reflections do not reside more than 2–3 mm from the edge of the vertebral bodies. In the presence of hemorrhage and edema, the lines will deviate laterally from the spine in a focal pattern indicating focal abnormality. Significant spinal cord compromise is unusual with this type of fracture. For deformities that result in 30% or more loss in height, the loss will likely be permanent, and resultant deformity may potentiate subsequent degenerative changes because of the altered biomechanics.

Quantitative computed tomography (CT) analysis is perhaps the most reliable imaging modality for the early assessment of osteoporosis, although it is relatively expensive and should not be ordered routinely.[51a] Even with this or any other advanced or even plain-film imaging modality, the findings should always be evaluated in light of the patient's clinical presentation, as the causes for osteoporosis are extensive.

### Lumbar spine and sacral radiographic series

A variety of radiographic views can be taken when evaluating the lumbosacral region (Fig. 4-23). The standard views consist of the A-P, lateral oblique and either a frontal or a lateral lumbosacral spot. Some facilities will add, subtract, or interchange views as part of their standard series, depending on what is to be evaluated and the age of the patient.[5,31,108]

### Lines of mensuration of the lumbar spine[69,137]

The following measurements are meant to be utilized as approximations of alignment and should not be considered exact measurements. Minor variations in patient positioning and mensuration techniques could alter the results of these measurements significantly. Patient positioning must always be considered when evaluating these lines. For example, excessive elevation of the arms could shift weight bearing posteriorly, while taking radiographs in the recumbent posture can decrease the lordosis. Additionally, a measurement that is outside a suggested range may still be normal for that individual. As such, clinical application is often tenuous, and the radiographic findings should not overshadow the clinical findings without sufficient reason.

**Angle of lumbar lordosis.** On a lateral lumbar film, one line is drawn along the superior end plate of L1,

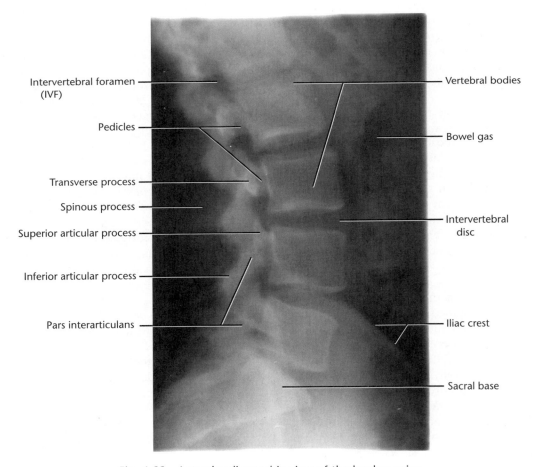

*Fig. 4-23*   Lateral radiographic view of the lumbar spine.

and another line is drawn along the inferior end plate of L5. Perpendicular lines are drawn from each of these lines, and the superior angle formed by the intersection of these lines is measured. The normal range is 35 to 45 degrees. A variation of this line uses the sacral base, rather than L5 as the inferior reference point. The normal range for this angle is 50 to 60 degrees.

A measurement in excess of these ranges could indicate hyperlordosis. Although the clinical significance of these findings is in question, it is suggested that hyperlordosis places more stress on the facet articulations, which could predispose a person to facet disease or "facet syndrome." A decrease in the angle suggests an antalgic posture.

**Lumbosacral disc angle.** On a lateral lumbar film, one line is drawn along the inferior end plate of L5 and another line is drawn along the sacral base. These lines should be extended posteriorly. This measurement can be evaluated in two ways: (1) The anterior angle formed by the lines should measure between 10 and 20 degrees and (2) The lines should intersect posterior to the IVFs.

An angle greater than 20 degrees or intersection of the lines in the IVFs suggest extension of L5 on S1. This may result in facet imbrication, which has been implicated by some as a cause of low back pain.[108] If the angle is less than 10 degrees or the lines fail to intersect, flexion of L5 on S1 is suggested, which may be seen in antalgic postures.

**Sacral base angle (Ferguson's angle).** On a lateral lumbar film, a line is drawn along the sacral base and a second line is drawn parallel to the bottom edge of the film so that it intersects the first line. The posterior angle is then measured. There is a wide variation in ranges of normal depending on the source. Yochum and Rowe[137] list the range at 26 to 57 degrees.

The significance of a measurement outside the normal range has not been proved, although it is suggested that an increase in the angle places greater stress on the posterior joints, which could cause low back pain.[70]

**Meyerdings's grading system for spondylolisthesis.** On a lateral or lateral spot film, the sacral base is divided into four equal segments, which are numbered from back to front (grades 1 to 4). The posteroinferior corner of the L5 body is then evaluated as to the segment it lines up with. Normally, the posterior aspects of the L5 and S1 levels are evenly aligned. This method can also be used at other levels of the lumbar spine.

This system is used to categorize the degree of anterior slippage (anterolisthesis, spondylolisthesis) of one level on another (see Case 14). If the posterior corner of the L5 body lines up over the third segment of the sacral base, this would be termed a "grade 3" spondylolisthesis. It should be noted that alignment is always determined by the position of the level above in relation to the level below, never conversely (that is, S1 does not slide posterior under L5, L5 slides anterior or posterior on S1).

## Radiology of the sacroiliac joint

Although an x-ray examination would seem unnecessary in Case 15, radiographic evaluation could play an important role in ruling out an inflammatory arthritis. Conditions such as ankylosing spondylitis (Case 17) can have a clinical presentation similar to that in Case 15, with referral of pain into the hip and gluteal regions.[103a] The patient is in the correct age range, and although the pain seems to have been brought on mechanically, this does not rule out the possibility of coincidental development of sacroilitis. After pregnancy, conditions such as osteitis condensans ilii can also be identified with plain films. In this case, the soft tissue findings cannot be evaluated with plain films.

## REFERENCES

1. Apps BK, Cohen BB, Steel CM: *Biochemistry, a concise text for medical students,* ed 5, Iowa City, 1992, Bailliere Tindall.
2. Arnoldi CC, et al: Lumbar spinal stenosis and nerve root entrapment syndromes, *Clin Orthop* 115:4, 1976.
3. Bakkum B, Cramer G: Muscles that influence the spine. In Cramer G, Darby S: *Basic and clinical anatomy of the spine, spinal cord, and ANS,* St. Louis, 1995, Mosby.
4. Bakland O, Hanse J. The axial sacroiliac joint, *Anatomica Clinica* 6:29, 1984.
5. Ballinger PW, editor: *Merrill's atlas of roentgenographic positions and standard radiologic procedures,* ed 7, St. Louis, 1990, Mosby.
6. Basmajian JV, Slonecker CE: *Grant's method of anatomy: a clinical problem-solving approach,* ed 11, Baltimore, 1989, Williams & Wilkins.
7. Behrsin JF, Briggs CA: Ligaments of the lumbar spine: a review, *Surg Radiol Anat* 10:211, 1988.
8. Bergmann TF, Peterson DH, Lawrence DJ: *Chiropractic technique,* New York, 1993, Churchill Livingstone.
9. Bernard T, Cassidy D: The sacroiliac joints revisited. Report from the San Diego congress on the sacroiliac joint, *The Chiropractic Report* 7:1, 1993.
10. Bhagavan NV: *Medical biochemistry,* Boston, 1992, Jones & Bartlet.
11. Blakney MG: The cervical spine. In Hertling D, Kessler RM, editor: *Management of common musculoskeletal disorders,* ed 2, Philadelphia, 1990, Lippincott.
12. Bogduk N: The anatomy of the lumbar intervertebral disc syndrome, *Med J Aust* 1:878, 1976.
13. Bogduk N: The innervation of the lumbar spine, *Spine* 8:286, 1983.
14. Bogduk N, Twomey LT: *Clinical anatomy of the lumbar spine,* London, 1991, Churchill Livingstone.
15. Bogduk N, Tynan W, Wilson A: The nerve supply to the human lumbar intervertebral discs, *J Anat* 132:39, 1981.
16. Bogduk N, Wilson A, Tynan W: The human lumbar dorsal rami, *J Anat* 134:383, 1982.
17. Bolton PS, Stick PE, Lord RSA: Failure of clinical tests to predict cerebral ischemia before neck manipulation, *JMPT* 12:304, 1989.
18. Bose K, Balasubramaniam P: Nerve root canals of the lumbar spine, *Spine* 9:16, 1984.
19. Buckwalter J: Spine update: aging and degeneration of the human intervertebral disc, *Spine* 20:1307, 1995.
20. Buckwalter JA, et al: Articular cartilage and intervertebral disc proteoglycans differ in structure: an electron microscope study, *J Orthop Res* 7:146, 1989.

21. Buckwalter JA, et al: Proteoglycans of human infant intervertebral disc: electron microscopic and biochemical studies, *J Bone Joint Surg* 67A:284, 1985.

22. Buckwalter JA, et al: Articular cartilage and intervertebral disc proteoglycans differ in structure, *J Orthop Res* 7:146, 1989.

23. Butler D, Gifford L: The concept of adverse mechanical tension in the nervous system. Part 1: Testing for "dural tension," *Physiotherapy* 75(11):622, 1989.

24. Cassidy JD, Mierau DR: Pathophysiology of the sacroiliac joint. In Haldeman S, editor: *Principles and practice of chiropractic,* ed 2, Norwalk, 1992, Appleton & Lange.

25. Cassidy JJ, Hiltner A, Baer E: Hierarchical structure of the intervertebral disc, *Connect Tissue Res* 23:75, 1989.

26. Chusid JG: *Correlative neuroanatomy and function neurology,* ed 7, Los Altos, 1979, Lange.

27. Cipriano J: *Photographic manual of regional orthopaedic and neurological tests,* ed 2, Baltimore, 1991, Williams & Wilkins.

28. Cramer G: The lumbar region. In Cramer G, Darby S: *Basic and clinical anatomy of the spine, spinal cord, and ANS,* St. Louis, 1995, Mosby.

29. Cramer G, et al: Generalizability of patient profiles from a feasibility study, *J Can Chiropractic Assoc* 36:84, 1992.

30. Crock HV: Normal and pathological anatomy of the lumbar spinal nerve root canals, *J Bone Joint Surg* 63:487, 1981.

31. Cullinan AM: *Optimizing radiographic positioning,* Philadelphia, 1992, Lippincott.

31a. Daffner RH, et al: The radiology assessment of post-traumatic vertebral stability, *Skeletal Radiol* 19:103, 1990.

32. Darby S: The autonomic nervous system. In Cramer G, Darby S: *Basic and clinical anatomy of the spine, spinal cord, and ANS,* St. Louis, 1995, Mosby.

33. de Peretti F, et al: Biomechanics of the lumbar spinal nerve roots and the first sacral root within the intervertebral foramina, *Surg Radiol Anat* 11:221, 1989.

34. Dodd J, Role LW: The autonomic nervous system. In Kandel ER, Schwartz JH, Jessell TM: *Principles of neural science,* ed 3, New York, 1991, Elsevier.

35. Dommisse GF, Louw JA: Anatomy of the lumbar spine. In Floman Y, editor: *Disorders of the lumbar spine,* Rockville and Tel Aviv, 1990, Aspen Publishers, Inc. and Freund Publishing House, Ltd.

36. Dupuis PR: The anatomy of the lumbosacral spine. In Kirkaldy-Willis W, editor: *Managing low back pain,* ed 2, New York, 1988, Churchill Livingstone.

37. Dussault R, Lander P: Imaging of the facet joints, *Radiol Clin North Am* 28:1033, 1990.

38. Dvorak J, et al: Age and gender related normal motion of the cervical spine, *Spine* 17:S393, 1992.

39. Dvorak J, et al: Clinical validation of functional flexion/extension of the normal cervical spine, *J Orthopaed Res* 9:828, 1991.

40. Edgar M, Ghadially J: Innervation of the lumbar spine, *Clin Orthop* 115:35, 1976.

41. Engel R, Bogduk N: The menisci of the lumbar zygapophyseal joints, *J Anat* 135:795, 1982.

42. Eyre D, et al: The intervertebral disk: basic science perspectives. In Frymoyer JW, Gordon SL, editors: *New perspectives on low back pain,* Park Ridge, 1989, American Academy of Orthopaedic Surgeons.

43. Fahrini WH: Observations on straight leg-raising with special reference to nerve root adhesions, *Can J of Surg* 9:44, 1966.

44. Fechtel S: Examination. In Gatterman MT, editor: *Chiropractic management of spine related disorders,* Baltimore, 1990, Williams & Wilkins.

45. Floyd WF, Silver PHS: Function of the erectro spinae in flexion of the trunk, *Lancet* 20:133, 1950.

46. Foreman SM, Croft AC: *Whiplash injuries: The cervical acceleration/deceleration syndrome,* ed 2, Baltimore, 1995, Williams & Wilkins.

47. Freeman MD, Fox D, Richards T: The superior intracapsular ligament of the sacroiliac joint: confirmation of Illi's ligament, *J Manipulative Physiol Ther* 13:374, 1990.

48. Frymoyer JW, Gordon SL, editors: *New perspectives on low back pain,* Park Ridge, 1989, American Academy of Orthopaedic Surgeons.

49. Gaenslen FJ: Sacro-iliac arthrodesis: indications, author's technic and end-results, *JAMA* 89:2031, 1927.

50. Gatterman MI: Disorders of the pelvic ring. In Gatterman MI, editor: *Chiropractic management of spine-related disorders,* Baltimore, 1990, Williams & Wilkins.

51. Gatterman MI, Panzer DM: Disorders of the cervical spine. In Gatterman MI, editor: *Chiropractic management of spine related disorders,* Baltimore, 1990, Williams & Wilkins.

51a. Genant HK: Quantitative bone mineral analysiss. In Resnick D, Niwayama G, editor: *Diagnosis of bone and joint disorders,* Philadelphia, 1988, Saunders.

52. Ghosh P, et al: A comparison of the high buoyant density proteoglycans isolated from the intervertebral discs of chondrodystrophoid and nonchondrodystrophoid dogs, *Matrix* 12:148, 1992.

53. Giles LGF: *Anatomical basis of low back pain,* Baltimore, 1989, Williams & Wilkins.

54. Giles LGF: Human zygapophyseal joint inferior recess synovial folds: a light microscopic examination, *Anat Rec* 220:1124, 1988.

55. Giles LGF, Taylor JR: Human zygapophyseal joint capsule and synovial fold innervation, *Br J Rheumatol* 26:93, 1987.

56. Goddard MD, Reid JD: Movements induced by straight leg raising in the lumbo-sacral roots, nerves and plexus, and in the intrapelvic section of the sciatic nerve, *J Neuro Neurosurg Psychiatry* 28:12, 1965.

56a. Goldstein LA, Waugh TR: Classification and terminology of scoliosis, *Clin Orthop Rel Res* 1973; 93:10.

57. Greenman PE. *Principles of manual medicine,* Baltimore, 1989, Williams & Wilkins.

58. Greenstein GM, Summers DJ. Biomechanics. In: Lawrence DJ, editor: *Fundamentals of chiropractic diagnosis and management,* Baltimore, 1991, Williams & Wilkins.

59. Grenier N, et al, Normal and disrupted lumbar longitudinal ligaments: correlative MR and anatomic study, *Radiology* 171:197, 1989.

60. Groen G, Baljet B, Drukker J: Nerves and nerve plexuses of the human vertebral column, *Am J Anat* 188:282, 1990.

61. Guebert GM, Yochum TR, Rowe LJ: Congenital anomalies and normal skeletal variants. In: Yochum TR, Rowe LJ, editors: *Essentials of skeletal radiology,* vol 1, Baltimore, 1987, Williams & Wilkins.

62. Hasue M, et al: Anatomic study of the interrelation between lumbosacral nerve roots and their surrounding tissues, *Spine* 8:50, 1983.

63. Hornel SE, Eyre DR: Collagen in the aging human intervertebral disc: an increase in covalently bound fluorophores and chromophores, *Biochem et Biophys Acta* 1078(2):243, 1991.

64. Hutton WC: The forces acting on a lumbar intervertebral joint, *J Manual Medicine,* 5:66, 1990.

65. Jackson HC, et al: Nerve endings in the human lumbar spinal column and related structures, *J Bone Joint Surg* 48:1272, 1966.

66. Jeffries B: Facet joint injections, *Spine* 2:409, 1972.

67. Johnstone B, et al: Identification and characterization of glycanated and non-glycanated forms of biglycan and decorin in the human intervertebral disc, *Biochem J* 292:661, 1993.

68. Keats TE. *Atlas of normal roentgen variants that may simulate disease,* ed 5, St. Louis, 1992, Mosby.

69. Keats TE, Lusted LB: *Atlas of roentgenographic measurements,* ed 6, St. Louis, 1990, Mosby.

70. Keats TE, Smith TH: *An atlas of normal developmental roentgen anatomy,* ed 2, Chicago, 1988, Yearbook Medical Publishers, Inc.

71. Kelley WN, et al: *Textbook of Rheumatology,* ed 4, vol I, Philadelphia, 1993, Saunders.

72. Deleted in galleys.

73. Kirkaldy-Willis WH, et al: Pathology and pathogenesis of lumbar spondylosis and stenosis, *Spine* 3:319, 1978.

74. Kirkaldy-Willis W: The pathology and pathogenesis of low back pain. In Kirkaldy-Willis W, editor: *Managing low back pain,* ed 2, New York, 1988, Churchill Livingstone.

75. Korkala O, et al: Immunohistochemical demonstration of nociceptors in the ligamentous structures of the lumbar spine, *Spine* 10:156, 1985.

76. Kraemer M, Patris A: Radio-functional analysis of the cervical spine using the Arlen method. Part II. Paradoxical tilting of the atlas, *J of Neuroradiol* 16:65, 1989.

77. Krag MH, et al: Internal displacement: distribution from in vitro loading of human thoracic and lumbar spinal motion segments: experimental results and theoretical predictions, *Spine* 12:1001, 1987.

78. Lancourt JE, Glenn WV, Wiltse LL: Multiplanar computerized tomography in the normal spine and in the diagnosis of spinal stenosis. A gross anatomic-computerized topographic correlation, *Spine* 4:379, 1979.

79. Lazorthes C: Les branches postérieures des nerfs preluders et le plan articulaire vertebral postérieur, *Am Med Phys* 15:192, 1972.

80. Lee CK, Rauschning W, Glenn W: Lateral lumbar spinal canal stenosis: classification, pathologic anatomy and surgical decompression, *Spine* 13:313, 1988.

81. Lind B, et al: Normal range of motion of the cervical spine, *Arch Phys Med Rehabil* 70:692, 1989.

82. Lippitt AB: The facet joint and its role in spine pain: Management with facet joint injections, *Spine* 9:746, 1984.

83. Liyang D, et al: The effect of flexion-extension motion of the lumbar spine on the capacity of the spinal canal: an experimental study, *Spine* 14:523, 1989.

84. Magarey ME: Examination of the cervical and thoracic spine. In Grant R editor: *Clinics in physical therapy: physical therapy of the cervical and thoracic spine,* New York, 1988, Churchill Livingstone.

85. Magee DJ: *Orthopedic physical assessment,* ed 2, Philadelphia, 1992, Saunders.

86. Maldonaldo BA, Oegema TR: Initial characterization of the metabolism of the intervertebral disc cells encapsulated in microspheres, *J Orthopaedic Res* 10:677, 1992.

87. McNab I: Negative disc exploration: an analysis of the causes of nerve-root involvement in sixty-eight patients, *J Bone Joint Surg* 53A:891, 1971.

88. Möller TB, Reif E, Stark P: *Pocket atlas of radiographic anatomy,* New York, 1993, Thieme Medical Publishers, Inc.

89. Montgomery R, Conway TM, Spector AA: *Biochemistry: a case oriented approach,* ed 5, St. Louis, 1990, Mosby.

90. Moore KL: *Clinically oriented anatomy,* ed 3, Baltimore, 1992, Williams & Wilkins.

91. Mosner EA, et al: A comparison of actual and apparent lumbar lordosis in black and white adult females, *Spine* 14:310, 1989.

92. Murray RK, et al: *Harper's biochemistry,* ed 23, Norwalk, 1993, Appleton-Lange.

93. Nachemson AL: The lumbar spine: an orthopedic challenge, *Spine* 1:59, 1976.

93a. Nash CL, Moe JH: A study of vertebral rotation, *J Bone Joint Surg* 51A:223, 1969.

94. Nicholson AA, Roberts GM, Williams LA: The measured height of the lumbosacral disc in patients with and without transitional vertebrae, *Br J Radiol* 61:454, 1988.

95. Norman GP, May A: Sacroiliac condition simulating intervertebral disc syndrome, *WJSO & G* (Aug):401, 1956.

96. Olsewski JM, et al: Evidence from cadavers suggestive of entrapment of fifth lumbar spinal nerves by lumbosacral ligaments, *Spine* 16:336, 1991.

97. Olczyl K: Age-related changes in collagen of human intervertebral disks, *Gerontology* 38:196, 1992.

98. Osterbauer PJ, et al: Three-dimensional head kinematics and clinical outcome of patients with neck injury treated with spinal manipulative therapy: A pilot study, *J Manipulative Physiol Ther* 15:501, 1992.

99. Panjabi MM, et al: Biomechanics of healing posterior cervical spinal injuries in a canine model, *Spine* 13:803, 1988.

100. Paris S: Anatomy as related to function and pain, Symposium on Evaluation and Care of Lumbar Spine Problems, 1983.

101. Penning L: Normal movements of the cervical spine, *Am J Roentgenol* 130:317, 1979.

102. Pitkin HC, Pheasant HC: Sacroarthrogenic telalgia, *J Bone Joint Surg* 18A:111, 1936.

103. Rahlmann JF: Mechanisms of intervertebral joint fixation: a literature review, *J Manipulative Physiol Ther* 10:177, 1987.

103a. Rangel GS: Ankylosing spondylitis simulating hip bursitis, *CDI Roengten Brief* 6(90126), 1989.

104. Rauschning W: Normal and pathologic anatomy of the lumbar root canals, *Spine* 12108, 1987.

104a. Risser JC: The iliac apophysis: an invaluable sign in the management of scoliosis, *Clin Orthop* 11:111, 1958.

105. Ro CS: Sacroiliac joint. In Cox JM: *Low back pain: mechanism, diagnosis and treatment,* ed 5, Baltimore, 1990, Williams & Wilkins.

106. Ro CS, Cramer G: The sacrum, sacroiliac joint, and coccyx. In Cramer G, Darby S: *Basic and clinical anatomy of the spine, spinal cord, and ANS,* St. Louis, 1995, Mosby.

107. Rothman RH, Simeone FA, editors: *The spine,* ed 3, vol 1, Philadelphia, 1992, Saunders.

108. Rowe LJ, Yochum TR: Radiographic positioning and normal anatomy. In Yochum TR, Rowe LJ, editors: *Essentials of skeletal radiology,* vol 1, Baltimore, 1987, Williams & Wilkins.

109. Saamanen AM, et al: Effect of running exercise on proteoglycans and collagen content in the intervertebral discs of young dogs, *International J Sports Med* 14:48, 1993.

110. Scham S: Tension signs in lumbar disc prolapse, *Clin Orthop* 75:195, 1971.

110a. Shapiro R, Youngberg AS, Rothman SLG: The differential diagnosis of traumatic lesions of the occipito-atlanto-axial segment, *Rad Clin North Am* 11:505, 1973.

111. Simons DG: Muscle pain syndromes, *J Manual Medicine* 6:3, 1991.

112. Smith EL, et al: *Principles of biochemistry,* ed 7, New York, 1983, McGraw-Hill.

113. Stathopoulos P, Cramer G: The microscopic anatomy of the zygapophyseal joints and intervertebral discs. In Cramer G. Darby S: *Basic and clinical anatomy of the spine, spinal cord, and ANS,* St. Louis, 1995, Mosby.

114. Stratton SA, Bryan JM: Dysfunction, evaluation, and treatment of the cervical spine and thoracic inlet. In Donatelli R, Wooden MJ, editors: *Orthopedic physical therapy,* Edinburgh, 1989, Churchill Livingstone.

115. Taylor JR: The development and adult structure of lumbar intervertebral discs, *J Manual Med* 5:43, 1990.

116. Taylor JR, Twomey LT: Age changes in lumbar zygapophyseal joints: observations on structure and function, *Spine* 11:739, 1986.

117. Teasell RW, Shapiro AP, editors: Cervical flexion-extension/whiplash injuries, *Spine: State of the Art Reviews,* Philadelphia, 1993, Hanley & Belfus, Inc.

118. Thiel HW. Gross morphology and pathoanatomy of the vertebral arteries, *J Manipulative Physiol Ther* 14:133, 1991.

119. Twomey L, Taylor JR: Structural and mechanical disc changes with age, *J Manual Med* 5:58, 1990.

120. Urban JPG: The effect of physical factors on disc cell metabolism. In Buchwalter JA, Goldberg VM, Woo SL-Y editors: *Musculoskeletal soft tissue aging: Impact on mobility,* Rosemont, 1993, American Academy of Orthopaedic Surgeons.

121. Van Schaik J, Verbiest H, Van Schaik F: The orientation of laminae and facet joints in the lower lumbar spine, *Spine* 10:59, 1985.

122. Viikari-Juntura E, Porras M, Laasonen EM: Validity of clinical tests in the diagnosis of root compression in cervical disc disease, *Spine* 14:253, 1989.

123. Vital JM, et al: Anatomy of the lumbar radicular canal, *Anat Clin* 5:141, 1983.

124. Weisl H: The ligaments of sacroiliac joint examined with their particular reference to their function, *Acta Anat* 20:301, 1954.

125. White AA, Panjabi MM: *Clinical biomechanics of the spine,* ed 2, Philadelphia, 1990, Lippincott.

126. Wicke L: *Atlas of radiologic anatomy,* ed 5, Philadelphia, 1994, Lea & Febiger.

127. Wienir MA, editor: Spinal segmental pain and sensory disturbance, *Spine: State of the Art Reviews,* vol 2, Philadelphia, 1988, Hanley & Belfus, Inc.
128. Wilder DG: The biomechanics of vibration and low back pain, *Am J Ind Med* 23:577, 1993.
129. Williams PL et al, editors: *Gray's Anatomy,* ed 37, Edinburgh, 1989, Churchill Livingstone.
130. Winters JM, et al: Three-dimensional head axis of rotation during tracking movements: A tool for assessing neck neuromechanical function, *Spine* 18:1178, 1993.
131. Worth DR: Biomechanics of the cervical spine. In Grant, R editor: *Clinics in physical therapy: physical therapy of the cervical and thoracic spine,* New York, 1988, Churchill Livingstone.
132. Wyke B: Articular neurology and manipulative therapy. In Glasgow EF, et al, editors: *Aspects of manipulative therapy,* ed 2, London, 1985, Churchill Livingstone.
133. Xu GL, et al: Normal variations of the lumbar facet joint capsules, *Clin Anat* 4:11122, 1991.
134. Yang CL, et al: Collagen II from articular cartilage and annulus fibrosus: structural and functional implications of tissue specific post translational modifications of collagen molecules, *Eur J Biochem* 213:1297, 1993.
135. Yasuma T, et al: Histological changes in aging lumbar intervertebral discs: their role in protrusions and prolapses, *J Bone Joint Surg* 72A:220, 1992.
136. Yasuma T, Arai K, Yamauchi Y: The histology of lumbar intervertebral disc herniation: the significance of small blood vessels in the extruded tissue, *Spine* 18:1761, 1993.
137. Yochum TR, Rowe LJ: Measurements in skeletal radiology. In Yochum TR, Rowe LJ, editors: *Essentials of skeletal radiology,* vol 1, Baltimore, 1987, Williams & Wilkins.

## SUGGESTED READINGS

Bergmann TF, Peterson DH, Lawrence DJ: *Chiropractic technique,* New York, 1993, Churchill Livingstone.
Cramer G, Darby S: *Basic and clinical anatomy of the spine, spinal cord, and ANS,* St. Louis, 1995, Mosby.
Magee DJ: *Orthopedic physical assessment,* ed 2, Philadelphia, 1992, Saunders.
White AA, Panjabi MM: *Clinical biomechanics of the spine,* ed 2, Philadelphia, 1990, Lippincott.
Yochum TR, Rowe LJ, editors: *Essentials of skeletal radiology,* Baltimore, 1987, Williams & Wilkins.

# *The extremities*

## FUNCTIONAL ANATOMY AND BIOMECHANICS OF THE UPPER EXTREMITIES

BRUCE CARR (Functional Anatomy)
GARY M. GREENSTEIN (Biomechanics)

This section will focus on the functional anatomy and biomechanics as it pertains to common impingement syndromes (Case 19) and common joint articulation problems. Impingement syndromes involve anatomic structures that pass through areas that are surrounded by bone, ligament, or retinaculum. The neurovascular compression syndrome (thoracic outlet syndrome) can cause compromise of the brachial plexus or subclavian artery as they pass from the intervertebral foramen (IVFs) of the cervical and thoracic spine (C5 to T1) to the axilla. Shoulder impingement is most commonly found between the acromion and the head of the humerus. Mid-arm impingement usually affects the radial nerve in the radial groove of the humerus (for example, Saturday night palsy). At the elbow the ligament of Struther's, ulnar notch, or pronator teres can cause impingement on the peripheral nerves that pass through these areas. At the wrist, which is the most common area of impingement in the upper extremities, carpal tunnel syndrome (Case 21) and tunnel of Guyon impingements are found. In this section, the neurologic supply and its maladies are discussed, followed by the anatomy and biomechanics of the articulating joints of the upper extremities as they relate to the cases.

The clinician's responsibility is to locate the lesion. When solving nerve lesion problems, five rules of muscle innervation must be followed: (1) A muscle receives its nerve supply at the muscle belly, the proximal aspect, close to its origin; (2) Muscles are innervated by more than one root; (3) A peripheral nerve may have a lesion anywhere along its course and objective signs are found distal to the lesion; (4) If a nerve has a lesion it will affect motor, sensory, or both functions depending upon the type of nerve and its components; and (5) If a muscle is innervated by two or more peripheral nerves (composite), a loss of one of the nerves produces an overall weakness of that muscle.

## Neurovascular compression syndrome: thoracic outlet syndrome

Starting from the thoracic inlet and continuing to the axilla sit the neurovascular structures that feed the upper extremities. The thoracic inlet is surrounded by the manubrium anteriorly, the first thoracic vertebra posteriorly, and the first pair of ribs and their costal cartilages anterolaterally. A change in the area of the inlet caused by a cervical rib, scalenus anticus syndrome (compression of the subclavian artery or vein as it passes over the first rib) or costoclavicular syndrome can cause a neurologic or vascular compression of the anatomic structures (subclavian artery and vein and brachial plexus) that pass through this area.[15] A hyperabduction injury to the pectoralis minor can cause compression against the subclavian artery or brachial plexus as these structures approach the axilla. The patient's symptoms are described as paresthesias, dysesthesias with or without radicular pain to multiple dermatomes (neurologic compromise), or fatigue and a diffuse aching pain, when it is vascular in origin (see Case 10). The symptoms are always presented distal to the lesion.

**Brachial plexus.** The brachial plexus is a network of nerves that innervate all the muscles of the upper extremities. An injury (lesion) to any location along the plexus will produce a distinctive pain or muscle weakness pattern. The plexus originates in the cervical and thoracic spine and travels along with the subclavian artery through the *thoracic inlet* to the axilla (Fig. 5-1). At the axilla, it divides into the major nerves that innervate the upper extremities.

The brachial plexus is formed by the union of the ventral primary rami of nerves C5 to T1, commonly called the *roots of the brachial plexus*. After the cervical roots leave the IVF the ventral primary rami enter the posterior triangle of the neck and unite to form the *trunks* that split into the anterior and posterior divisions. The anterior division supplies the upper extremity flexor muscles and the posterior division supplies the posterior aspect (extensors) of the upper limb. The divisions then unite to form the lateral (C5 to C7), medial (C8 to T1), and posterior cords (C5 to T1).

At the inferolateral border of the pectoralis minor muscle the cords divide into two terminal branches: the lateral cord becomes the *musculocutaneous nerve and the lateral root of the median nerve;* the medial cord becomes the *ulnar nerve and the medial root of the median nerve;* and the posterior cord becomes the *axillary and radial nerve.* Table 5-1 presents the sensory and motor innervations of the brachial plexus.

### Ulnar, median, and radial nerves

**Ulnar nerve (nerve of the hand).** The ulnar nerve leaves the brachial plexus medial to the axillary and brachial arteries (medial cord). It has no muscle inner-

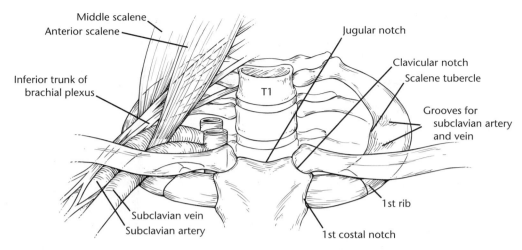

*Fig. 5-1*   The brachial plexus in the thoracic inlet.

*Table 5-1*   Common nerves of the brachial plexus and their motor and sensory innervations

| Nerve and level | Motor innervation | Sensory innervation |
|---|---|---|
| Medial cord | | Medial brachial cutaneous nerve and medial cutaneous nerve |
| Supraclavicular branches | | |
|   Dorsal scapular nerve (C5) | Rhomboid and levator scapulae | |
|   Long thoracic nerve (C5 to C7) | Serratus anterior | |
|   Nerve to subclavius (C5 to C6) | Subclavius muscle | |
|   Suprascapular nerve (C5 to C6) | Supraspinatus and infraspinatus | |
| Infraclavicular branches | | |
|   Medial cord | | |
|     Medial pectoral nerve (C8 to T1) | Pectoralis major (sternal) and minor | Medial brachial cutaneous nerve plus medial cutaneous nerve (medial antebrachial cutaneous nerve) |
|     Ulnar nerve (C8 to T1) | Flexor digitorum profundus (ulnar half), and flexor carpi ulnaris | Direct innervation |
|       Deep ulnar nerve (T1) | Abductor digiti minimum, lumbricales 3 and 4, palmar interosseous, and dorsal interosseous, adductor pollicis, opponens digiti minimi, and flexor digiti minimi | |
|       Medial root of median nerve (C5 to T1) | Pronator teres, flexor carpi radialis, flexor digitorum superficialis, palmaris longus, lumbricales 1 and 2 | Direct innervation |
|         Anterior interosseous nerve | Flexor pollicis longus, pronator quadratus, flexor digitorum profundus (radial one half) | |
|         Recurrent median nerve (T1) | Abductor pollicis brevis, flexor pollicis brevis, opponens pollicis | |
| Posterior cord | | |
|   Upper subscapular nerve (C5 to C6) | Subscapularis | |
|   Thoracodorsal nerve (C6 to C8) | Latissimus dorsi | |
|   Lower subscapular nerve (C5 to C6) | Subscapularis and teres major | |
|   Axillary nerve (C5 to C6) | Deltoid and teres minor | Lateral brachial cutaneous nerve |
|   Radial nerve (C5 to T1) | Triceps brachii, brachioradialis, extensor carpi radialis longus, and anconeus | Posterior brachial cutaneous nerve Posterior antebrachial cutaneous nerve Superficial radial nerve |
|     Deep radial nerve | Supinator and extensor carpi radialis brevis | |
|     Posterior interosseous nerve | Extensor carpi ulnaris, extensor digitorum, extensor pollicis longus, extensor pollicis brevis, extensor indicis, abductor pollicis longus, and extensor digiti minimi | |
| Lateral cord | Same as medial root of median nerve (C5 to T1) | Direct innervation |
|   Lateral pectoral nerve (C5 to C7) | Pectoralis major (clavicular head) | |
|   Musculocutaneous nerve | Biceps brachii, brachialis, and coracobrachialis | Lateral antebrachial cutaneous nerve |
|   Lateral root of median nerve | | |
|     Anterior interosseous nerve | | |
|     Recurrent median nerve (T1) | | |

*Adapted from Moore KL: Clinically oriented anatomy, ed 3, Baltimore, 1992, Williams & Wilkins, p 514, with permission.*

vations in the arm; however, its impingement in the ulnar notch can limit the flexibility of the nerve and cause sensory or distal motor changes in the forearm during flexion of the elbow.

As the ulnar nerve descends the ulnar side of the forearm, it lies sandwiched between the flexor digitorum superficialis and the flexor carpi ulnaris muscles. Along most of its course it accompanies the ulnar artery. In the distal forearm it becomes superficial and passes over the flexor retinaculum to enter the hand.

The motor branches of the ulnar nerve innervate the flexor carpi ulnaris and the ulnar half of the flexor digitorum profundus.

As the ulnar nerve enters the palm of the hand it lies superficial to and alongside the lateral border of the pisiform bone. Just proximal to entering the *tunnel of Guyon*, palmar and dorsal cutaneous branches of the ulnar nerve supply the ulnar aspect of the hand. The ulnar nerve and artery enter the tunnel of Guyon. Just distal to the tunnel the ulnar nerve gives off a superifical and deep branch. The superficial branch gives rise to the common palmar digital nerves that are sensory nerves to the fifth digit and the ulnar half of the fourth digit. When compression of this nerve occurs, the patient complains of paresthesias of one half of the fourth digit and the entire fifth digit. The deep branch of the ulnar nerve sends motor innervation to the hypothenar muscles, the lumbrical muscles of the fourth and fifth digits, all the interossei muscles, and the adductor pollices.[34]

**Median nerve (nerve of the anterior forearm).** The median nerve leaves the brachial plexus anterior to the axillary artery and travels with the brachial artery. It descends in the midline of the arm (the ligament of Struther's holds the median nerve in place in 0.5% to 1% of the population) to the cubital fossa where it lies deep to the bicipital aponeurosis.[27] It has no branches in the arm except for a small vasomotor nerve to the brachial artery.

The median nerve enters the forearm from the arm by passing between the two heads of the pronator teres. The median nerve gives off the anterior interosseous nerve that travels along the interosseous membrane and travels with the ulnar artery. This nerve continues down the forearm between the flexor digitorum profundus and the flexor pollices longus muscles and ends at the pronator quadratus muscle. It is the motor supply to the pronator quadratus, flexor pollices longus, and the radial half of the flexor digitorum profundus. The median nerve descends the forearm by passing down the midline between the flexor digitorum profundus and the flexor digitorum superficialis (Fig. 5-2).

An injury to the pronator teres (pronator teres syndrome) can cause impingement of the median nerve or the anterior interosseus nerve. Being a mixed nerve the Median nerve will present paresthesias, dysesthesias,

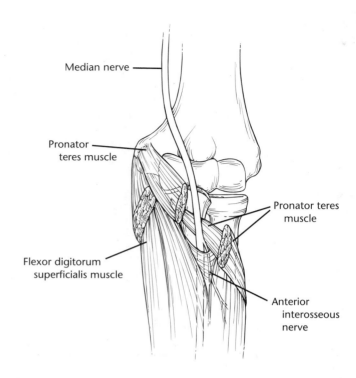

*Fig. 5-2*   The median nerve as it pierces the pronator teres and branches into the anterior interosseous nerve at the anterior aspect of the forearm just distal to the elbow. Anterior view of the elbow.

and radicular pain to the C6 to C7 dermatomes before muscle weakness appears. If impingement is persistent, muscle weakness will be present in the thenar muscles. The direct motor branches of the median nerve in the forearm are to the flexor digitorum superficialis, pronator teres, palmaris longus, and the flexor carpi radialis muscles. Impingement of the anterior interosseus nerve will cause motor changes only. The classic sign of anterior interosseus nerve impingement is the inability of the patient to perform thumb and forefinger opposition (the patient is able to perform apposition) and weakness in forearm pronation (Fig. 5-3).

The median nerve continues and enters the palm of the hand deep to the flexor retinaculum and through the *carpal tunnel* (Fig. 5-4). Compression of the median nerve in this area can be caused by fibrosis of the flexor retinaculum, fluid retention, or injury to the wrist by overuse or trauma and produces the *carpal tunnel syndrome* (see Case 21). The median nerve immediately splits after leaving the carpal tunnel into the motor and the digital branches. These branches are (1) the *common palmar digital nerves*—cutaneous nerves to digits 1, 2, 3, and the radial half of digit 4; (2) the *recurrent branch*—motor nerve to the muscles of the thenar eminence; and (3) the motor branches to the lumbricales 1 and 2. The carpal tunnel syndrome consists of paresthe-

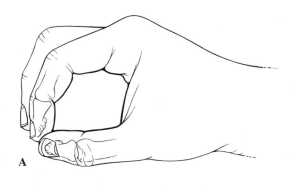

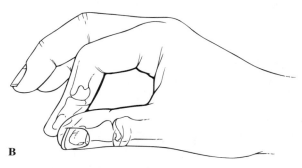

**Fig. 5-3** Hand opposition (**A**) and apposition (**B**); Note the position of the interphalangeal joints of the thumb and index finger in each position.

sias, anesthesias, and radicular pain to the area innervated by the common palmar digital nerve. Further nerve compression, or persistent compression, can cause signs of muscle weakness in the thenar eminence and lumbricals.

**Radial nerve (nerve and the posterior arm, forearm, and hand).** The radial nerve leaves the posterior cord and pierces the medial intermuscular septum to enter the posterior arm and travels down the arm in the radial groove with the profunda brachial artery. Nerve compression in this area produces wrist drop with paresthesias into the lateral forearm (Saturday night palsy). When it reaches the distal lateral arm (just above the lateral epicondyle), it pierces the lateral intermuscular septum to reenter the anterior compartment of the arm. It continues distally by passing anterior to the lateral epicondyle as it enters the forearm.

The *motor* branches in the proximal end of the radial groove of the arm feed the triceps brachii and the anconeus. At the *lateral supracondylar ridge* of the humerus the radial nerve supplies the *brachioradialis* and *extensor carpi radialis longus muscles,* which are muscles commonly involved in lateral epicondylitis (see Case 20). The most commonly involved muscle in lateral epicondylitis is the *extensor carpi radialis brevis* coming off the lateral epicondyle (common extensor tendon).

In the axilla, the sensory branches of the radial nerve give rise to the posterior cutaneous nerve of the arm that supplies the skin of the posterior arm. The sensory branches in the radial groove give rise to the posterior cutaneous nerve of the forearm that supplies the middle of the posterior forearm down to the wrist (Fig. 5-5).

At the elbow the radial nerve crosses anterior to the lateral epicondyle of the humerus and divides into the

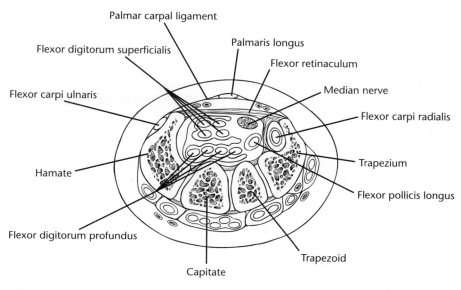

Palmar carpal ligament

Flexor digitorum superficialis

Palmaris longus

Flexor retinaculum

Flexor carpi ulnaris

Median nerve

Flexor carpi radialis

Hamate

Trapezium

Flexor pollicis longus

Flexor digitorum profundus

Trapezoid

Capitate

**Fig. 5-4** The carpal tunnel and its contents. Illustration is at the midcarpal joint.

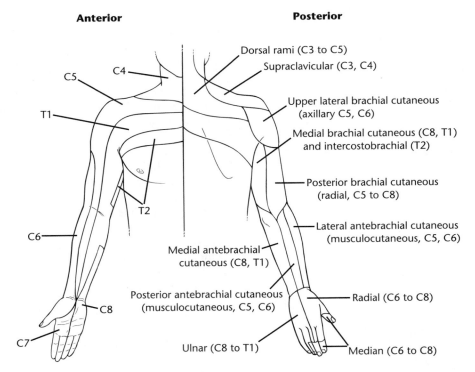

**Fig. 5-5** The cutaneous innervation of the upper extremity. Dermatomal levels are depicted in the anterior view and peripheral nerve cutaneous innervation is presented in the posterior view.

deep and the superficial radial nerve. The deep radial nerve gives motor branches to the supinator and extensor carpi radialis brevis muscles. The nerve then pierces the supinator muscle and winds laterally around the neck of the radius, and when it exits the supinator in the posterior compartment of the forearm it becomes the posterior interosseous nerve (Fig. 5-6).

The superficial radial nerve (general sensory nerve only) runs distally under the cover of the brachioradialis muscle and is accompanied by the radial artery. In the distal forearm it leaves the radial artery, passes posteriorly and enters the posterior compartment where it supplies the skin on the radial side of the dorsum of the wrist, hand, thumb, and the middle of the third finger.

## Neurologic levels of the upper extremities

In evaluating nerve lesions of the upper extremities, the clinician must be able to distinguish between a spinal nerve root lesion and a lesion of a named peripheral nerve. This is accomplished by understanding differences between these nerves (1) areas of cutaneous sensory nerve innervation; (2) muscle strength tests; and (3) deep tendon reflex evaluation (Table 5-2).

When the patient's history indicates a possible lesion to a peripheral nerve the corresponding innervated muscles need to be tested. For instance, in Case 19, muscle

testing of shoulder abduction and external rotation revealed muscle weakness. These muscles are innervated by the motor part of specific peripheral nerves that are branches of the brachial plexus (that is, axillary nerve intervates the deltoid [abduction] and teres minor [external rotation]).

## Reflex levels of the brachial plexus

A deep tendon reflex is used clinically to establish the intactness of the components of the reflex arc. In the cases presented, deep tendon reflexes are tested in each patient. The doctor strikes a tendon that, in turn, causes a contraction of a group of muscles that cause the extremity to jerk (for example, the knee jerk reflex). This test is used to test a monosynaptic reflex arc. The components that make up a monosynaptic reflex are (1) a quick stretch of a tendon, followed by a stretch within the muscle spindle and (2) the afferent neurologic supply to the spindle sending a signal to the dorsal horn that relays it directly to the ventral horn cell. The ventral neuron sends the stimulus via its efferent axons to the muscle group and spindle and causes a reflexive contraction of that muscle group and an inhibitory relaxation of the antagonist muscle group. A nonintact reflex arc indicates a dysfunction in at least one of the following three parts of the reflex arc: (1) the afferent limb;

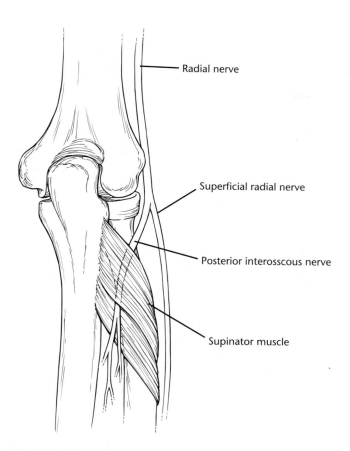

- Radial nerve
- Superficial radial nerve
- Posterior interosscous nerve
- Supinator muscle

***Fig. 5-6*** The radial nerve as it pierces the supinator muscle, travels around the head of the radius, and branches to the posterior interosseus nerve at the elbow. Posterior elbow view.

(2) the reflex center in the spinal cord (central nervous system [CNS]); or (3) the efferent limb. A hyporeflexive response will indicate a lower motor neuron lesion (LMNL). A hypereflexive response is indicative of a CNS lesion and is called an upper motor neuron lesion (UMNL).

## Distribution of dermatomes in the upper extremities

A dermatome is an area of skin that receives sensory innervation from a specific spinal nerve root. When di-agnosing the location of a peripheral nerve lesion, the area of cutaneous sensory anesthesias or paraesthesias may direct the clinician toward a possible dysfunction at the spinal level or in a peripheral named nerve. There are two dermatomal charts, each one being slightly different. It is important to realize that there is overlap between dermatomes. An area of the skin is rarely completely innervated by only one nerve root. Dermatomal mapping only depicts areas that are predominantly innervated by a nerve from a specific spinal nerve level. If the peripheral nerve that gives sensory innervation to a certain area of the skin is severed, the patient will experience total loss of sensation. If a nerve root is the only structure involved, then the patient will experience a change in sensation denoted as a paresthesia (for example, numbness and tingling).

### Shoulder joint

The examining clinician should be familiar with the functional anatomy and biomechanics of the shoulder in order to evaluate patients with shoulder problems (see Case 19).

The shoulder consists of four interrelated joints that are made up of five bony structures: (1) The head of the humerus and glenoid cavity of the scapula join together to form the *glenohumeral joint*; (2) The distal end of the clavicle and the acromion of the scapula join to form the *acromioclavicular joint*; (3) The proximal end of the clavicle joins with the manubrium of the sternum to form the *sternoclavicular joint*; and (4) The posterior aspect of the thoracic ribs join with the anterior aspect of the scapula to form the *scapulothoracic joint*. All are synovial, or diarthrodial, joints except for the scapulothoracic joint that is a bone-muscle-bone articulation. Each of these joints are freely movable and have 6 degrees of freedom.

**Glenohumeral joint.** The glenohumeral (GH) joint is a *ball and socket joint* that consists of the large hemispheric humeral head and a smaller glenoid fossa of the scapula (one third to one fourth the size of the humeral head). The bony structures have a poor surface area fit and are therefore supported by soft tissue structures. This disproportionate fit allows large degrees of freedom in all directions (6 degrees of freedom).[39]

***Table 5-2*** Neurologic levels of the upper extremities and their corresponding motor, reflex, and sensory responses

| Level | Motor test | Reflex | Dermatomal area |
|-------|-----------|--------|-----------------|
| C5 | Shoulder abduction<br>Forearm flexion | Biceps | Lateral arm |
| C6 | Wrist extension | Brachioradialis | Lateral forearm and thumb |
| C7 | Wrist flexion<br>Finger extension | Triceps | Middle finger |
| C8 | Finger flexion | None | Medial forearm and little finger |
| T1 | Finger abduction and adduction | None | Medial arm |

The bony structures of the glenoid cavity and humeral head are covered by a sheet of hyaline cartilage. The hyaline cartilage is thickest in the middle of both the humeral head and the glenoid cavity. The glenoid cavity increases its depth by a fibrocartilage ring called the *glenoid labrum.* The labrum consists of a fibrocartilaginous reflection of the joint capsule, the GH ligaments (superior, middle, and inferior), and the tendon of the long head of the biceps brachii muscle. The purpose of the glenoid labrum is to enhance the curvature of the glenoid fossa and to deepen the socket to give more stability to the joint but not to interfere with joint mobility.[57] The glenoid fossa is slightly retrotilted (by approximately 8 degrees) and in the resting position (arm in anatomic position) is tilted downward 5 degrees.[39] The humeral head is also retroverted about 32 degrees. The anatomic positions of the humeral head and the glenoid fossa allow the humeral head to have a snug fit when the humerus is externally rotated in the GH joint.

Synovial fluid bathes the GH joint and its internal structures. The synovial fluid is produced by synovium, which adheres to the capsule. The capsule is a large, broadened structure that loosely surrounds the GH joint. It attaches medially around the rim of the glenoid cavity proximal to the labrum, and extends to the root of the coracoid process enclosing the proximal attachment of the long head of the biceps. A capsular sleeve is extended along the bicipital groove and surrounds the long head of the biceps brachii. This capsular sleeve (*tenosynovium*) bathes the long tendon in synovial fluid and limits frictional forces in disturbing its function. Tenosynovium is located around any long tendon and is also found in the hand and foot.

The GH capsule attaches laterally at the anatomic neck of the humerus. The capsule is loosely folded, with the arm positioned in its anatomic position, at the inferior aspect and attaches to the surgical neck of the humerus (Fig. 5-7).[31,41] The attachment of the inferior aspect of the capsule allows for the extensive range of motion in the glenohumeral joint without allowing a great amount of stress to be applied to the capsule.

### Ligamentous structures of the glenohumeral joint.
The capsule is reinforced superiorly and anteriorly by the *glenohumeral ligaments,* and superiorly by the *coracohumeral ligament.* The superior, middle, and inferior GH ligaments appear as capsular thickenings at the superior, anterior, and anterior-inferior aspects of the capsule. The coracohumeral ligament attaches from the base of the coracoid process to the proximal end of the bicipital groove. These ligaments check external rotation of the humerus within the glenohumeral joint.[39,57]

At the superior aspect of the glenohumeral joint, but not directly attached to the capsule, is the coracoacromial ligament. This ligament attaches from the acromion to the coracoid process of the scapula. It, along with the acromion, forms an arch that prevents excessive upward displacement of the humeral head and serves as protection from direct trauma to the superior aspect of the GH joint.

The anatomic structures between the acromion and humeral head are of utmost importance to the clinician when evaluating the shoulder. These structures, when injured, produce pain from 60 degrees to 120 degrees of shoulder abduction. This pain presentation pattern is known as the *painful arc* of the GH joint (see Case 19). The structures that are located between the acromion and humeral head are presented in Table 5-3.

During the evaluation of a peripheral joint, the clinician will evaluate active and passive ranges of motion and apply the general rule that if the patient's pain complaints are reproduced during passive range of motion and not during active range of motion, then the injured anatomic structures are the noncontractile components. If the patient's pain complaints are present during active range of motion and not during passive range of motion evaluation, then the contractile components are considered to be the cause of the pathology. However, this rule does not hold true in the shoulder. The noncontractile and contractile structures are so interrelated in the shoulder that motion causes all anatomic structures to be involved.

### Acromioclavicular joint.
The acromioclavicular (AC) joint is classified as a plane type of articulation that consists of a small synovial articulation between the convex facet of the distal clavicle and the concave facet of the proximal acromion of the scapula. The bony structures of the joint are surrounded by fibrocartilage and are bathed in synovial fluid and the entire structure is enclosed in a joint capsule. A wedge-shaped, incomplete articular disc projects into the joint from the superior aspect of the joint capsule and partially divides the joint into two.[32]

The fibrous joint capsule is attached to the margins of the articular surfaces of the acromion and the clavicle. The capsule is supported superiorly and inferiorly by the superior and inferior acromioclavicular ligaments and by the trapezius muscle. The stability of the joint is provided mainly by two sections of the *coracoclavicular ligament,* the conoid and the trapezoid ligaments, which suspend the scapula from the clavicle. The conoid ligament sits medial to the trapezoid ligament. Neither of these ligaments is directly related to the AC capsule. Their location and direction help stabilize the AC joint during motion.

### Sternoclavicular joint.
The sternoclavicular (SC) joint is a saddle type of joint and is a synovial, diarthrodial articulation that exists between the shallow socket of the superolateral part of the manubrium of the sternum and the medial part of the first costal cartilage and the

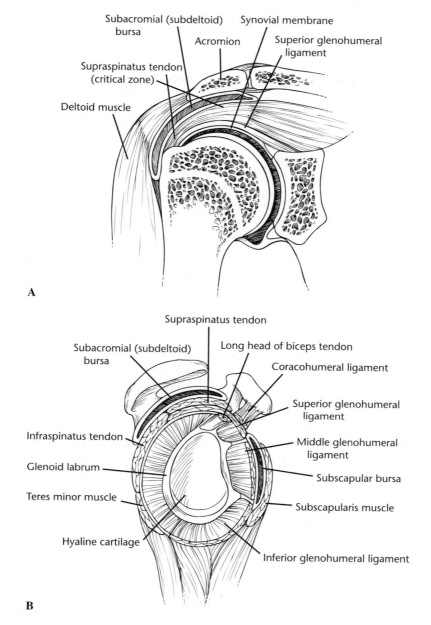

Subacromial (subdeltoid) bursa

Acromion

Synovial membrane

Superior glenohumeral ligament

Supraspinatus tendon (critical zone)

Deltoid muscle

**A**

Supraspinatus tendon

Subacromial (subdeltoid) bursa

Long head of biceps tendon

Coracohumeral ligament

Superior glenohumeral ligament

Infraspinatus tendon

Middle glenohumeral ligament

Glenoid labrum

Subscapular bursa

Teres minor muscle

Subscapularis muscle

Hyaline cartilage

Inferior glenohumeral ligament

**B**

***Fig. 5-7***   The glenohumeral joint of the shoulder. **A,** Anterior view showing the anatomical structures that are located between the acromion and the head of the humerus. **B,** Scaption view showing the rotator cuff muscles (SITS muscles: supraspinatus, infraspinatus, teres minor, and subscapularis) and surrounding ligamentous structures.

enlarged medial end of the clavicle.[32] Because of the difference in sizes of the articular bony surfaces of the clavicle and the manubrium, medial dislocation of the clavicle can occur. The principal stabilizing structure of the SC joint is the *costoclavicular ligament*. This ligament attaches the proximal end of the clavicle to the first rib. The ligament acts as a fulcrum for the gliding motion that occurs during shoulder movement.[29]

Unlike other synovial joint articulations, the articular surfaces of the SC joint are encapsulated by fibrocartilage. A fibrocartilaginous disc (meniscus) exists within the joint. The disc in the SC joint attaches to three structures and divides the joint into two functional units. The three structures are the clavicle, superiorly, and the manubrium and the cartilage of the first rib, inferiorly. The articular disc is continuous with the anterior and

*Table 5-3*   Anatomic structures between the acromion of the scapula and the head of the glenohumeral joint*

| |
| --- |
| Subacromial bursa (subdeltoid bursa) |
| Supraspinatus muscle |
| Glenohumeral ligaments |
|   superior |
|   medial |
|   inferior |
| Coracohumeral ligament |
| Capsule |

*\* All structures have nociceptive fibers and can produce pain.*

posterior SC ligaments that are thickenings of the surrounding fibrous capsule[32] and that reinforce the capsule. The anterior SC ligament prevents excessive movement of the clavicle posteriorly and the posterior SC ligament checks anterior clavicular motion. The interclavicular ligament is a thickening of the superior aspect of the capsule and traverses the length of the jugular notch of the sternum.

The capsule is composed of fibrous tissue that surrounds the entire joint, including the epiphysis of the clavicle. It is supported by anterior and posterior sternoclavicular ligaments and by the interclavicular ligament, superiorly. The inferior aspect of the capsule is thin.

**Shoulder kinematics.** The shoulders move the upper extremities in all the planes of motion. These movements are (1) elevation in the coronal (frontal) plane (abduction and adduction); (2) flexion and extension in the sagittal plane; (3) horizontal adduction and abduction in the transverse (horizontal) plane; and (4) internal and external rotation (torque around the humerus). The shoulder's total range of external and internal rotation is described as 180 degrees (external rotation 108 degrees [60%] and internal rotation 72 degrees [40%]) with the arm placed at anatomic position. With the arm at 90 degrees of abduction the total rotational arc is 120 degrees (more internal rotation) and at full flexion, minimal internal and external rotation is possible. The reason for the change in external and internal rotation motion at different shoulder elevations is GH capsular tightness. As the arm is elevated, the capsule becomes more taut, limiting rotation about the long axis of the humerus.[20,41] The greatest amount of abduction occurs along the plane of the scapula and is called scaption. The unfolding of the inferior part of the joint capsule along this plane allows at least 180 degrees of shoulder motion to occur. Three motion types are involved in a ball-and-socket joint: rotation, translation (gliding), and rolling. These motions combine to produce the concave-convex rule.

The kinematics of the shoulder demonstrates that the humeral head elevates and rotates in the *same* direction during the first 90 degrees of abduction. There is approximately 3 mm of elevation occurring during the first 90

degrees of rotation.[57] After 90 degrees the humeral head descends approximately 0.5 mm for every 30 degrees of continued abduction over 90 degrees. At 180 degrees of abduction, the humeral head has cumulatively ascended 1.5 mm from its resting anatomic position.[41] As is presented in Case 19, inflammation caused by injury to any of the anatomic structures located between the acromion and the ascending humeral head during shoulder abduction will cause a *painful arc* between 60 and 120 degrees.[48] From 0 degrees to 90 degrees, the humeral head has elevated approximately 3 mm. The decrease in area between the acromion and humeral head at 60 degrees appears to be enough to produce pain. At approximately 120 degrees the humeral head has descended enough to allow sufficient space to be produced between the acromion and the humeral head, causing the patient to experience a decrease in pain (Fig. 5-8). Depending on which anatomic structures are injured, the humeral head may not descend after 90 degrees but may ascend irregularly (for example, in rotator cuff tear or injury). This warrants evaluation of the inferior glide of the GH joint.

The production of scapular motion is a major component of shoulder abduction. During the first 60 degrees of shoulder abduction the scapula is settling in position.[20,31,32] After the first 60 degrees of shoulder abduction, the scapula begins to protract at a ratio of 1 degree for every 2 degrees of humeral motion (2:1 ratio). The ratio between humeral motion and scapular protraction continues until abduction is completed. This ratio can change. If a weight is held in the hand of the abducting shoulder, the ratio changes to 3:2. Other research[11,57] indicates that the ratio may be 1.5:1 (1.5 degrees of humeral abduction and 1 degree of scapula protraction). The rhythm that is presented between the humerus and the scapula is known as *scapulohumeral rhythm.*

External rotation of the humerus accompanies shoulder abduction. This prevents the greater tubercle of the humerus from contacting the acromion of the scapula and allows the 2:1 ratio between humeral motion and scapular protraction to continue. External rotation also allows the humeral head to make better contact with the glenoid fossa by increasing the contact surface area between these two structures. The anterior ligaments of the glenohumeral joint also become taut during external rotation. This, along with the increase in the area of surface contact between the head of the humerus and the glenoid fossa, increases joint stability and is called the *closed-packed position* of the shoulder. The closed-packed position for the other extremity joints are listed in Table 5-4.

## Motions of acromioclavicular and sternoclavicular joints

The greater part of the AC joint motion occurs in the first 20 degrees and the last 45 degrees of shoulder

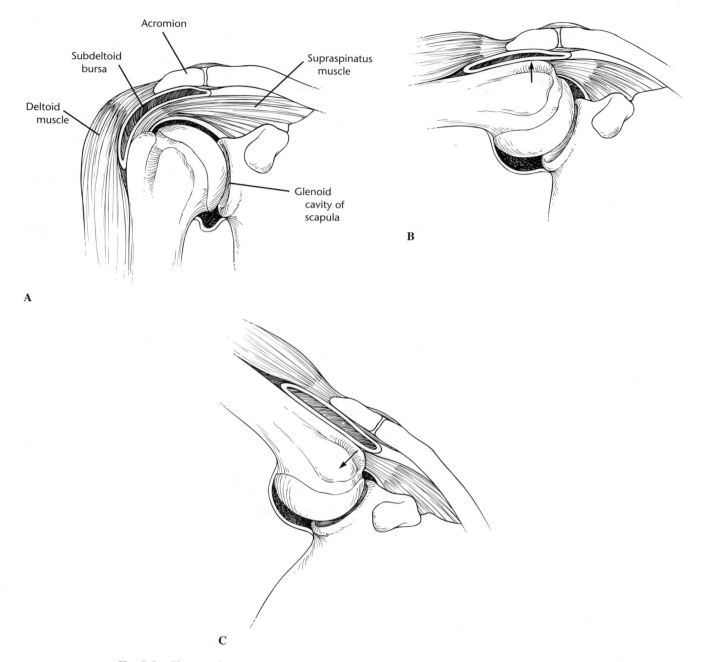

*Fig. 5-8* The translatory motion of the glenohumeral joint during shoulder abduction. **A,** The shoulder in anatomical position. **B,** At 90 degrees. **C,** At 170 degrees. Note that the head of the humerus translates upward during the first 90 degrees of shoulder abduction and translates in a downward direction after 90 degrees to 180 degrees (see text).

abduction. The AC joint elevates from its anatomic position by a total of 20 degrees. At the end of elevation, approximately 40 degrees of backward rotation occurs. This backward rotation causes the scapula to complete protraction. There are six degrees of freedom within the AC joint. The scapula, during shoulder abduction, rotates in the frontal plane, wings in the horizontal plane, and tips in the sagittal plane.[11,57] The motions

that occur between the clavicle and the scapula in the AC joint during shoulder abduction are: elevation (accompanied with scapular protraction), clavicular backward rotation with scapular tipping, and scapular rotation along the frontal plane. The conoid ligament is the axis of rotation (at 30 degrees) during scapular protraction and retraction and clavicular elevation. The trapezoid ligament is the axis of rotation (at 60 degrees)

*Table 5-4*    The closed-packed position of the common joints of the upper and lower extremities

| Joint | Position |
|---|---|
| Shoulder | Combined horizontal abduction and external rotation |
| Elbow | Extension |
| Wrist | Extension with radial deviation |
| Hip | Internal rotation with extension and abduction |
| Knee | Extension with external rotation |
| Ankle | Dorsiflexion |

*Table 5-5*    Shoulder joint motion involved in abduction*

| Joint | Type of motion | Total range of motion |
|---|---|---|
| Glenohumeral | Elevation and rotation | 120 degrees of total motion |
| Acromioclavicular | Elevation | First 20 degrees and last 45 degrees |
|  | Backward rotation | 40 degrees of total motion |
| Sternoclavicular | Depression | First 20 degrees and last 45 degrees |
|  | Backward rotation | 40 degrees of total motion |
| Scapulothoracic | Protraction | 60 to 180 degrees 60 degrees of total motion (2:1 ratio) |

*\* The total range of motion of the shoulder (180 degrees) is an accumulation of the motions of all the joints.*

for the scapula during tipping and clavicular backward rotation, and the AC joint is the axis of rotation (at 30 degrees) during scapular rotation along the frontal plane.[11]

Inman[20] describes SC motion as 4 degrees of clavicular depression, relative to the manubrium for every 10 degrees of shoulder abduction. This occurs during the first 90 degrees of shoulder abduction. Beyond 90 degrees depression is minimal, and at the end of abduction, backward rotation occurs. The two functional units of the SC joint are between the sternum and the meniscus and the clavicle and the meniscus. Anterior-posterior gliding (clavicular protraction and retraction) occurs between the sternum and the meniscus and superoinferior gliding (clavicular elevation and depression) occurs between the clavicle and the meniscus. The meniscus adds to the stability of the SC joint by absorbing shock transmitted to the clavicle from its lateral end and checks the tendency for medial dislocation of the clavicle.[57] The poor fit between the clavicle and manubrium encourages medial dislocation of the clavicle. In addition to the meniscus compensating for this disadvantage, the ligamentous structures are also thickened at the anterior aspect of the joint and attach to other surrounding structures. The costoclavicular ligament that attaches to the clavicle and first rib is the principal stabilizing structure of the SC joint.[57] This ligament acts as an axis of rotation for the significant gliding movement (protraction/retraction) that occurs between the clavicle and manubrium during shoulder motion[28,32] and limits clavicular elevation.[32,57] The anterior and posterior SC ligaments reinforce the capsule by checking the anterior and posterior movements at the clavicle upon the manubrium, and the interclavicular ligament checks depression of the clavicle (Table 5-5).

## Kinetics of the shoulder

This section will concentrate on shoulder abduction and will present the participating muscles according to their different phases.

There are 17 muscles involved in shoulder motion. Three important aspects of muscle function are involved in shoulder motion: (1) A muscle that exerts an effect on the humerus must act in concert with other muscles to avoid producing dislocating forces at the joint; (2) A single muscle may span several joints, exerting an effect on each joint; and (3) The extensive range of shoulder motion causes muscle function to vary depending on the position of the arm in space. Usually, the action of any muscle may be inferred from its origin and insertion, but this is not the case in the shoulder. For example, when the arm is at the side, contraction of the middle deltoid muscle lifts the humerus along its axis but does not produce abduction because the line of action of the middle deltoid fibers is essentially parallel to the long axis of the humerus (Fig. 5-9).[57] However, if the action of the middle portion of the deltoid is coupled with other muscle actions, abduction can occur. Shoulder abduction is initiated by the supraspinatus muscle and

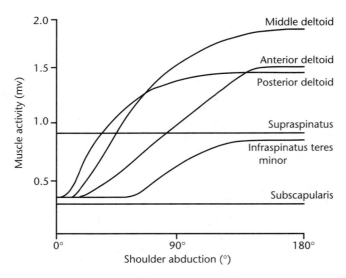

*Fig. 5-9*    Muscle action during shoulder abduction.

the other rotator cuff muscles (the infraspinatus, teres minor, and subscapularis muscles) act to stabilize and bring the humeral head into the glenoid cavity, thereby providing a fixed fulcrum for shoulder abduction.[57] The rotator cuff muscles are oriented so that their contraction may not only result in a desired motion but also resist displacement of the humeral head. In this way they act as a *dynamic stabilizer* of the glenohumeral joint.

Muscle sequencing during shoulder abduction is controversial. The discussion centers around which muscles initiate abduction. As described, the deltoid muscle alone cannot initiate shoulder abduction because of its fiber orientation. The supraspinatus muscle is required to participate in the motion. Perry[39] states that shoulder abduction is initiated by the cocontraction of the supraspinatus and the deltoid muscles, and that cocontraction produces a fulcrum around which rotation occurs. Celli et al.[8] state that shoulder abduction is initiated by the supraspinatus and the deltoid muscle is active at 20 degrees of shoulder abduction. Of further interest is the activity of the middle, posterior, and anterior deltoid muscles. All these muscles are active during abduction. The primary activity of the anterior deltoid is shoulder flexion and internal rotation, and it is a secondary shoulder abductor. The primary activity of the posterior deltoid is shoulder extension and external rotation, and it, also, is a secondary abductor.[11,57] The synchrony of these muscles assists in the motion of shoulder abduction without flexion and extension or internal and external rotation occurring simultaneously because their primary motions are canceled by each other.

The trapezius muscle demonstrates constant activity at the beginning of motion (it acts as a stabilizer) and then increases its activity at approximately 60 degrees of shoulder abduction. It acts to stabilize scapular motion for the first 60 degrees and to participate in scapular protraction from 60 degrees to 180 degrees.

As discussed earlier, shoulder abduction is accompanied by external rotation of the humerus. Activity of the infraspinatus and teres minor muscles cause external rotation of the humerus that, in turn, moves the greater tuberosity in a direction that prevents it from making contact with the acromion of the scapula.[8] The infraspinatus muscle increases in activity from 0 to 90 degrees of external rotation. After 30 degrees of humeral external rotation, the teres minor muscle increases its activity and participates in the motion.[8] As is illustrated in shoulder abduction, not only do the infraspinatus and teres minor muscles participate in glenohumeral joint stability (they act as dynamic stabilizers) but they also produce forces that cause external rotation of the shoulder.

## Anatomy and biomechanics of the elbow

The elbow acts as a lever system that, along with the other joints, changes the direction of the upper extremity to put the hand in the most effective functional position. The elbow consists of three bones: the distal end of the humerus and the proximal ends of the radius and the ulna. The distal end of the humerus is formed by the hyperboloid trochlea medially and the convex capitellum laterally (Fig. 5-10).

The proximal end of the ulna consists of the olecranon process, posteriorly, and the coronoid process, anteriorly. The concave trochlear fossa lies between the two processes, and the radial notch is on the lateral proximal surface of the ulna. The proximal end of the radius consists of a cup-shaped articular surface called the radial head.

Three separate synovial-diarthrodial articulations form the elbow joint. The *humeroulnar* joint consists of the articulation of the trochlea of the humerus and the trochlear fossa of the ulna, the *humeroradial* joint comprises the capitellum of the humerus and the radial head; and the proximal *radioulnar* joint consists of the head of the radius and the radial notch on the humerus. Each bony surface is covered with hyaline cartilage, bathed in synovial fluid, and encapsulated by the fibrous joint capsule. The humeroulnar and humeroradial articulations are ginglymoid (hinged) joints that permit flexion and extension. The proximal radioulnar articulation is a trochoid joint that permits forearm pronation and supination. The elbow joint is therefore classified as a trochoginglymoid joint. Case 20 illustrates a patient who has a problem with the elbow. Pain elicited during palpation of the joint and its surrounding structures informs the clinician about anatomic structures that need further evaluation. In this case pain is elicited at the lateral condyle of the humerus. The description and location of the pain indicate that the soft tissue structures of the wrist extensors and the elbow flexors are involved. The elbow is further evaluated for its range of motion (flexion and extension, and supination and pronation). In this case, no pain is elicited during passive range of motion of the elbow, indicating that the internal joint is not injured. The presence of pain during active range of motion, provocative maneuvers, and muscle tests indicate that the surrounding muscles are causing the patient's chief complaint.

**Articular surface area of the elbow.** The articular surface of the trochlea of the humerus is 330 degrees in circumference. This surface fits snugly with the trochlear fossa of the ulna, which is 190 degrees in circumference. The range of motion that can occur between these two surfaces is the difference in their combined circumferen-

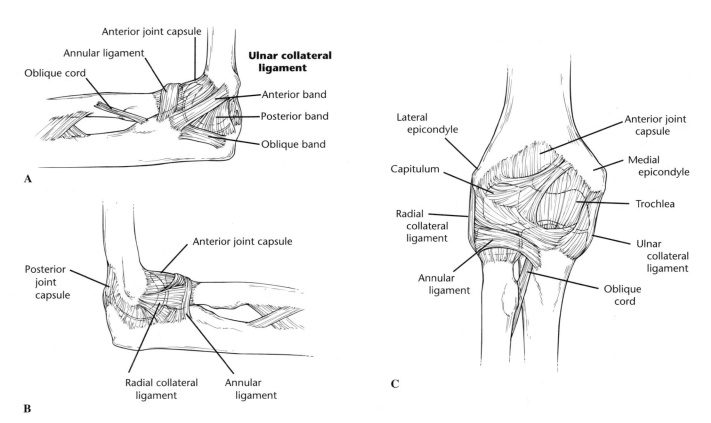

*Fig. 5-10* The anatomical structures of the elbow joint. **A,** Medial view. **B,** Lateral view. **C,** Anterior view. Note the extent of the capsular and ligamentous coverage of the elbow.

tial areas, namely, 140 degrees. The joint surface area of the capitellum is 180 degrees and the joining surface of the proximal radial head is 40 degrees, again giving a total surface area of 140 degrees.[35] Gliding is the major motion that occurs between the joint surfaces of the elbow during flexion and extension. Rolling becomes the major motion at the end of flexion and extension. At the end of flexion, the coronoid process of the ulna comes into contact with the coronoid fossa; in extension, the olecranon of the ulna makes contact with the humeral olecranon fossa. Contact of these structures results in rolling being the major joint motion.[33]

Unlike the situation with the shoulder joint, the concave-convex rule is followed during flexion and extension in the elbow. The movement of the concave trochlea of the ulna on a fixed humerus (convex condyle) causes translation and rotation to occur in the same direction. This motion occurs during flexion or extension of the elbow. During a push-up or pull-up when the ulna and radius are fixed (concave structures), the humerus will translate in the opposite direction of rotation.

**Elbow stabilization.** The elbow is stabilized by the interlocking configuration of the articulating surfaces.

The main contributor to bony stability is the articulation between the trochlea and the trochlea fossa.[46] The coronoid process provides a block to posterior displacement as the elbow flexes, whereas the humeroradial articulation provides resistance to valgus stress across the elbow and inhibits posterior dislocation at 90 degrees or more of flexion. The proximal radioulnar articulation does not provide significant elbow stability but simply allows forearm pronation and supination to occur.[46]

Soft tissue stability of the elbow is provided by the ligamentous structures that support the joint capsule. The medial collateral ligament is the major stabilizer against valgus stress. The medial collateral ligament has fibers moving in two directions—an anterior oblique direction and a posterior oblique fiber direction. The posterior oblique fiber direction is the more important stabilizing component of the elbow medial collateral ligament.[46]

The elbow does not possess a true lateral collateral ligament. The anatomic structure that acts as a lateral collateral ligament originates on the lateral epicondyle of the distal humerus and attaches to the annular ligament but does not attach directly to bone. The anconeus muscle provides additional stability against varus elbow stress.[3] The valgus and varus orthopedic provocative tests are used to evaluate the medial and lateral collateral ligaments, respectively. The annular ligament surrounds the radial head and holds it securely in place to articulate with the capitellum. The ligament allows the radial head to rotate along its long axis and cross over the ulna during forearm pronation. In children younger than 7 years of age and up to 10 years of age, there is a tendency of the radial head to subluxate out of the annular ligament support. At birth to approximately 7 years of age, the annular ligament is round. At approximately 7 years of age the annular ligament becomes cone shaped with the distal diameter being smaller than the proximal diameter. The cone shape increases the stability of the radial head in the annular ligament and snugly holds the radial head in position. Before 7 years of age, if the forearm is forcibly pulled, the radial head may slip out of the ligament and will produce severe pain and an inability of the child to pronate or supinate the forearm (Malgaigne's luxation or pulled-elbow syndrome).

**Carrying angle of the elbow.** Anatomically, the medial lip of the trochlea extends more distally than does its lateral lip. The trochlea also extends more distally than does the capitellum. This difference in length and shape produces a carrying angle when the arm and forearm are in the anatomic position. The valgus angle of the elbow ranges from 10 to 15 degrees. The purpose of the angle is to allow the forearm to extend beyond the width of the pelvis and to be able to sustain high tensile stresses on its medial aspect. The clinician needs to be aware that the carrying angle is a normal finding and is not indicative of an elbow occult fracture. Of interest, the knee and elbow both present with a valgus angle in the anatomic position. In the knee, this angle is measured by the quadriceps angle (the Q angle). The stresses that are applied are primarily on the medial aspect of both these joints. In both cases degeneration and arthritic changes present primarily on the medial aspect.

**Cubital fossa.** The cubital fossa is a triangle-shaped area in front of the elbow and distal to the skin crease. It has the following boundaries: lateral—brachioradialis muscle; medial—pronator teres muscle; superior—imaginary line drawn between two epicondyles (forms the base of the triangle); the floor—supinator and brachialis muscles; and the roof—the bicipital aponeurosis and deep fascia.

The cubital fossa contains the biceps brachii tendon, brachial artery, the median nerve, the bifurcation of the brachial artery into the radial and ulnar arteries, the radial nerve, and the deep radial nerve. The median cubital vein crosses the roof of the fossa. The clinical significance of the fossa is that the brachial artery is close to the surface and is easily palpable. Blood pressure is most commonly taken in this area using the brachial pulse.

**Kinetics of elbow function.** The muscles that produce elbow flexion and extension originate on the proximal aspect of the humerus or on the scapula. The major muscles of elbow flexion and extension are the brachialis and the triceps brachii, respectively. The brachialis muscle and the lateral and medial heads of the triceps muscle traverse one joint (elbow) and are considered power muscles. The long head of the triceps affects two joints, the GH joint (it assists in shoulder extension) and the elbow joint. A muscle that crosses more than one joint is an endurance muscle and produces a wide range of joint motion. During concentric action, the brachialis flexes and the triceps extends the elbow. During eccentric action these muscles will change joint angle and resist gravity. The brachialis muscle will contract eccentrically when the elbow is being extended against gravity.

In Case 20 muscle tests revealed no change in strength during elbow flexion when the forearm was supinated or pronated. Muscles are labelled either primary (major) movers or secondary (minor) movers. A primary mover's main function is to cause the motion described. A secondary mover assists the primary mover in the described motion. During elbow flexion the primary mover is the brachialis, regardless of the position the forearm is in. The biceps brachii muscle assists the brachialis muscle in elbow flexion only when the forearm is supinated. The biceps brachii muscle is not a primary mover in any of the motions it participates in. It is a secondary mover in both elbow flexion and forearm supination in which it assists the supinator muscle.[3]

### Anterior antebrachial muscles

The anterior antebrachial muscles are divided into six layers, layer 1 being the deepest and layer 6 the most superficial (Table 5-6). The common flexor tendon of the medial epicondyle is the origin of the muscles involved in wrist and hand flexion. Of this group, the flexor carpi ulnaris and flexor carpi radialis are the major

*Table 5-6*   The anterior antebrachial muscles and their respective layers

| Layer | Muscles |
| --- | --- |
| 1 (deep) | Supinator and pronator quadratus |
| 2 | Flexor pollicis longus and flexor digitorum profundus |
| 3 | Pronator teres |
| 4 | Flexor digitorum superficialis |
| 5 | Palmaris longus, flexor carpi radialis, and flexor carpi ulnaris |
| 6 (superficial) | Brachioradialis |

wrist flexors. The palmaris longus and flexor digitorum superficialis muscles assist wrist flexion and are major contributors to hand flexion (making a fist).[3] During eccentric muscle activity these muscles will move the wrist from the flexed position to the extended position.

When a concentric muscle action occurs, the insertion moves closer to the muscle origin. The force produced is parallel to the origin and insertion of the muscle. Muscles, however, are not always in direct alignment with the joints they move. Therefore, secondary motion occurs when each muscle contracts. In the case of the flexor carpi ulnaris muscles, wrist flexion is accompanied with ulnar deviation. In accordance, the flexor carpi radialis muscle simultaneously flexes and radially deviates the wrist. Simultaneous concentric contraction of the flexor carpi ulnaris and flexor carpi radialis muscles produce a net result of wrist flexion, with ulnar and radial deviation nullifying each other.

The other muscle whose origin is located at the medial epicondyle of the humerus is the pronator teres. It also has an origin at the coronoid process of the ulna. During concentric action, the pronator teres assists the brachialis muscle during elbow flexion and assists the pronator quadratus muscle during forearm pronation.

The flexor digitorum profundus muscle originates along the proximal three fourths of the medial and anterior surface of the ulna. It is the only muscle that flexes the distal interphalangeal joints and is innervated by the anterior interosseous nerve, a branch of the median nerve. The flexor pollices longus originates along the anterior surface of the radius and the anterior interosseous membrane. It inserts into the base of the distal phalanx of the thumb and is innervated by the anterior interosseous nerve. An impingement of the anterior interosseous nerve will affect hand opposition and forearm pronation.

**Cutaneous nerve supply of the anterior forearm.** Sensory innervation of the forearm is supplied by the medial and lateral antebrachial cutaneous nerves. The dermatomal innervation of the medial area of the forearm is from C8 at the distal aspect and from T1 at the proximal aspect. The lateral dermatomal area of the forearm is innervated by C6 (see Fig. 5-5).

### Forearm extensors and the back of the hand

**Posterior antebrachial compartment.** The posterior (extensor) region of the forearm contains 11 muscles (Table 5-7) that are organized into four functional groups. The majority of the muscles of the superficial extensor layer originate at the common extensor tendon of the lateral epicondyle of the humerus. The exceptions are the brachioradialis and the extensor carpi radialis longus muscles. These originate at the supracondylar ridge of the lateral epicondyle. The concentric action of the majority of the superficial muscles is to extend the wrist and to stabilize the wrist during forceful twisting (for example, twisting jar caps) by static contraction with the wrist flexors. The exception is the brachioradialis muscle, which inserts onto the ulnar styloid and assists in elbow flexion. When testing the deep tendon reflex of the brachioradialis (C6) the motion response is elbow flexion not wrist extension (see Cases 19 to 22).

All of the muscle groups of the extensor forearm compartment are innervated by the radial nerve or by its branches, the deep radial or the posterior interosseous nerves. The radial nerve divides into the deep radial and the superficial radial nerves just after it enters the forearm. The superficial radial nerve is entirely sensory and innervates the skin on the dorsum of the wrist, hand, thumb, and lateral one and one-half digits (thumb, second finger, and radial one-half of third finger).[34] The deep radial nerve is entirely motor refraction and supplies the extensor carpi radialis brevis and supinator muscles. It then pierces the supinator muscle and curves around the lateral side of the radius, entering the posterior fascial compartment of the forearm and providing

*Table 5-7* Innervations, muscles, and actions of the posterior compartment of the forearm

| Innervation | Muscle(s) | Concentric action |
|---|---|---|
| Radial nerve (C5 to C7) | Brachioradialis | Flexes forearm |
| | Extensor carpi radialis longus | Extend and abduct wrist |
| | Anconeus | Stabilizes elbow joint on full extension |
| Deep branch of the radial nerve (C5 to C6) | Supinator | Supinates forearm |
| | Extensor carpi radialis brevis | Extends and abducts wrist |
| Posterior interosseous nerve (C7 to C8) | Extensor digitorum | Extends medial four digits at metacarpophalangeal joints |
| | Extensor carpi ulnaris | Extends and abducts wrist |
| | Extensor digiti minimi | Extends fifth digit at metacarpophalangeal joint |
| | Abductor pollicis longus | Abducts thumb at carpometacarpal joint |
| | Extensor pollicis longus | Extends distal phalanx of thumb at metacarpophalangeal and interphalangeal joints |
| | Extensor pollicis brevis | Extends thumb at carpometacarpal joint |
| | Extensor indicis | Extends second digit and assists in extending hand |

many branches to the wrist extensor muscles.[34] In the posterior fascial compartment, the deep radial nerve gives off the posterior interosseous nerve that travels with the posterior interosseous artery and supplies the deep extensor muscles.

Fractures to the head and neck of the radius can lead to injury of the deep radial nerve. In this case, there would be no sensory loss or total wrist drop. The radial nerve innervates the extensor carpi radialis longus before it penetrates the supinator and wraps around the radial neck. The patient, however, would have difficulty with extension of the thumb and fingers at the metacarpal phalangeal joint, with thumb abduction and opposition, and with wrist extension. An injury to the superficial radial nerve would cause a sensory loss over the dorsum of the hand.

**Synovial tunnels of the dorsum of the wrist.** There are six synovial tunnels over the dorsum of the wrist through which the tendons of the posterior forearm muscles pass in order to enter the dorsum of the hand. Tunnel 1 contains the abductor pollices longus and extensor pollices brevis tendons. These muscles surround the anatomic snuffbox. Injury to the tenosynovium or tendons produces stenosing tenosynovitis (de Quervain's disease, see Case 22). Finkelstein's test is used to evaluate this area. Passing through the tunnel 2 are the tendons of the extensor carpi radialis longus and brevis muscles. Tunnel 3 consists of the extensor pollices longus tendon that turns 45 degrees at Lister's tubercle and is the posterior boundary of the anatomic snuffbox. The extensor digitorum and extensor indices tendons pass through tunnel 4 and the extensor digiti minimi tendon is in tunnel 5. Tunnel 6 consists of the extensor carpi ulnaris tendon. Any one of these tunnels may produce an impingement causing pain in the dorsum of the wrist and hand and into the lateral posterior aspects of the forearm.

**Cutaneous nerves of the posterior forearm and hand.** The cutaneous nerve innervation to the posterior forearm is from three nerves: the medial antebrachial cutaneous nerve from the brachial plexus; the lateral antebrachial cutaneous nerve from the musculocutaneous nerve; and the posterior antebrachial cutaneous nerve from the radial nerve in the radial groove.

The cutaneous nerve innervation over the dorsum of the hand is also from three nerves: the superficial radial nerve, the ulnar nerve, and the median nerve.

## Functional anatomy and biomechanics of the wrist

The position of the wrist is essential for proper functioning of the digital flexor and extensor muscles to cause an effective hand grasp.[52] The wrist is considered a two-joint system. The midcarpal joint and the intercarpal joint allow for large ranges of motion with less exposed articular surfaces and less tendency for structural pinch at extremes of wrist range of motion and also allow for flatter multiple joint surfaces that are more capable of withstanding imposed pressures. The wrist consists of eight carpal bones, with the distal radius; the structures of the ulnocarpal space; and the proximal end of the metacarpal bones (Fig. 5-11). There are two distinct rows of carpal bones (proximal and distal). The proximal row is very movable and consists of the scaphoid, lunate, and triquetrum bones. These bones articulate with the radius and an intraarticular disc to form the radiocarpal joint. The distal row consists of the trapezium, trapezoid, capitate, and hamate bones, is immobile, and is supported by the interosseous ligaments. The pisiform bone functions as a sesamoid bone for the flexor carpi ulnaris and enhances this muscle's mechanical advantage.

The palmar surface of the carpus is concave and is the floor for the carpal tunnel. The distal aspect of the radius, lunate, and triquetrum bones articulate with the distal ulna to form the ulnocarpal complex that allows a large range of motion of the wrist and hand without compromising hand prehension. The ulnocarpal complex consists of a meniscus homologue (radiotriquetral ligament) that dissipates stresses, a triangular fibrocartilage (articular disc), the ulnolunate ligament, the ulnar collateral ligament, and poorly distinguishable dorsal and palmar radioulnar ligaments. Between the meniscus and the triangular fibrocartilage is the prestyloid recess that is filled with synovium.

The wrist consists of flexion and extension and abduction (radial) and adduction (ulnar) deviations. These

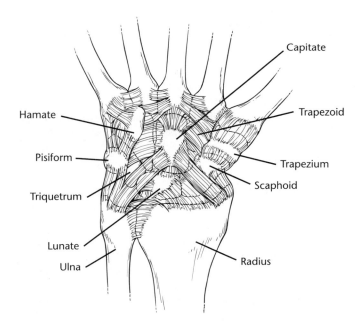

*Fig. 5-11*  The anatomical structures of the wrist joint.

motions occur in the midcarpal and radiocarpal joints. Approximately 60% of total wrist flexion occurs at the midcarpal joint and 40% of total flexion occurs at the radiocarpal joint; 60% of total extension occurs at the radiocarpal joint and 40% of total extension occurs at the midcarpal joint.

Radial and ulnar wrist deviations consist of the proximal carpal row moving in the opposite direction. Coupled motion also occurs in the proximal row. During radial deviation the trapezoid compresses the scaphoid onto the radial styloid. The distal pole of the scaphoid rotates toward the palm. During ulnar deviation the triquetrum glides distally on the hamate and causes the distal aspect of the hamate to move dorsally.

Supination and pronation are not considered wrist motions but do play an important role in hand positioning. From pronation to supination the ulnar head glides in the radial sigmoid notch from a dorsal distal position to a palmar proximal position.

The position of the wrist determines the strength of a hand grasp. By positioning the wrist in a direction opposite to the fingers, the functional length of the digital tendons are altered so that maximal finger movement can be attained.[52] Twenty degrees of wrist extension and slight ulnar deviation are needed for maximal hand grasp (power grasp) strength. Wrist extension is accompanied with finger flexion and finger extension accompanies wrist flexion.

Kinetically, the main function of the wrist is to transmit compressive loads from the hand to the forearm. Compressive loads are directed across the carpus along a vector force pattern that passes through the head of the capitate bone to the scapholunate junction and to the distal radioulnar triangular fibrocartilage surfaces.[54] The major forearm muscle that is pertinent to the integrity of wrist stability is the flexor carpi ulnaris. Its function controls the wrist in slight ulnar deviation and co-contracts with the extensor carpi ulnaris to stabilize the wrist during a power grasp. During a precision hand grasp the wrist does not have a fixed position. The forearm muscles put the hand in a position to achieve the task needed (that is, the wrist is in a different position when writing than when picking up a coin with precision grasp).

## Functional anatomy and biomechanics of the hand

In Cases 21 and 22 a thorough hand examination is performed. The hand can inform the clinician as to the condition of the peripheral nerves, muscles, and sensory innervation of the entire upper extremities. This section will focus on the functional anatomy and biomechanics of the hand with relevance to the physical examination.

There are 19 bones and 14 joints in the hand. The hand has five metacarpal bones and 14 phalanges. Each finger is made up of three phalanges and two joints, with the thumb having only one joint. All are synovial diarthrodial joints. Three arches are formed by the bony structures of the hand, two transverse and one longitudinal arch. The *proximal transverse arch,* with the capitate as its keystone, lies at the level of the distal carpus and is fixed. The *distal transverse arch,* with the head of the third metacarpal as its center, passes through all the metacarpal heads and is more mobile than the proximal transverse arch. The longitudinal arch is composed of the four digital rays and the proximal carpus. The second and third metacarpal bones form the central pillar of this arch.[54]

The finger rays are numbered from the radial side to the ulnar side. Ray I is the thumb and rays II to V are the fingers from the index finger to the little finger.

**Shape and motion of the joints of the hand.** There are three joint shapes in the hand. The carpometacarpal (CMC) joints are saddle shaped and allow primarily flexion and extension, the metacarpophalangeal (MCP) joints are unicondylar and allow all ranges of motion, whereas the interphalangeal (IP) joints are bicondylar and allow mostly flexion and extension.

The second and third metacarpals are linked to the trapezoid and capitate bones and to each other by tight-fitting joints that are basically immobile. The second and third metacarpal joints are considered the *immobile unit of the hand* and function to support objects during a power grasp allowing the rest of the hand to wrap around the object. The fourth and fifth metacarpal joints articulate with the hamate and permit approximately 10 to 15 degrees of flexion and extension at the fourth CMC joint and 20 to 30 degrees at the fifth CMC joint. When a fist is made, the metacarpals will displace in a palmar direction. This allows cupping of the hand and is essential for gripping (Fig. 5-12).

As was stated earlier, the MCP joints of the four fingers are unicondylar diarthrodial joints. These joints allow motion in three planes: flexion and extension, abduction and adduction, and rotation along the long axis (torque) that is coupled with abduction and adduction. Average flexion at the MCP joints of the fingers is approximately 90 degrees. The MCP joint of the fifth finger is the most mobile and flexes 95 degrees, whereas the MCP joint of the second (index) finger will flex 70 degrees.[54] Abduction averages a 10-degree variance from the third (middle) finger and adduction places the fingers in parallel with the third finger. The thumb web allows the thumb to abduct, flex, and rotate more freely from the rest of the fingers of the hand. The adductor pollices muscle is located within the web.

The proximal interphalangeal (PIP) and distal interphalangeal (DIP) joints of the four digits are bicondylar hinge joints (tongue-and-groove fit articulating surfaces).[34] Flexion and extension are the only motions

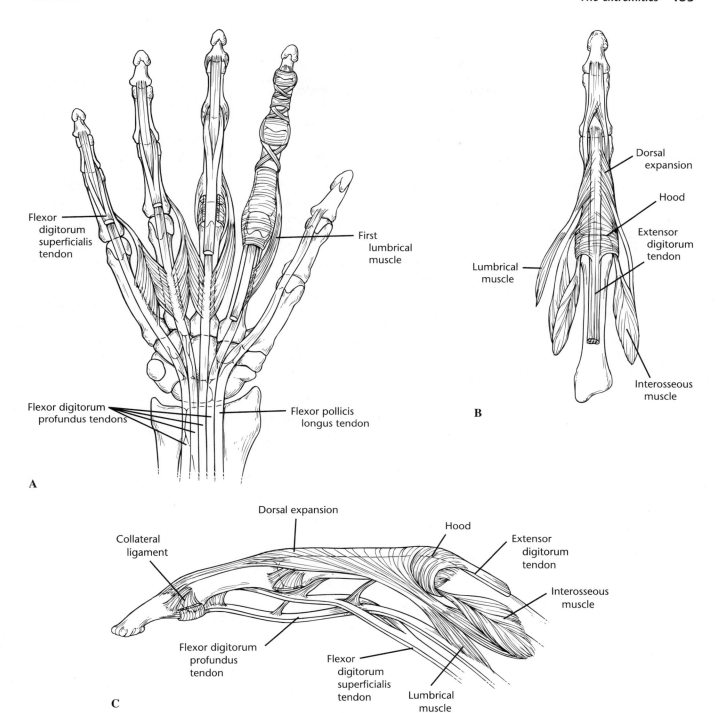

*Fig. 5-12*   The anatomical structures of the hand. **A,** Palmar view. **B,** Dorsal view of the index finger, and **C,** Lateral view of the index finger. Note the presence of the extensor hood on the dorsal aspect of the finger and the intricate retinacular network of the palmar aspect of the hand on the palmar view.

that occur in these joints. On average, 110 degrees of flexion occurs at the PIP joint and 90 degrees of flexion occurs at the DIP joint.

**Prehension (hand grasp).** The unique orientation of the thumb, the large web space, and the special configuration of the CMC joint of the thumb afford this digit great mobility and versatility. The CMC joint of the thumb is a saddle joint that meets with the trapezium. The most unique feature of the human hand is the ability of the thumb to oppose the finger. *Opposition* is part of human development that separates humans from their closest ancestor, the ape. An ape can appose the thumb but cannot oppose it. Apposition is the ability to put the flat part of the distal tuft of a finger in contact with the flat part of the distal tuft of the thumb. Opposition is the ability to put the tips of the distal tufts of the thumb and finger in contact by simultaneously flexing the DIP of the contact finger and the IP of the thumb. This maneuver gives humans the ability to grasp objects with precision. The use of hand opposition is called *precision grasp.*

There are two categories of hand grasp: the power and the precision grasp. Power grasp is the ability of the hand to hold an object snug against the immobile first and second rays; the third, fourth, and fifth rays wrap around the object, and the thumb is in line with the radius and is adducted against the object. The wrist is in 20 degrees of extension as well and slightly ulnar deviated (Fig. 5-13). In a precision grasp the thumb is abducted, internally rotated, and flexed. In thumb opposition the CMC joint allows abduction and slight internal rotation.[4] Further internal rotation and slight flexion of the thumb occurs at the MCP joint and flexion occurs at the PIP and DIP joints.

Prehensile movements of the hand are those in which an object is seized and held partly or wholly within the compass of the hand. Bejjani[4] describes efficient prehensile function as depending on a multitude of factors, the most important of which are (1) mobility of the CMC joint of the thumb and the MCP joints of the fourth and fifth fingers; (2) relative rigidity of the second and third CMC joints; (3) stability of the longitudinal finger and thumb arches; (4) balanced synergism and antagonism between the long extrinsic muscles and the intrinsic muscles; (5) wrist angle during grasp; and (6) adequate sensory input from all areas of the hand including the precise relationships of the length, mobility, and position of each ray.

**Power grip versus precision grip.** Power grip (power grasp), described above, is performed with the fingers flexed at all three joints and the object held securely between the finger and palm of the hand with the thumb. The wrist is extended 20 degrees and is slightly ulnar deviated. The long axis of the thumb aligns with the long axis of the forearm. Precision grip (precision handling) involves the manipulation of the hand to hold small objects. The objects are finely controlled by the hand with the thumb and the flexor aspects of the fingers. The wrist position varies so as to increase the hand range. The fingers are generally semiflexed, and the thumb is abducted and opposed.

Included in a precision grip is the dynamic tripod wherein the thumb, index finger, and middle finger work in close synergy, and the ring and little fingers are used largely for support and static control. Another example of precision grip is pinching a small object between the thumb and index finger. This is called tip pinch or palmar pinch. The ability of the fingers to pinch incorporates the *extensor release mechanism* of the extensor hood of the fingers. If a finger is flexed to 90 degrees at the PIP joint the extensor hood is pulled forward and the extensor digitorum, lumbricals, interossei, and flexor digitorum profundus muscles are placed at a biomechanical disadvantage. The muscle control of the DIP joint is forfeited, and the pressure applied by the opposed thumb can manipulate the position of the distal phalanx

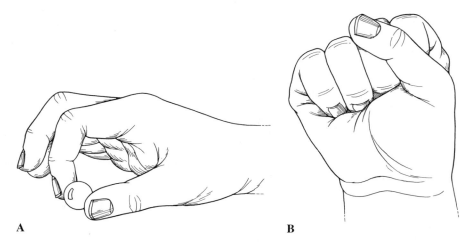

**A**        **B**

*Fig. 5-13*   **A,** Precision grasp and **B,** power grasp of the hand.

causing the pinch. The pinching mechanism allows an individual to pick up very small objects such as a paper clip or a dime and is the most precise type of grip.

**Wrist and hand as diagnostic tools.** In Cases 20, 21, and 22 thorough muscle testing of the wrist and hand is conducted. The wrist is positioned in flexion, extension, and ulnar and radial deviation. In each position the patient is asked to hold and resist a force applied by the examiner. The force is applied for 6 seconds. Any resistance deviation presented by the patient is recorded by the clinician. The patient is then asked to resist a force throughout a range of motion.

General muscle function of the hand is first evaluated by a handshake. Any gross weakness can be determined at this time. A thorough muscle evaluation of the thumb is then conducted (Table 5-8). By placing the thumb in different static positions, muscles of the thenar eminence and forearm can be evaluated. The thumb is first abducted and a resistance is applied by the clinician. The concentric muscle actions of the abductor pollicis longus and abductor pollicis brevis are tested. The former muscle is innervated by the radial nerve and the latter, by the recurrent branch of the median nerve. Any weakness in performing this task informs the examiner that either nerve may have a lesion. The lesion may be located by testing other muscles that are innervated by the same peripheral nerves. Thumb internal rotation, thumb MCP flexion, and thumb IP flexion are also tested. Thumb internal rotation is performed by concentric action of the opponens pollicis located in the thenar eminence and innervated by the recurrent branch of the median nerve. Flexion of the MCP joint is caused by concentric action of the flexor pollicis brevis in the thenar eminence that is also innervated by the recurrent branch of the median nerve. Interphalangeal joint flexion is produced by concentric action of the flexor pollicis longus in the anterior compartment of the forearm with innervation from the anterior interosseous nerve just distal to the elbow. Other motions that are not involved in opposition of the thumb are extension and adduction. The extensor pollicis brevis extends the CMC joint and the extensor pollicis longus extends the MCP and IP joints. Both are innervated by the radial nerve via the posterior interosseous nerve. Thumb adduction is caused by concentric action of the adductor pollicis innervated by the ulnar nerve.

In summary, an understanding of the kinesiology of the upper extremities helps the clinician determine functional problems and develop protocols for treatment. Nerve root lesions cause muscle weakness of only the muscles innervated by the nerve root, whereas peripheral nerve lesions can produce gross weakness or flaccidity of muscle groups. Tests that determine hand motor function include the bilateral handshake that determines overall hand weakness. The inability to flex the IP of the thumb during hand opposition informs the clinician that a lesion may be present at the pronator teres with the anterior interosseous nerve. The inability of the patient to oppose the thumb but still be able to flex the IP joint is indicative of a lesion in the carpal tunnel (see Case 21). Changes in touch or the presence of pain helps the clinician locate lesions in sensory nerves.

## THE LOWER EXTREMITIES

This section will focus on the joints and the common impingement syndromes affecting the lower extremities. The piriformis syndrome (Case 16) and the anatomic deviation of the sciatic nerve will be presented. This section will begin with an introduction to hyaline cartilage and bone healing (see Case 23).

### General histological features of cartilage
EMILE GOUBRAN

Cartilage plays a major role within every synovial diarthrodial articulation. The most common type of cartilage is hyaline cartilage. The human body contains three types of cartilage: *hyaline cartilage, elastic cartilage,* and *white fibrocartilage.* All cartilaginous structures are spe-

***Table 5-8***   Muscles and nerves involved in thumb movements

| Thumb motion | Muscles | Innervation |
| --- | --- | --- |
| Flexion | Flexor pollicis brevis | Recurrent median nerve |
| | Flexor pollicis longus | Anterior interosseous nerve from the median nerve |
| Extension | Extensor pollicis longus | Posterior interosseous nerve from radial nerve |
| | Extensor pollicis brevis | Posterior interosseous nerve from radial nerve |
| Adduction | Adductor pollicis | Ulnar nerve |
| Abduction | Abductor pollicis longus | Radial nerve |
| | Abductor pollicis brevis | Recurrent median nerve |
| Opposition | Abductor pollicis longus, abductor pollicis brevis, opponens pollicis, and flexor pollicis brevis and flexor pollicis longus | Radial nerve |
| | | Recurrent median nerve |
| | | Recurrent median nerve |
| | | Anterior interosseous nerve from the median nerve |

cialized, avascular connective tissue.[14] Cartilage is made up of a matrix of ground substance composed chemically of glycoproteins and proteoglycans. The main proteoglycan in cartilage is chondroitin sulfate, which is responsible for the firm consistency of the cartilage matrix.[21,55] The matrix does not demonstrate any apparent fibers under the light microscope (LM). However, under the electron microscope, the matrix is seen to be composed of fine collagen fibrils that help to enforce the structure of the cartilage matrix.[10]

Cartilage cells are called *chondrocytes.* They may occur singly as flat to round cells or in groups called cell nests or isogenous groups. These nests, or groups, contain multiple chondrocytes that are widely separated and surrounded by matrix.

The surface of most cartilage is covered by a fibrocellular, vascular membrane called the *perichondrium.*[50] The perichondrium is composed of an outer dense fibrous layer and an inner cellular or chondrogenic layer. Because of the inner layer, the perichondrium is important in the nutrition growth, and regeneration of cartilage.[22]

The growth of cartilage occurs through two mechanisms: (1) by appositional growth in which layers of cartilage are added to the surface by the perichondrium and (2) by interstitial growth through cellular division of chondrocytes in the matrix resulting in the development of cell nests.[21,50,55] Hyaline cartilage is of main concern to this section because it is the cartilage that covers synovial joint surfaces.

**Adaptation of hyaline cartilage to articular surfaces.** Hyaline cartilage covering bony articular surfaces located within joints is called *articular cartilage.* The perichondrium does not cover the articular hyaline cartilage and thus there is a smooth articulating surface with minimal friction.[16] The synovial fluid in synovial joints supplements for the loss of the perichondrium by providing nutrients to the articular cartilage[30] and by reducing the friction between articulating surfaces.

The articular hyaline cartilage consists of five zones resting on the subchondral bone (Fig. 5-14). Starting from the most peripheral zone, the articular surface consists of the superficial tangential zone that makes up 10% to 20% of the total cartilage. The articular surface is an extremely smooth surface that is bathed in synovial fluid. The chondrocytic cells are tangential because of the shearing forces that occur on the articular surface when joint motion occurs.[21]

The middle zone comprises of 40% to 60% of the total hyaline cartilage thickness and consists of cuboid chondrocyte cells. The deep zone is 30% of the total cartilage thickness and lies on the tidemark that separates the deep zone from the calcified cartilage zone. The calcified cartilage zone is a zone of transition from cartilage to bone and protects the subchondral bone.

**Histology of meniscal structures of the knee.** The meniscal structures found inside the synovial cavity of the knee joint are two semilunar pieces of cartilage made up almost completely of white fibrocartilage.[45] The histology of white fibrocartilage is characterized by abundant collagen bundles that run in various directions in the matrix and enclosed between them are rows of single chondrocytes (Fig. 5-15). The abundance of collagen in the matrix gives fibrocartilage the ability to withstand tension applied to its surfaces.[6] As with articular hyaline cartilage, there is no perichondrium covering the surfaces of fibrocartilage because it exists between articulating surfaces.[25]

### General histologic features of bone

In Case 23, the diagnosis was a fractured femoral neck. A knowledge of normal bone development is necessary to understand the healing properties of bone. This section discusses the histology of bone along with its healing properties.

Bone is a specialized connective tissue (CT) belonging to the skeletal system. It is hard in consistency because

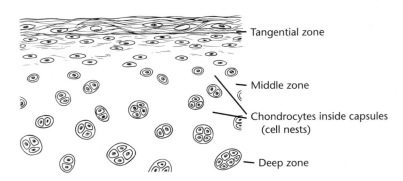

*Fig. 5-14*    Three zones of hyaline cartilage.

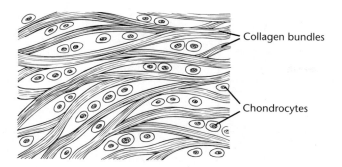

*Fig. 5-15* Fibrocartilage.

of mineral salts in its matrix.[6] Compact bone tissue has the following components:

1. The bone matrix. Bone matrix is produced in the form of thin sheets known as bone lamellae, which have organic and inorganic components. The organic matrix is similar to that of hyaline cartilage, with more collagen fibers that are arranged parallel to each other within the lamella. The collagen fibers in one lamella run at right angles to those of the adjacent lamella (Fig. 5-16).[14] This arrangement of collagen fibers allows bone to withstand a higher degree

of mechanical stresses. the inorganic matrix consists largely of calcium phosphate deposited as *hydroxyapatite*. This mineral deposit is what gives the bone its bony consistency.

2. Bone cells. There are four basic types of bone cells. (a) *Osteocytes* are oval cells with processes existing within lacunae, which are bone spaces between lamellae. Osteocytes extend their processes into bony canaliculi that connect lacunae together and serve as channels for passage of interstitial fluid.[9] Osteocytes function to maintain the bone matrix. (b) *Osteogenic or osteoprogenitor* cells are found on bone surfaces and resemble fibroblasts in appearance. They are undifferentiated bone cells that give rise to osteoblasts. (c) *Osteoblasts* are bone-forming cells found on bone surfaces. They are large cuboidal cells with interconnected processes that function to produce the organic bone matrix and later help in the process of its calcification.[14] (d) *Osteoclasts* are bone destroying cells found on bone surfaces. They cause bone resorption that entails decalcification of bone matrix and causes a breakdown of the organic matrix. Osteoclasts are large, giant cells with multiple nuclei and vacuolated cytoplasm. They are found against bone surfaces undergoing resorption and appear to fill up

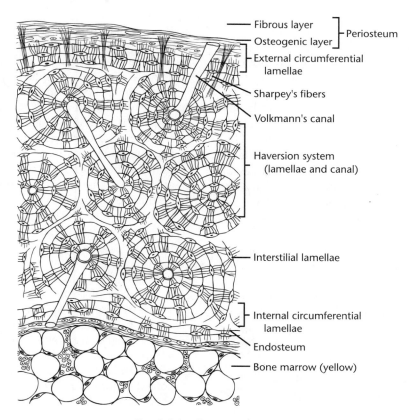

*Fig. 5-16* Compact bone.

deep concavities called Howship's lacunae.[22] During menopause, osteoblastic activity decreases and osteoclastic activity remains the same. Estrogen normally binds with the osteoblast and facilitates its activity. Without estrogen, osteoblastic activity decreases leading to bony resorption and osteoporosis (see Case 12). All women will lose approximately the same amount of bone because of menopause. The factor that determines whether bone fracture will occur is the bone mass of the woman before the start of menopause.

3. The *periosteum* is a membrane on the outer surface of bone that is made up of outer fibrous and an inner osteogenic layer that is rich in blood vessels. The osteogenic layer consists of osteogenic cells that include osteoprongenitor cells and osteoblasts.[30] The periosteum is important in the nutritive, growth, reconstructive, and regenerative functions of healing bone. On the inner part of cortical bone is the *endosteum*. The endosteum is a membrane lining with bone marrow cavities and has one layer of osteogenic cells.

**Types of bone.** There are two types of bone: *compact* (cortical), or ivory, bone and *cancellous,* or spongy, bone. Compact bone is found in the shafts of long bones. In cross section, a long bone has a large marrow cavity filled with yellow (inactive) bone marrow and lined with endosteum. The bone lamellae are located in two areas of bone: the external circumferential (periosteal) lamellae are located under the periosteum and the internal circumferential (endosteal) lamelae are juxtaposed to the endosteum. Other lamellae between the periosteum and the endosteum are arranged in concentric layers around blood vessels and are called Haversian lamellae. The canal occupied by the blood vessel is called a Haversian canal. Both the canal and the surrounding lamellae constitute the *Haversian system.*[21] The blood vessel of the Haversian canal supplies nutrients and oxygen to the osteocytes via the bony canaliculi. Interstitial lamellae are lamellae that occupy areas between the Haversian systems (Fig. 5-17).

*Volkmann's canals* are bony channels that contain blood vessels and nerves.[25] They carry vessels and nerves to Haversian canals from the periosteum and the endosteum. Sharpey's fibers are collagen fibers that extend from the periosteum into the external circumferential and interstitial lamellae of bone. They strengthen muscle attachments to bone and keep the periosteum attached firmly to the bone.[25]

**Bone growth.** Bones grow in length through the activity of the epiphyseal cartilage disc.[10] Like hyaline cartilage, the epiphyseal disc has different zones that represent a sequence of events in the process of intracartilaginous ossification (Fig. 5-18). Intracartilaginous os-

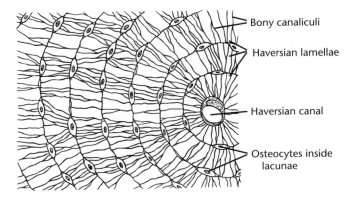

**Fig. 5-17** Haversian system of bone.

sification adds bone at each end of the diaphysis, thereby increasing the length of the diaphysis.

The epiphyseal disc shows the following zones starting the epiphysis and proceeding toward the diaphysis:

1. Zone of resting cartilage. This zone looks like typical hyaline cartilage with cells and cell nests scattered in the matrix.

2. Zone of proliferating or arranged cartilage. This zone shows flattened chondrocytes in longitudinal columns arranged like a pile of coins. Cartilage cells in this zone proliferate with minimal cartilage matrix between them.

3. Zone of mature cartilage cells. This zone shows longitudinal columns of cartilage cells that appear large and rounded or cuboidal. These cells produce the enzyme alkaline phosphatase that gradually brings about the calcification of cartilage matrix.

4. Zone of calcified and degenerating cartilage. Cartilage matrix becomes calcified and appears darkly basophilic. The cartilage cells imprisoned inside their lacunae undergo degeneration as a result of lack of nutrition because of inability of tissue fluid to permeate through the calcified cartilage matrix. As a result of this degeneration of cartilage cells, the lacunae become empty and usually open into one another, especially those that are vertically aligned, because there is little matrix separating them, thus creating multiple longitudinal tunnels. In a cross-sectional view, this zone has a honeycomb appearance.

5. Zone of ossification. The tunnels soon become invaded by vascular osteogenic tissue from the marrow cavity. Ostoblasts then line up over the calcified tunnel walls and lay down bone. The first bone to develop is cancellous; the central part of this bone will resorb to add to the medullary cavity and the outer zone develops into compact bone by being filled with Haversian systems as previously described.

The process of ossification and the increase in length of bones occurs through the activity of the epiphyseal

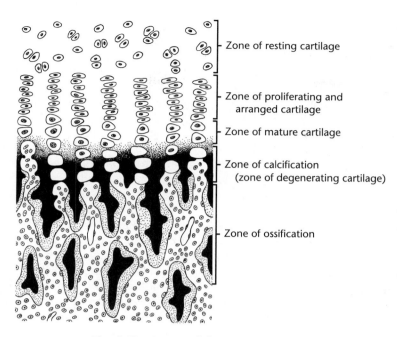

Zone of resting cartilage

Zone of proliferating and arranged cartilage

Zone of mature cartilage

Zone of calcification (zone of degenerating cartilage)

Zone of ossification

*Fig. 5-18*   Layers of the epiphyseal disc.

disc. Cartilage cells are formed at the proliferation zone, whereas other cartilage cells degenerate and disappear at the calcification zone, thus keeping the thickness of the epiphyseal disc constant while forming and adding bone to the length of the diaphysis.

This process, however, does not continue through life. The growth of most long bones ceases by the age of 20 years (bones of the spine continue to grow till the age of 25 years approximately). This is because proliferation of cartilage in epiphyseal discs is inhibited by high levels of gonadal hormones.[14] There is, therefore, no growth at the zone of proliferation to compensate for the degenerating cartilage. The result is a gradual diminution in thickness of the epiphyseal disc until it becomes completely replaced by bone; the epiphyses of bones become fused with the diaphysis (physis).

**Bone growth in width.** Increase in bone width occurs through the osteogenic activity of the periosteum which, by intramembranous ossification, adds circumferential lamellae to the outer surface of bone.[14] Addition of bone to the outside causes increase in the width of bones, however, the thickness of bone does not increase much because of bone resorption taking place inside (medullary side). The endosteum, after resorption occurs, adds few circumferential lamellae by membranous ossification.

**Remodeling and reconstruction of bone.** In response to mechanical stress, bones undergo continuous reconstruction and remodeling.[30] In this process, the primary Haversian systems, as well as the circumferential lamellae at a later stage undergo resorption at certain areas through vascular buds invading from the periosteum or the endosteum. In deeper parts of bone, resorption may occur as a result of some osteocytes assuming a resorptive activity, a process known as osteolysis.[30] In all cases, cavities are created in bone and appear as longitudinal tunnels. These tunnels become invaded by vascular osteogenic tissue from periosteum or endosteum, and osteoblasts start laying down concentric lamellae to convert the cavities into Haversian systems with a central canal containing blood vessels.

The remaining portions of the old Haversian systems constitute the interstitial lamellae. After reconstruction is completed, periosteum and endosteum lay down new circumferential lamellae. Some of the fibers of the periosteum become incorporated into the outer circumferential lamellae as Sharpey's fibers.

The process of absorption and reconstruction may be repeated several times and old Haversian systems become replaced by new ones.

### Anatomy and biomechanics of the lower extremities
GARY M. GREENSTEIN

The functional anatomy and biomechanics of the lower extremity for this text are best explained by describing common impingement syndromes and the functions of the joints of the lower extremities as they relate to the cases in Chapter 1.

**Common entrapments of the lower extremities.** Few impingement syndromes exist in the lower extremities. The more common maladies are presented in this section. The major nerves of the lower extremities are the femoral, the sciatic, and the obturator nerves. Their cutaneous branches are shown in Figure 5-19).

The cutaneous branches of the femoral nerve are usually entrapped at the level of the inguinal ligament. The lateral femoral cutaneous nerve innervates the lateral aspect of the thigh and can be impinged upon as it passes the inguinal ligament (*meralgia paresthetica*). On rare occasion the femoral nerve is impinged upon as it passes between the inguinal ligament and the hip. A patient with this condition complains of anterior and medial thigh pain.

The *piriformis syndrome* (see Case 16) is most commonly confused with the lumbar intervertebral disc syndrome with sciatic radiculopathy (see Case 14).[16] Subtle differences can affect the working diagnosis. Usually, in a peripheral nerve radiculopathy the pain travels to multiple dermatomes, and muscle weakness, if present, is more diffuse than in a nerve root radiculopathy. The anatomic basis for the piriformis syndrome is that, on occasion, the common peroneal part of the sciatic nerve pierces through the piriformis muscle (Fig. 5-20). When injury or tightness occurs in this muscle the patient complains of radicular pain along this nerve (see Case 16). Orthopedic provocative tests are usually negative because the contributing factor is not in the lumbar spine.[13,16]

The obturator nerve sends cutaneous branches to the medial portion of the thigh above the saphenous zone. Pain from *obturator nerve impingement* is usually located in the medial aspect of the thigh, and muscle weakness involves the adductor muscles. Impingement may occur in the obturator canal and is usually caused by a hernia in this area. The pathognomonic symptom for this impingement is pain into the medial aspect of the thigh when intraabdominal pressure is increased (Valsalva's maneuver).[27,34]

Another fairly common entrapment, the *tarsal tunnel entrapment,* occurs at the medial aspect of the ankle. The tibial nerve passes through this tunnel and causes radicular pain into the dorsum of the foot and, at times, up into the calf.

**Functional anatomy and biomechanics of the lower joints of the extremities.**

*Hip.* The bony structures of the iliofemoral joint (the hip) is depicted by a ball that fits within a socket. The

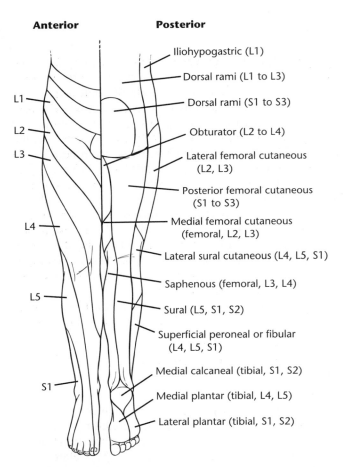

**Anterior**    **Posterior**

Iliohypogastric (L1)

Dorsal rami (L1 to L3)

Dorsal rami (S1 to S3)

Obturator (L2 to L4)

Lateral femoral cutaneous (L2, L3)

Posterior femoral cutaneous (S1 to S3)

Medial femoral cutaneous (femoral, L2, L3)

Lateral sural cutaneous (L4, L5, S1)

Saphenous (femoral, L3, L4)

Sural (L5, S1, S2)

Superficial peroneal or fibular (L4, L5, S1)

Medial calcaneal (tibial, S1, S2)

Medial plantar (tibial, L4, L5)

Lateral plantar (tibial, S1, S2)

**Fig. 5-19** Cutaneous distribution of the lower extremity. Dermatomal levels are presented in the anterior view and peripheral nerve cutaneous innervation is presented in the posterior view.

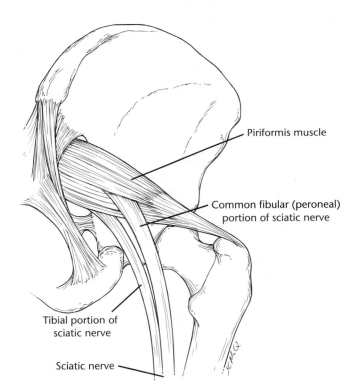

Piriformis muscle

Common fibular (peroneal) portion of sciatic nerve

Tibial portion of sciatic nerve

Sciatic nerve

**Fig. 5-20** The atypical position of the sciatic nerve and its relationship to the piriformis.

ball is the head of the femur and the socket is the acetabulum of the pelvis (Fig. 5-21). The femoral head is a spherical structure that fits snugly into the acetabulum. The acetabulum consists of three bones: the ilium, the ischium, and the pubis. The epiphyseal line of the acetabulum is triradiate and fuses by 17 years of age. The hyaline cartilage of the femoral head and the acetabulum is the thickest in its respective joint areas to resist joint reaction forces that center at the superior aspect of the femoral head.[36]

The femoral head has a thin cortical shell that surrounds the cancellous bone. The cancellous bone of the femoral head presents two distinctive trabecullar patterns: a medial trabecular pattern that forms in re-

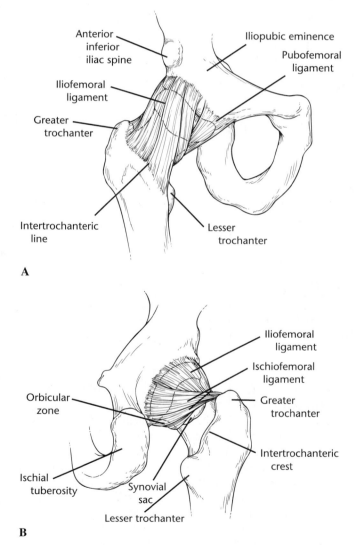

**A**

**B**

*Fig. 5-21*    The anatomical structures of the hip joint. **A,** Anterior view. **B,** Posterior view. The ligaments of the hip are strong bands that support the hip joint.

sponse to the reactive forces applied to the hip and the lateral trabecular pattern that is formed by the activity of the lateral muscular group.[36]

A distinctive limp is present in 85% of patients who have hip injuries. The patient leans toward the injured hip when walking (*trendelenburg gait*).[25a] The limp moves the center of mass toward the center of rotation of the involved hip, which concomitantly decreases the length of the moment arm causing a decrease in total moment applied to the hip (Fig. 5-22). Other pathologies can also cause this limp in the hip. The two most common are (1) hip pathology (see Case 23) and (2) weakness of the tensor fascia lata, gluteus medius, and gluteus minimus muscles.[36]

Two angles are measured between the femoral neck and head, and the femoral shaft. The *angle of inclination* is measured in the coronal plane and has a range of 90 to 135 degrees (average, 125 degrees); the angle of *anteversion* is measured in the sagittal plane and is 12 degrees on average.[24,36]

Any change in the angle of inclination will cause a valgus or varus presentation of the hip. An angle greater than 125 degrees will produce *coxa valga,* whereas an angle less than 125 degrees will produce *coxa vara.* In response to the valgus or varus deformity at the hip, a concomitant angular change occurs at the knees. Coxa valga produces genu varum (bowlegs) and coxa varum produces genu valgum (knock-knees). Early detection of coxa valga or vara can prevent the possible occurrence of other pathologic conditions such as slipped capital femoral epiphysis, Legg-Calve-Perthes disease, or hip dislocation.[36]

An increase in the anteversion angle of the femur can cause lower extremity internal rotation, and conversely, too little anteversion (retroversion) produces lower extremity external rotation. A more common finding is coxa vara with an increase in anteversion.

### Articular capsule of the iliofemoral joint (hip)

The fibrous hip joint capsule attaches from the brim of the acetabulum to the intertrochanteric line and anatomic neck posteriorly. The capsule is a strong, thick cylindrical sleeve that is supported by large ligaments (Fig. 5-21). The collagen fibers of the capsule course obliquely or spirally. Some of the deep fibers of the joint capsule pass around the neck of the femur to produce the *orbicular zone.* These fibers form a collar that constricts the capsule and helps hold the femoral head in the acetabulum.[34] Some of the deep longitudinal fibers of the capsule form retinacula that support the blood vessels that supply the head and neck of the femur.

The iliofemoral joint is surrounded by three large, strong ligaments. They are the iliofemoral ligament, the pubofemoral ligament, and the ischiofemoral ligament.

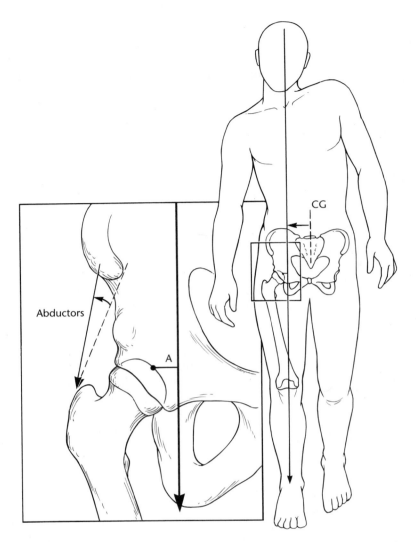

***Fig. 5-22*** The affect of moment and its explanation of trendelenburg gait. When injury to the hip occurs, the patient will lean toward the bad hip during gait, moving the center of gravity (CG) closer to the axis of hip rotation. This decreases the lever arm distance (A) between the center of gravity and the hip axis, therefore decreasing the total moment about the hip joint. The abductor muscles' direction of force is also changed, decreasing total forces about the hip.

The *iliofemoral ligament,* called the Y ligament because of its attachments, is a very strong ligament that covers the anterior aspect of the joint capsule. The dual function of the iliofemoral ligament functions via a *screw-home mechanism* to prevent overextension and to secure the femoral head in the acetabulum. In support of the screw-home mechanism are the other ligaments that support the iliofemoral joint: the *pubofemoral* and *ischiofemoral* ligaments. The pubofemoral ligament prevents excessive extension and abduction of the hip and the ischiofemoral ligament reinforces the capsule posteriorly.[34] It assists the iliofemoral ligament during extension by securing the femoral head into the acetabulum and prevents hyperextension.

## Muscles and fascia that surround the hip joint

**Gluteal region.** The fascia of the lateral compartment of the gluteal region becomes thickened and forms a wide band that develops to form the iliotibial tract (band). The iliotibial tract begins at the iliac crest tubercle and traverses the length of the thigh to the lateral aspect of the tibia (Gerty's tubercle) and head of the fibula. The tract passes directly over the greater trochanter of the femur and a bursa prevents direct contact of the tract with the trochanter. The tract envelops the tensor fascia lata muscle at its proximal end and receives fibers from the gluteus maximus muscle. The muscles of the posterior and lateral compartments are presented in Table 5-9.

*Table 5-9*   Muscles and their peripheral nerve supply in the gluteal region

| Nerve | Muscle | Concentric action |
|---|---|---|
| **Posterior compartment** | | |
| Obturator nerve (L3 to L4) | Obturator externus | External rotation of the hip |
| Nerve to quadratus femoris (L4 to S1) | Inferior gemellus and quadratus femoris | External rotation of the hip<br>External rotation of the hip |
| Inferior gluteal nerve (L5 to S2) | Gluteus maximus | Extension of hip |
| Nerve to obturator internus (L5 to S1) | Obturator internus and superior gemellus | External rotation of hip, abduction of flexed thigh, |
| Nerve to piriformis (S1 to S2) | Piriformis | steadying of femoral head in acetabulum |
| **Lateral compartment** | | |
| Superior gluteal nerve (L4 to S1) | Gluteus medius, gluteus minimus, and tensor fascia lata | Abduction of hip and medial rotation |

## Compartments of the thigh

**Fascial compartments.** There are three fascial compartments of the anterior thigh. They are separated by intermuscular septa that pass from the fascia lata to the linea aspera of the femur. The three fascial compartments are identified according to their anatomical location on the thigh. They are the anterior, posterior, and medial compartments.

The anterior compartment contains the femoral triangle, femoral sheath, adductor canal, and muscles that cause hip flexion and knee extension during concentric action. The posterior compartment of the thigh contains muscles that, during concentric action, produce hip extension and knee flexion; and the medial compartment of the thigh produce hip adduction during concentric action (Table 5-10).

The contents of the *femoral triangle* are the femoral nerve, artery, vein, and lymphatic vessels. The *femoral sheath* is located in the femoral triangle and is an extension of the internal investing layer of the deep fascia of the anterior and posterior abdominal wall. There are three compartments in the sheath. The lateral compartment contains the femoral artery, the intermediate compartment contains the femoral vein, and the medial compartment contains the lymphatic vessels. The medial compartment is also known as the *femoral canal.* The femoral nerve is not located in the sheath or canal of the femoral triangle.

The femoral pulse can be readily palpated from this area. Any lesion that occurs within this area can lead to arterial and neurologic sequelae. As is illustrated in Case 23, the femoral pulse is taken during an evaluation of the lower extremities. Mrs. Esther P. complains of pain located over the inguinal canal, femoral triangle, and posterior aspect of the buttocks. These pain locations are a common presentation for a patient who has some type of hip pathology. Further evaluation of this patient reveals that she has a limited range of hip motion and x-ray films reveal a fracture of the femoral neck with some necrosis of the head. The necrosis is probably caused by damage to either the femoral circumflex arteries or the obturator artery. Elderly women are more prone to bone fracture because of the development of osteopenia after menopause. This is presented in Esther's case by the loss of bone density observed on x-ray films.

The *adductor canal* is a narrow fascial tunnel that begins at the apex of the femoral triangle and ends at the *adductor hiatus.* The adductor hiatus is an opening in the tendinous insertion of the adductor magnus that is covered by the sartorius muscle. The contents of the adductor canal are the femoral artery and vein, saphenous nerve, and branches of the obturator nerve as it travels to the knee. These structures pass through the hiatus to travel further down the lower extremity to the foot.

**Popliteal fossa.** The popliteal fossa is located at the posterior aspect of the knee. It is a diamond-shaped intermuscular area that is bounded by the biceps femoris and lateral head of the gastrocnemius and plantaris on the lateral aspect and by the semitendinosus, semimembranosus, and medial head of the gastrocnemius on the medial aspect. The contents of the popliteal fossa are presented in Table 5-11.

The peripheral nerves that travel through the popliteal fossa are the tibial nerve that gives off genicular branches to the knee and the sural nerve that is a general sensory nerve to the lateral aspect of the ankle and foot. The common peroneal nerve also travels through the popliteal fossa and gives off genicular branches to the knee and the peroneal communicating nerve that anastomose with the sural nerve.

## Knee

The knee is a hinge articulation that consists of the *tibiofemoral* and *patellofemoral* joints (Fig. 5-23). The bones that are part of the knee joint are the femur, the tibia, and the patella. The tibiofemoral joint is a synovial diarthrodial articulation that consists of interarticular ligaments and two large menisci. The medial condyle

*Table 5-10* Muscles of the lower extremities, their actions, and innervations

| Nerve and level | Motor innervation (muscle) | Concentric action |
|---|---|---|
| **Anterior thigh compartment** | | |
| (L1 to L3) | Psoas major | Hip flexion |
| Femoral nerve (L2 to L3) | Iliacus | Hip flexion |
| | Sartorius | Hip flexion |
| | | Hip external rotation |
| | | Knee flexion |
| | Pectineus | Hip flexion |
| | | Hip adduction |
| Femoral nerve (L2 to L4) | Rectus femoris | Hip flexion |
| | | Knee extension |
| | Vastus lateralis | Knee extension |
| | Vastus medialis | Knee extension |
| | Vastus intermedius | Knee extension |
| **Posterior thigh compartment** | | |
| Sciatic nerve (L5 to S2) | | |
| Tibial division (L5 to S2) | Semitendinosis | Hip extension knee flexion, knee rotation medially |
| | Semimembranosus | Hip extension, knee flexion, knee rotation medially |
| | Long head of biceps femoris | Hip extension, knee flexion, lateral rotation of knee |
| Common peroneal division (L5 to S2) | Short head of biceps femoris | Hip extension, knee flexion, external rotation of knee |
| **Lateral thigh compartment** | | |
| Greater gluteal nerve (L4 to S1) | Tensor fascia lata | Hip abduction and internal rotation, hip flexion |
| | Gluteus medius | Hip abduction and internal rotation |
| | Gluteus minimus | |
| **Medial thigh compartment** | | |
| Obturator nerve (L2 to L4) | Adductor longus | Hip adduction |
| | Adductor brevis | Hip adduction |
| | Adductor magnus | Hip adduction and flexion |
| | Gracillis | Hip adduction, knee flexion, knee medial rotation |
| Femoral nerve (L2 to L4) | Pectineus | Hip adduction and flexion |
| **Anterior leg compartment** | | |
| Deep peroneal nerve (L4 to S1) | Tibialis anterior | Ankle dorsiflexion, foot inversion |
| | Extensor hallicus longus | Big toe extension, weak ankle dorsiflexion, foot inversion |
| Deep peroneal nerve (L5 to S1) | Extensor digitorum longus | Extension of toes (2 to 5), weak ankle dorsiflexion |
| | Extensor digitorum brevis | Extension of all toes |
| | Peroneus tertius | Weak ankle dorsiflexion and foot eversion |
| **Posterior leg compartment** | | |
| Tibial nerve (L5) | Popliteus | Knee flexion, medial rotation of tibia on femur |
| Tibial nerve (L5 to S1) | Tibialis posterior | Ankle plantar flexion, foot inversion |
| | Flexor digitorum longus | Toe flexion (2 to 5), ankle plantar flexion |
| | Flexor hallicus longus | Big toe flexion, ankle plantar flexion |
| Tibial nerve (S1 to S2) | Gastrocnemius | Ankle plantar flexion, knee flexion |
| | Soleus | Ankle plantar flexion |
| | Plantaris | Ankle plantar flexion, knee flexion |
| **Lateral leg compartment** | | |
| Superficial peroneal nerve (L5, S1, S2) | Peroneus longus | Calcaneal eversion and weak ankle plantar flexor |
| | Peroneus brevis | Calcaneal eversion and weak ankle plantar flexor |

of the femur is larger in surface area and projects more distally than does the lateral condyle. However, the lateral condyle projects more anteriorly. They are oval-shaped structures that help guide the patella and tibia during knee motion. Each condyle is surrounded by hyaline cartilage and is bathed in synovial fluid. The tibial plateaus are large, slightly concave surfaces that are situated along the horizontal plane. The medial plateau is approximately 50% larger than the lateral plateau

in order to make contact with the larger medial condyle.[26] The articular hyaline cartilage on the medial plateau is three times thicker than the lateral plateau and sustains greater forces during knee motion.[26]

The knee capsule consists of fibrous tissue that joins the tibia, femur, coronary ligaments, medial collateral ligament, and patellar ligament. It is reinforced anteriorly by the aponeurotic expansions of the vastus medialis and vastus lateralis; medially by the sartorius, graci-

*Table 5-11*  Contents of the popliteal fossa at the posterior aspect of the knee

Popliteal artery (continuation of the femoral aretery in the popliteal fossa)
    medial superior genicular artery
    lateral superior genicular artery
    middle genicular artery
    medial inferior genicular artery
    lateral inferior genicular artery
    sural artery
    anterior tibial artery
    posterior tibial artery
Popliteal veins
Common peroneal nerve
Tibial nerve
Posterior femoral cutaneous nerve
Small saphenous vein
Popliteus muscle

lis, semitendinosis; and laterally by the biceps femoris and iliotibial band. At the posterior aspect of the capsule, the fibers are parallel with the popliteus muscle and the oblique popliteal ligament that is attached to the semimembranosus tendon.

Because the knee is a superficial joint, many anatomic structures can be palpated. The clinician should be able to palpate the anatomic structures that may be injured with fairly good accuracy.

**Collateral ligaments of the knee.** There are two collateral ligaments that give support to the capsule: the medial (tibial) and the lateral (fibular) collateral ligaments. When the knee is flexed, both ligaments are slack and permit medial and lateral rotation and valgus and varus motions. When the knee is extended, both ligaments are taut, adding support on the lateral aspect of the knee, preventing valgus and varus stress, and limiting tibial long axis rotation. The medial collateral ligament has two layers, deep and superficial. The superficial part of the ligament is a long band that bridges the femoral epicondyle and the tibial condyle. The deeper part is deltoid and anchors the femoral condyle to the margin of the medial meniscus and to the tibial condyle. One or more bursae lie deep to the long superficial band. The band is crossed by the tendinous expansion of the sartorius, gracilis, and semitendinosus (*pes anserinus*). They help reinforce the medial side of the knee capsule and are part of the medial patellar retinaculum.

The lateral collateral ligament is a cordlike structure that is not attached to the lateral meniscus and is partly overlapped by the biceps femoris tendon. A bursa is located between the biceps femoris tendon and the lateral collateral ligament.

**Cruciate ligaments of the knee.** The two cruciate ligaments are intra-articular structures but are extracap-

sular because a tenosynovium surrounds each ligament. The two cruciate ligaments are named according to their location on the tibia. The anterior cruciate attaches the anterior aspect of the tibial eminence to the medial aspect of the lateral condyle of the femur. The posterior cruciate attaches the posterior aspect of the tibial eminence to the medial aspect of the medial condyle of the femur. The crossing of the two cruciate ligaments help support the *screw-home mechanism* and tibial displacement during knee extension. The anterior cruciate ligament prevents excessive anterior motion of the tibia and excessive posterior motion of the femur, whereas the posterior cruciate ligament prevents the opposite motions.

**Patellofemoral joint.** The patella is a sesamoid bone that has two facets and is covered with hyaline cartilage on its posterior aspect. It contacts the femoral condyles of the femur to make up the patellofemoral joint. It is a synovial diarthrodial joint that is an extension of the tibiofemoral joint described above. The patella provides for a mechanical advantage for the quadriceps muscle group during knee flexion and extension. The joint-functions like a pulley system in which its motion is determined by the quadriceps muscle and the position of the patellar tendon and its attachment to the tibial tuberosity. Located in the quadriceps tendon, the patella moves superiorly and slightly laterally during knee extension.

When the knee is fully extended, the patella sits in the trochlear surface of the femur. On flexion of the knee, the patella moves downward approximately 7 cm and slightly medially to make contact with the medial condyle and sits in the intercondylar groove.

The patella has two important biomechanical purposes. First, it aids in knee extension by producing anterior displacement of the quadriceps tendon throughout the entire range of motion (changing the distance of the lever arm to control quadriceps muscle contraction); and second, it prevents stress risers from developing on the femur by distributing the stresses between the patellar tendon and the femur. Improper tracking, or motion, of the patella can lead to patellofemoral pain. Overuse injuries, chondromalacia patella, and vastus medialis weakness are just a few of the more common causes of a patellar tracking problem (see Case 24). Table 5-12 lists the common anatomic structures that control patellar motion during knee flexion and extension and that can lead to a patellar tracking problem.

### Fascial compartments of the leg

**Anterior compartment of the leg.** The leg is divided into three compartments by the anterior, the posterior, and the lateral intermuscular septum. The muscles of the anterior, posterior, and lateral compartments are listed in Table 5-10. Concentric actions of the muscles

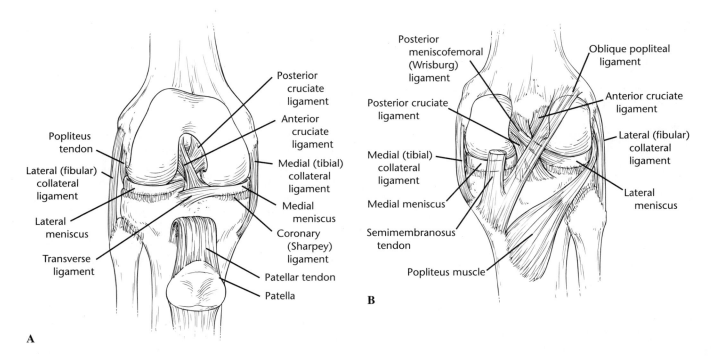

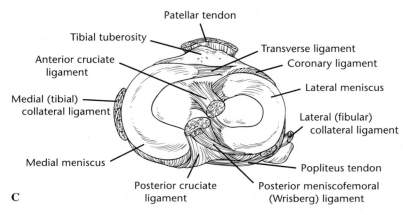

***Fig. 5-23*** The anatomical structures of the knee joint. **A,** Anterior view. **B,** Posterior view. **C,** View of the tibial plateau.

in the anterior, posterior, and lateral compartments produce dorsiflexion (extension) at the ankle (mortise) joint plantar flexion (flexion) at the mortise joint, and calca-

neal eversion and ankle plantar flexion, respectively (Fig. 5-24).

The common peroneal nerve passes posteriorly to the neck of the fibula and divides into the deep and superficial peroneal nerves. The deep peroneal nerve innervates the muscles of the anterior compartment of the leg and continues into the dorsum of the foot where it is general sensory nerve to the skin between the first and second toes.

**Lateral compartment of the leg.** The lateral compartment of the leg consists of the peroneus longus and peroneus brevis muscles that are innervated by the su-

***Table 5-12*** Anatomic structures that control patellar motion

| |
|---|
| Vastus medialis (oblique fibers) |
| Medial and lateral patellar retinaculum |
| Anterior aspect of lateral condyle |
| Trochlear groove |
| Posterior facets of patella |
| Patellar tendon and ligament |

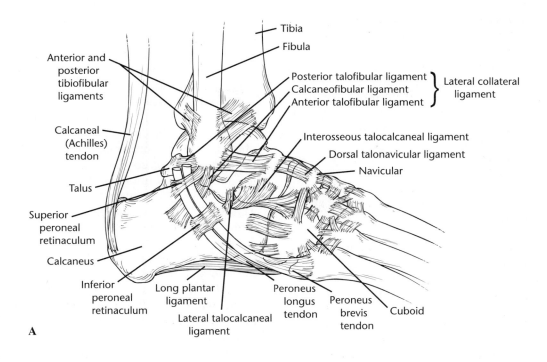

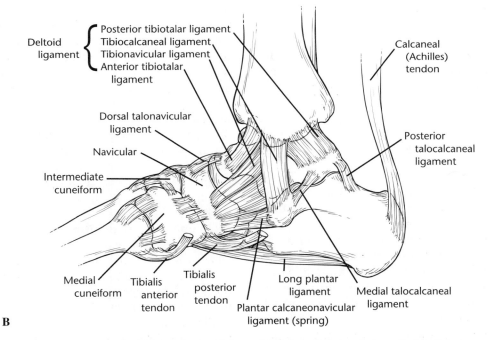

*Fig. 5-24*  The anatomical structures of the ankle joint. **A,** Lateral view. **B,** Medial view.

perficial peroneal nerve, which, in addition to being a motor nerve to the muscles of the lateral compartment, is also a sensory nerve to the skin on the lower lateral aspect of the leg and dorsum of the foot at the second to the fourth toes.

The peroneus longus insertion acts as a pulley by passing inferior to the tubercle of the cuboid bone and obliquely crossing the sole of the foot. Not only does this muscle produce foot pronation (calcaneal eversion) and assist in plantar flexion at the ankle, it is also a major muscle that helps support the longitudinal arch of the foot.

**Posterior compartment of the leg.** The posterior compartment of the leg is the major plantar flexor of the foot at the ankle. The muscles that are located in this area are listed in Table 5-10. Many of these muscles assist in supporting the longitudinal arch of the foot.

Evaluation of the anterior and posterior compartments of the leg is conducted by asking the patient to perform a heel walk and a toe walk. Heel walk evaluates level L4 and toe walk evaluates nerve root level S1. Level L5 is evaluated by the strength of the extensor hallicus longus. To differentiate muscle weakness in the gastrocnemius muscle from that in the soleus muscle in the posterior compartment of the leg, knee flexion is also evaluated. When the knee is extended, the gastrocnemius muscle is evaluated primarily. When the knee is flexed, the soleus muscle is isolated because the gastrocnemius muscle is put at a mechanical disadvantage. If the patient's complaints occur in both positions, then the soleus muscle is the problem. If the problem only occurs when the knee is extended, then the gastrocnemius muscle is primarily involved. This phenomenon can be explained by the origin of these two muscles. The origin of the gastrocnemius crosses the knee joint whereas the origin of the soleus does not. Depending on the angle of the knee joint, the gastrocnemius muscle may extend the knee.

The tibial nerve of the sciatic nerve innervates the muscles of the posterior compartment of the leg. As the nerve enters the plantar surface of the foot through the tarsal tunnel, it divides into the medial and lateral plantar nerves that provide both motor and sensory innervation to the sole of the foot. Cutaneous innervation of the posterior compartment of the leg is supplied by sensory branches of the tibial nerve.

### Ankle (mortise joint)

**Retinacula at the ankle.** The deep fascia of the leg becomes thickened to form a series of retinacula that keep the long tendons of the muscles of the leg in position so that they may act as pulleys. At the dorsum of the ankle, the superior extensor retinaculum connects the distal tibia and fibula and encloses the tendon of the tibialis anterior. The inferior extensor retinaculum is a Y-shaped band that connects the calcaneus, medial malleolus, and plantar aponeurosis. It encloses the tendons of all the anterior compartment muscles. At the lateral aspect of the ankle, the superior peroneal retinaculum attaches to the lateral malleolus and the calcaneus and binds the tendons of the peroneus longus and peroneus brevis. The inferior peroneal retinaculum connects from the calcaneus bone to the peroneal tendons and holds the peroneus longus and peroneus brevis in place as they curve around the lateral malleolus. At the medial aspect of the ankle, the flexor retinaculum attaches the medial malleolus to the calcaneus. It en-

closes the tendons of the tibialis posterior, flexor digitorum longus, and flexor hallucis longus muscles. The purpose of the retinaculum is to hold the tendons in place and provide leverage for the muscles to produce a moment with the application of as little force possible.

**Ankle joint articulation.** The mortise joint consists of three bones: (1) the distal end of the tibia (medial malleolus); (2) the distal end of the fibula (lateral malleolus); and (3) the proximal end of the talus. The three bones make up three joints: the tibiotalar, the fibulotalar, and the distal tibiofibular articulations. The tibiotalar and fibulotalar joints are synovial diarthrodial joints. The tibiofibular joint is joined by interosseous membrane and is a synarthrodial joint. The mortise joint is made up of the three bones, the corresponding joints, the joint capsule surrounded by the deltoid ligament, the lateral ligaments, and the interosseous ligaments. The lateral malleolus is located 2 cm distal to the level of the blunt end of the medial malleolus and the medial malleolus is more anterior than is the lateral malleolus. The talus is tortoise shaped with the body looking like the shell and the anterior aspect resembling the head and neck of the tortoise. The body is saddle shaped and articulates the tibia and fibula at its sides. The posterior surface of the body of the talus tapers to two tubercles separated by a groove for the flexor hallicus longus muscle. The head is rounded anteriorly to articulate with the navicular bone. The inferior aspect of the talus articulates with the calcaneus to form the subtalar joint. The talus is unique in that there it has no muscle attachments.

The trochlear aspect of the talus becomes more narrow in its posterior aspect and forms a frustrum (section of a cone). The anterior surface is wider by as much as 6 mm.[37] This shape adds to the stability of the joint during dorsiflexion, when the joint is in its closed-packed position.

**Ligamentous structures of the ankle.** The *deltoid ligament* is the medial collateral ligament of the ankle, which arises from the blunt end of the medial malleolus and has two distinct parts: The superficial and the deep portions. The superficial band passes posteroinferiorly to the sustentaculum tali. The deltoid portion fans out to the nonarticular section of the medial aspect of the talus and reaches as far as the navicular bone.[34]

The lateral collateral ligament of the ankle has three parts: the calcaneofibular ligament, the posterior talofibular ligament, and the anterior talofibular ligament. The calcaneofibular ligament attaches the fibula to the calcaneus; the posterior talofibular ligament lies deep and passes horizontally to the lateral tubercle of the talus; and the anterior talofibular ligament is a thin, weak band that traverses anteriorly from the fibula to the talus (see Case 25).

**Kinematics of the ankle.** The ankle is a unipolar hinge joint that is not pure in its motions. Motion occurs primarily in the sagittal plane as dorsal and plantar flexion. Because of the position of the malleolus and the shape of the talus body, the axis of rotation is not directly along the horizontal plane and a coupled motion occurs. Inversion of the foot occurs along with ankle plantar flexion and foot eversion is noted with dorsiflexion of the ankle.

Mortise joint stability is primarily maintained by the shape of the talus, tightness of its fit between the fibula and tibia, and the interosseous membrane between these two bones. The greatest stability occurs during dorsiflexion. Mortise joint stability during plantar flexion occurs primarily through the ligaments and the locations of the malleoli.

## Foot

The foot consists of 28 bones (two bones are sesmoid bones and are located under the first metatarsal head) (Fig. 5-25). There are a total of 57 joints that can be locked to make the foot a rigid lever or opened to make the foot flexible.

**Dorsum of the foot.** The foot is intersected by the midsagittal plane through the second ray, and each toe has a medial and lateral aspect. The medial aspect of the foot is along the medial longitudinal arch; however, the lateral aspect of the big toe is in the same area as the medial aspect of the foot.

At the dorsum of the foot are two muscles: the extensor digitorum brevis and the extensor halluces brevis. From their origins, they combine to interdigitate to all five toes. The extensor digitorum brevis is an easily palpable muscle that is located at the lateral aspect of the dorsum of the foot just distal to the lateral malleolus. When the toes of the foot are extended, this muscle is easily seen. These muscles act to extend all the toes, and they are innervated by the deep peroneal nerve (S1 to S2). The cutaneous nerve supply to the dorsum of the foot consists of the superficial peroneal nerve that innervates the medial side of the big toe and the dorsum of the foot, except for the area between the big toe and the second toe. The deep peroneal nerve innervates the skin between the big toe and the second toe and the sural nerve innervates the skin at the lateral side of the fifth metatarsal area.

**Plantar surface (sole) of the foot.** The deep fascia of the sole of the foot forms the plantar aponeurosis. This sheet is a very strong tissue that is triangular, with its apex located at the medial and lateral tubercles of the calcaneus. The base divides into five slips that attach to the fibrous digital sheaths and deep transverse ligaments in the phalanges. The purpose of the plantar aponeurosis is to protect the underlying anatomic structures from injury during walking, and it plays a major role in supporting the arch of the foot. Because it has an attachment on the calcaneus in common with the Achilles tendon, its synchronized action with that of the Achilles tendon is important in foot function (see Case 26 and Chapter 6).

The muscles of the sole of the foot collectively are significant for posture, locomotion, and arch support. They are divided into four layers. Table 5-13 illustrates these layers. The cutaneous nerve supply of the sole of the foot is from the tibial nerve at the heel and the lateral plantar nerve at the lateral one third of the sole and all of the toes to the medial half of the fourth toe. The saphenous and sural nerves supply sections of the medial and the lateral sole, respectively (see Fig. 5-19).

**Foot arches.** There are two significant arches of the foot: the transverse and the longitudinal arches. The arches act as shock absorbers, help support the weight of the body in the erect posture, and are important in propulsion during gait. The arches are located between the calcaneus and the six points of contact of the metatarsal heads. There are two points of contact under the first metatarsal head and one point under each other metatarsal head.

The longitudinal arch of the foot is subdivided into the medial and the lateral aspects. Both arches are formed by the five metatarsal bones, the seven tarsal bones, and the ligaments that give support. The medial longitudinal arch is higher and more important for weight distribution and shock absorption. It is composed of the calcaneus, talus, navicular, three cuneiforms, and three metatarsal bones with the head of the talus as the "keystone."[34] The staples that keep the arch in place, by holding the joints together, are the short and long plantar ligaments and the spring ligament; the tie beam of the arch is the flexor halluces longus and the suspension bridge is the peroneus longus.

The lateral part of the longitudinal arch is much flatter than the medial portion and rests on the ground when a person is standing. It consists of the calcaneus, cuboid, and the lateral two metatarsal bones.

The transverse arch runs from the medial aspect to the lateral aspect of the foot. It is formed by the cuboid bone, three cuneiform bones, and the bases of the metatarsal bones also known as the tarsal-metatarsal joint (*joint of Lisfranc*). The cuneiform bones, being wedge shaped, form the "keystone" of the arch, with the medial and lateral longitudinal arches acting as pillars. The arch is supported by the tendon of the peroneus longus muscle that crosses the foot obliquely, the interosseous muscles, and the plantar and dorsal ligaments.

From the viewpoint of biomechanics, the foot is divided into three units: the forefoot (anterior aspect) consisting of the phalanges and metatarsal bones; the midfoot (middle) consisting of the three cuneiforms, the navicular, and the cuboid bones; and the hindfoot (posterior) consisting of the talus and calcaneus bones.

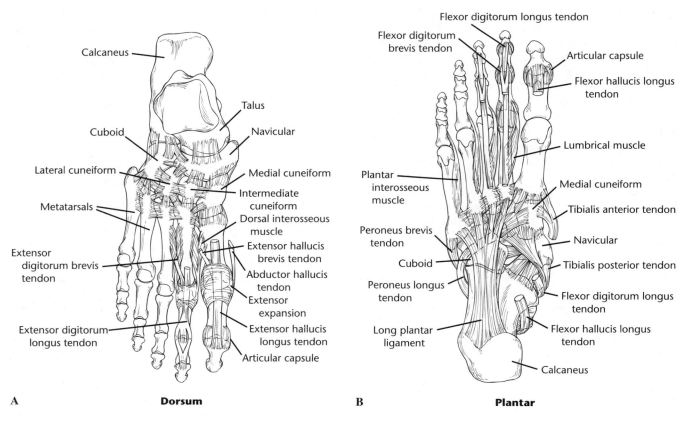

*Fig. 5-25* The anatomical structures of the foot. **A,** Dorsal view. **B,** Plantar view.

*Table 5-13* The sole of the foot: movements, muscles, and peripheral nerves

| Nerve | Muscle | Concentric action |
|---|---|---|
| **Layer 1** | | |
| Medial plantar nerve (S2 to S3) | Abductor hallucis, flexor digotorum brevis | Abduction of big toe<br>Flexion of toe at PIP joints 2 to 5 |
| Lateral plantar nerve (S2 to S3) | Abductor digiti minimi | Abduction of little toe |
| **Layer 2** | | |
| Lateral plantar nerve (S2 to S3) | Quadratus plantae | Adjustment of pull on flexor digitorum longus and aid in flexion of toes 3 to 5 |
| | Lumbricals (nos. 2 to 4) | Flexion of MTP joints 3 to 5 and extension PIP and DIP joints 3 to 5 |
| Medial plantar nerve (S1 to S2) | Lumbrical (no. 1) | Flexion of MTP joint of toe 2, extension of PIP and DIP joints of toe 2 |
| **Layer 3** | | |
| Medial plantar nerve (S1 to S2) | Flexor hallucis brevis | Flexion of MTP joint of big toe |
| Lateral plantar nerve (S2 to S3) | Adductor hallucis | Adduction of big toe |
| | Flexor digiti minimi brevis | Flexion of proximal phalanx of little toe |
| **Layer 4** | | |
| Lateral plantar nerve (S2 to S3) | Plantar interosseous | Adduction of toes 3 to 5, flexion of toes 3 to 5 at MTP, extension of toes 3 to 5 at PIP and DIP joints |
| | Dorsal interosseous | Abduction of toes 2 to 4, flexion of toes 2 to 4 at MTP, extension of PIP and DIP joints of toes 2 to 4 |

*DIP, distal interphalangeal; MTP, metatarsal phalangeal; PIP, posterior interphalangeal*

The calcaneus is the largest tarsal bone and is divided for identification purposes into thirds. The anterior two thirds supports the talus and the posterior one third forms the prominence of the heel that rests on the ground. The anterior aspect of the calcaneus articulates with the cuboid and is called the calcaneal cuboid joint. The posterior part of the calcaneus is the insertion point for the Achilles tendon of the tricep surae muscle group of the posterior compartment of the leg.

The posterior third of the superior surface of the calcaneus is saddle shaped and nonarticular. The intermediate third supports the body of the talus and is convex and faces obliquely to the coronal plane. A medial projecting shelf of bone is located on the calcaneus and is called the *sustentaculum tali.*

Kinematically, there are three major joints within the foot: *the subtalar joint,* the transverse tarsal joint (*Chopart's joint*), and the tarsalmetatarsal joint (*Lisfranc's joint*).

The subtalar joint is not a joint of the ankle but is considered a joint of the foot. The subtalar joint plays a major role in "ankle sprains." The majority of ankle sprains are caused by excessive inversion of the foot occurring at the subtalar joint, and the ankle is correspondingly plantar flexed. In the plantar-flexed position, the direction of forces is along the long axis of the anterior talofibular ligament. On forceful inversion of the foot a large inversion force is applied to the ankle causing injury to the anterior talofibular ligament and the traversing anterior retinaculum (see Case 25).

The combination of the movements of these three joints allows the foot to invert and evert (subtalar joint), abduct and adduct (Chopart and Lisfranc's joints), and flex and extend (Chopart and Lisfranc's joints). The toes of the foot flex and extend. Their kinematics will be further discussed in Chapter 6.

## Provocative testing of the extremities
WARREN HAMMER

In this section, the differences between active and passive ranges of motion and some of the provocative tests used to evaluate anatomic structures will be covered. The general rule is that active range of motion evaluates the contractile anatomic components, whereas passive range of motion evaluates passive components and the flexibility (stretch) and elasticity of the active and passive components of an anatomic structure. In striated muscle the active components are the actin and myosin fibrils and the passive components consist of the epimysium, the perimysium, the endomysium, and tendons. In other areas of the neuromusculoskeletal structure, the passive components are the joint capsule and bursae, the tensosynovium, the bone, all neurologic tissues, and blood vessels, etc.

When evaluating an anatomic joint, active range of motion evaluation informs the clinician about the active components.[19] In Case 19, the patient complains of a painful arc. This informs the clinician that the active components play a major role in this patient's problem. A passive range of motion determination allows the clinician to stress the tissues to determine whether the tissues have been injured, causing improper healing (for example, injured muscle tissue is usually replaced with fibrous tissue. Fibrous tissue is far less flexible and elastic and has a different end-feel on passive evaluation).[19]

Resisted isometric muscle testing (muscle testing) provides the clinician with information about muscle strength. These tests are performed with the muscle placed in a static position and the patient being asked to resist a force, which causes a concentric action that the clinician can evaluate to determine the presence of muscle weakness. Functional muscle testing involves the patient moving the limb through a range of motion and evaluating the ability of the muscles involved to perform the task. These tests can provide information about the integrity of the peripheral nerve and myoneuro junction. Electromyography (EMG) and nerve conduction velocity (NCV) tests also provide support for the location of a neurologic lesion.

Provocative tests incorporated in the cases involving the upper extremities are all designed to determine which anatomic structures could be causing the patient's problem. There are many tests to evaluate the more common shoulder maladies. These tests, whether performed passively or actively, indicate whether injury is present in the stressed anatomic tissues. In Case 19, a shoulder impingement test is positive indicating that the anatomic structure(s) between the acromion and head of the humerus is(are) inflamed.[13,17] Muscle testing of the rotator cuff muscles and the surrounding shoulder musculature also provide further information about muscle weakness caused by neurologic deficit.[13,17] With any provocative test the name of the test is not important. What is important is that the clinician should understand which anatomic structures are being tested and what a positive finding is.

In the elbow, active and passive ranges of motion tests provided the examiner with valuable information about the integrity of the anatomic structures surrounding the joint. The provocative tests performed on this joint evaluate the flexibility of the involved structures.[13,17] Mill's maneuver and valgus and varus stress determine the flexibility of the extensor tendinous sheath and the medial collateral ligament, respectively. Muscle tests on the elbow involves the muscles of the arm and forearm and the effects of these muscles on the elbow, wrist, and hand.

Muscle testing is an important aspect of proper hand evaluation. Passive and active joint testing are also used to determine if capsular or bony adhesions are present (for example, retinaculum test and Bunnel-Littler test). In all evaluations of neuromusculoskeletal injury the joints proximal to the area of chief complaint need to be evaluated. In many clinical presentations the lack of motion in an injured joint can be compensated for by other joints, causing diagnostic confusion and, in many cases, treatment of the wrong anatomic structures. A thorough evaluation of all joints involved is therefore imperative.

The same rules hold true for the lower extremities. Soft tissues as well as joint integrity need to be examined. There are many provocative tests that evaluate the joints of the lower extremities. There are so many tests for knee evaluation that it is difficult for the clinician to determine which tests to use. It is therefore crucial that the clinician understand the anatomy and biomechanics of the joint so that the tests that will provide the most information will be used. In the knee, the provocative tests can be divided into tests that determine one-plane stability and those that determine multiple-plane stability.[13,17,19] Table 5-14 lists the more common provocative tests of the extremities.

## RADIOLOGY OF THE EXTREMITIES
### The upper extremities

TIMOTHY MICK

**Shoulder.** The usual sequence of viewing a radiograph is to use the articulations-bone-cartilage-soft tissue (ABCS). Bone alignment, bone density, cartilage, and soft tissues are of major importance when evaluating any radiograph. In the shoulder there are three joints of major radiographic concern: the scapulothoracic, the acromioclavicular (AC), and the glenohumeral (GH) articulations. Only the latter two will be considered here because the scapulothoracic articulation is not a true joint and is not readily imaged with conventional plain film radiography. The sternoclavicular (SC) joint may be associated with shoulder dysfunction and pain, but it, too, is difficult to image adequately on plain x-ray films alone, and requires plain film tomography or computed tomography (CT).

Radiographic views of the glenohumeral joint involve an anteroposterior (A-P) view with internal and external rotation of the humerus and a "baby-arm" view (Fig. 5-26). Radiographic views needed to evaluate shoulder trauma also include an axillary view, a tangential (Y) view of the scapula, or a transthoracic view of the proximal humerus. If the suspected abnormality lies in the AC joint, the examination must employ weighted and non-weighted A-P views of both AC joints to allow comparison of the suspected abnormal joint with the presumed normal site. Radiographs of the asymptom-

*Table 5-14* Common provocative tests used to evaluate anatomic structures of the articulations of the extremities

| Provocative tests | Anatomic structures evaluated |
|---|---|
| **Shoulder** | |
| Supraspinatus test | Rotator cuff injury, supraspinatus tendinitis |
| Codman's drop arm test | Supraspinatus tear, roator cuff injury |
| Apley's scratch test | Shoulder range of motion |
| Impingement test | Rotator cuff injury, glenohumeral impingement |
| Apprehension test | Glenohumeral dislocation |
| Speed's test | Supraspinatus tendinitis |
| Transverse humeral ligament test | Transverse ligament rupture, bicipital tendinitis (long head) |
| Booth-Marvel test | Transverse ligament rupture, bicipital tendinitis (long head) |
| **Elbow** | |
| Mill's test | Lateral epicondylitis |
| Cozen's test | Lateral epicondylitis |
| Test for medial epicondylitis | Medial epicondylitis |
| Tinel's sign | Peripheral nerve entrapment |
| **Wrist** | |
| Phalen's test | Carpal tunnel |
| Prayer test | Carpal tunnel |
| Finkelstein's test | Stenosing tenosinovitis (de Quervain's disease) |
| Tinel's test | Peripheral nerve entrapment |
| **Hip** | |
| Patrick's test (sign of four) | Hip pathology |
| Ober's test | Trochanteric bursitis, lateral thigh compartment weakness |
| Trandelenberg's test | Lateral thigh compartment weakness, hip pathology |
| **Knee** | |
| Varus/valgus test | Lateral and medial collateral ligaments |
| Lachmann test | Anterior cruciate ligament |
| Anterior-posterior drawer | Anterior and posterior cruciate ligaments |
| Posterior sag sign | Posterior cruciate ligament |
| Slocum | Anterior cruciate and collateral ligaments |
| Lateral pivot shift (Macintosh test) | Anterior cruciate and collateral ligaments |
| Noble's compression | Iliotibial band compression rub |
| McMurry's test | Menisci |
| Apley's compression and distraction test | Menisci and collateral ligaments |
| Apprehension test | Patellar dislocation |
| Patellar grind test | Chondromalacia patella |
| **Ankle** | |
| Anterior-posterior drawer | Anterior and posterior talofibular ligament |
| Inversion displacement | Anterior-posterior talofibular ligament Calcanealfibular ligament |
| **Foot** | |
| Compression sign | Morton's neuroma |

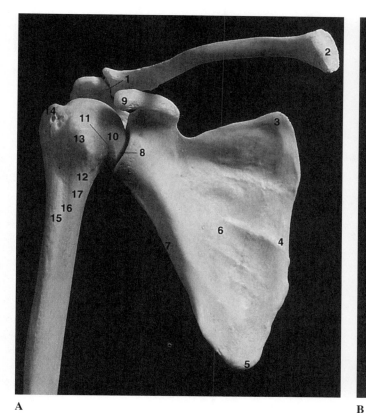
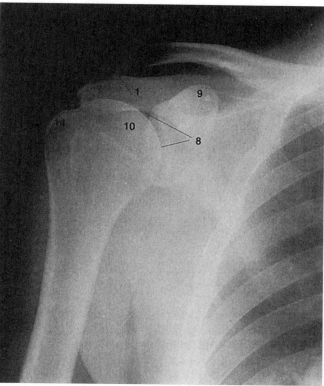

**A**                                                      **B**

*Fig. 5-26*   Bones of the right shoulder. **A,** Scapula, clavicle, and upper end of the humerus, from the front. **B,** External rotation radiograph. 1, Acromioclavicular joint; 2, sternal end of clavicle, for articulation with the sternum at the sternoclavicular joint; 3, superior angle of scapula; 4, vertebral (medial) border. Serratus anterior is attached along its whole length; 5, inferior angle; 6, subscapular fossa, for the origin of subscapularis; 7, axillary (lateral) border; 8, margin of glenoid cavity, the very shallow 'socket' of the shoulder joint—coracoid process—head of humerus, forming the shoulder joint with the glenoid cavity of the scapula; 11, anatomical neck, the margin of the smooth head; 12, surgical neck, the upper part of the shaft below the head (10) and the tuberosities (13 and 14); 13, lesser tuberosity, to which subscapularis is attached; 14, greater tuberosity. Supraspinatus is attached to the uppermost part shown here; farther back and lower down it receives infraspinatus and teres minor; 15, lateral lip of intertubercular (bicipital) groove, for the attachment of pectoralis major; 16, floor of intertubercular groove, for attachment of latissimus dorsi. The tendon of the long head of biceps is lodged in the groove; 17, medial lip of intertubercular groove, for attachment of teres major. (From: McMinn RM, Gaddum-Rosse P, Hutchings RT, Logan BM: *McMinn's functional and clinical anatomy.* St. Louis, 1995, Mosby, with permission.)

atic side act as an important control, especially in situations involving a possible AC separation.

A variety of pathologies involving the shoulder and brachial plexus are typically associated with negative results on plain x-ray films and require advance diagnostic imaging. Historically, shoulder arthrography was often the examination of choice, after plain film radiography. Today, however, magnetic resonance imaging (MRI) is used in the majority of cases to image this type of radiographically occult pathology, including rotator cuff abnormalities (see Case 19).

The acromiohumeral interspace should be measured to assess superior subluxation of the humeral head, which may be associated with abnormality of the rotator cuff. An acromiohumeral distance of less than 7 mm, measured on a well-positioned internal or external rotation view, provides presumptive evidence of a rotator cuff (supraspinatus) tear and may be associated with a shoulder impingement syndrome (see Case 19). A measurement of greater than 11 mm may also be abnormal, described as a "drooping shoulder."[1,31] Because of projectional distortion on the baby-arm view, this acromiohumeral interspace space should not be assessed on this film. This is also true of the acromioclavicular and coracoclavicular relationships.

The AC joint space should be measured. This is typically no greater than 4 mm, although there is considerable variation. Comparison to the contralateral side is useful, especially if there is history of trauma and concern for AC joint separation. A difference of more than 2 to 3 mm from one side to the other is suggestive of at least a grade II AC sprain.[40]

AC alignment is also assessed by observing the relationship of the inferior margin of the distal clavicle, relative to the inferior aspect of the acromion process. Normal alignment is present when the inferior margins of these structures are on the same plane. The superior margins do not provide reliable landmarks and should not be used in evaluation of the AC alignment. This tends to produce a false positive diagnosis of superior subluxation of the distal clavicle as seen in grade II or grade III AC sprain.[2,42]

The coracoclavicular interval may be assessed to provide additional information regarding the status of the AC joint. Again, a difference in measurement greater than 2 to 3 mm from one side to the other, is suggestive of at least grade II AC sprain on the side of the greater measurement.[2,42]

A line drawn along the axillary border of the scapula and continued laterally along the medial margin of the humeral head and neck should form a smooth, unbroken arc. Disruption of this arc on the internal or external rotation views may be an important sign of glenohumeral dislocation.

The only specific soft tissue structure to look for in the shoulder is the fat pad lying adjacent and parallel to the subacromial-subdeltoid bursa. Like the scaphoid and pronator fat pads in the wrist, this fat pad may be visualized normally but is not invariably seen. When it is, present, blurring or displacement of the pad may be secondary to trauma or inflammation related to arthritis or bursitis.

**Elbow.** Like other joints in the extremities, the elbow is a complex of several joints rather than a single joint. Plain films adequately visualize the humeroulnar, radiocapitellar, and proximal radioulnar joint. There are four views in a complete plain film study of the elbow: anteroposterior (A-P), lateral, oblique, and tangential (Jones) views (Fig. 5-27). A useful ancillary view is the radicapitellar view, which is especially valuable in evaluating elbow trauma and subtle fractures of the radial head.

The radiocapitellar relationship should be maintained on all standard elbow projections.[38] Loss of the normal close relationship of the radial head to the capitellum is always considered abnormal. On the lateral view, a line drawn through the shaft of the proximal radius (radicapitellar line) should intersect the capitellum, re-

gardless of the degree of flexion of the elbow.[49] This line may be useful if the patient is unable to flex the elbow to 90 degrees due to pain or restricted range of motion.

On an A-P view, the distal articular surface of the humerus is oriented with approximately 6 to 8 degrees of valgus tilt.[23] The neck of the radius is also angled approximately 15 degrees laterally with respect to the shaft.[12]

On a lateral view, the capitellum should be angled anteriorly such that it forms a 30-degree angle with the long axis of the humerus.[38] Decrease in this angle, especially in children, may indicate a supracondylar fracture of the distal humerus.

When a line is drawn on the lateral view along the anterior cortical margin of the distal humerus, the capitellum should project significantly anterior to this line. If only a small amount of capitellum or no capitellum at all is visible anterior to this line, a supracondylar fracture is suggested. No quantitative figures were provided in the original description of this line.[23]

The fat pads of the elbow are the most important soft tissue structures to observe. There are paired fat pads located in an intracapsular, extrasynovial location. The pads normally lie very close to the distal humerus and are not typically visible on a well-positioned lateral view of the elbow. Faint visualization of the anterior fat pad in proximity to the anterior cortex of the distal humerus on the lateral view is acceptable.

These fat pads may be displaced by distention of the joint capsule by abnormal fluid (blood, pus, or excess synovial fluid) within the joint. This elevation of the fat pads away from their shallow fossa on the distal humerus allows visualization as a subtle strip of lucency lying oblique to the humerus. This is a nonspecific finding that may indicate arthritis or trauma. Malpositioning of the lateral view of the elbow (especially insufficient or excessive flexion of the elbow) may produce a false-positive "fat pad sign."[5,38,43,44,49]

**Wrist.** There are four views in a complete radiologic study of the wrist: P-A, lateral, oblique, and P-A with ulnar deviation (Fig. 5-28). Ancillary views may be obtained in clinical settings in which specific pathology or subtle or occult fractures must be excluded. These include the scaphoid view (positioned like an ulnar deviation view, but with the addition of 45 degrees of tube tilt toward the elbow) and the reverse oblique view (valuable for visualizing the pisiform and pisiform-triquetral joint).

Three normal unbroken carpal arcs should be observed on the P-A view: Arc I is drawn along the proximal articular surfaces of the scaphoid, lunate, and triquetrum. Arc II is drawn along the distal articular surfaces of the scaphoid, lunate, and triquetrum. Arc

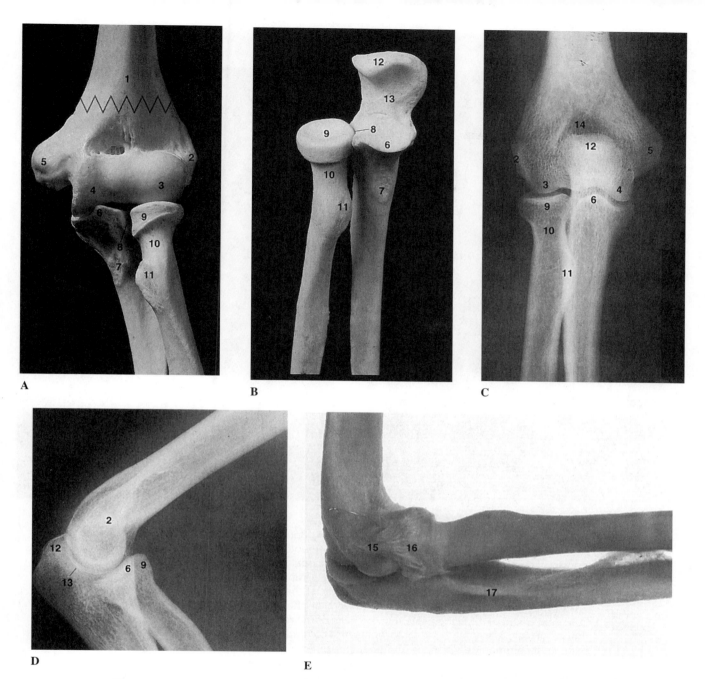

**Fig. 5-27** **A-C,** Anterior-posterior radiographs of the elbow. **D, E,** Lateral radiographs of the elbow. 1, lower end of shaft of humerus, with the common site for supracondylar fracture indicated by the jagged line; 2, lateral epicondyle, the "common extensor origin" for some extensor muscles of the forearm; 3, capitulum, the lateral part of the articular surface; 4, trochlea, the medial part of the articular surface, which has a prominent medial margin. The capitulum (3) and trochlea of the humerus form the elbow joint by articulating with the trochlear notch of the ulna (13) and the head of the radius (9); 5, medial epicondyle, the "common flexor origin" of some flexor muscles of the forearm. It forms a more prominent "knob" than the lateral epicondyle (2); 6, coronoid process of ulna, at the front of the trochlear notch (13); 7, tuberosity of ulna, below the coronoid process, for the attachment of brachialis; 8, radial notch of ulna. It articulates with the head of the radius (9) to form the proximal radioulnar joint; 9, head of radius; 10, neck of radius; 11, tuberosity of radius, on the ulnar side of the shaft below the neck for insertion of the tendon of biceps; 12, olecranon of ulna, at the back of the trochlear notch (13); 13, trochlear notch of ulna, bounded behind by the olecranon (12) and in front by the coronoid process (6); 14, olecranon fossa, on the posterior surface of the humerus; 15, lateral ligament, fusing with the annular ligament (16); 16, annular ligament, embracing the head of the radius (9); 17, supinator crest of ulna, for part of the origin of the supinator muscle. (From: McMinn RM, Gaddum-Rosse P, Hutchings RT, Logan BM: *McMinn's functional and clinical anatomy,* St. Louis, 1995, Mosby, with permission.)

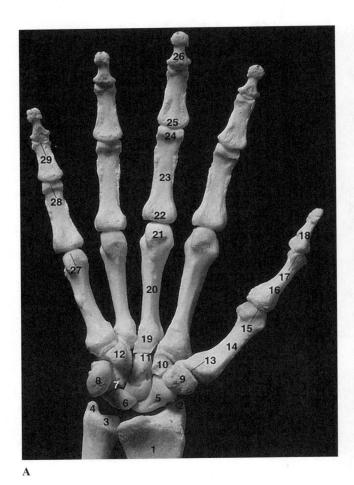

**A**

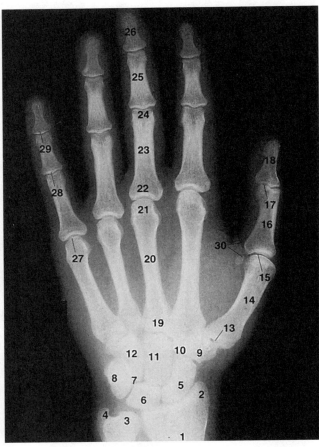

**B**

*Fig. 5-28* Right wrist and hand, from the front. **A,** Bones of the wrist and hand, palmar surface. **B,** Radiograph. The wrist contains three smooth carpal arcs: Arcs I, II, and III. A zig-zag configuration exists along the carpometacarpal row. Fracture or arthritis are the most common causes of the arcs or configuration disruptions. 1, Lower end of radius, the most commonly fractured bone of the whole body, at the site indicated by the jagged line; 2, styloid process of radius, lying at a lower level than the ulnar styloid (4); 3, head of ulna, at the lower end of the bone. Note that the head of the radius is at its upper end; 4, styloid process of ulna; 5, scaphoid, the carpal bone most commonly fractured; 6, lunate, the carpal bone most commonly dislocated; 7, triquetral; 8, pisiform; 9, Trapezium; 10, Trapezoid; 11, capitate; 12, hamate; 13, first carpometacarpal joint; 14, first metacarpal; 15, metacarpophalangeal (MP) joint of the thumb; 16, proximal phalanx of thumb; 17, interphalangeal (IP) joint of the thumb; 18, distal phalanx of thumb; 19, base of third metacarpal; 20, shaft of third metacarpal; 21, head of third metacarpal; 22, base of proximal phalanx of middle finger; 23, shaft of proximal phalanx of middle finger; 24, head of proximal phalanx of middle finger; 25, middle phalanx of middle finger; 26, distal phalanx of middle finger; 27, metacarpophalangeal (MP) joint of little finger; 28, Proximal interphalangeal (IP) joint of little finger; 29, distal interphalangeal (IP) joint of little finger; 30, sesamoid bones. (From: McMinn RM, Gaddum-Rosee P, Hutchings RT, Logan BM: *McMinn's functional and clinical anatomy.* St. Louis, 1995, Mosby, with permission.)

III is drawn along the proximal articular surfaces of the capitate and hamate.[18]

The distal radial articular surface should angle approximately 20 degrees (in the direction of the ulnar) relative to the long axis of the radius. This angle ranges from 15 to 25 degrees.[18]

The distal radial articular surface should be on the same plane as that of the distal radial ulnar surface. An ulna that is shorter or longer than the radius, developmentally, is described as demonstrating a negative or a positive ulnar variance, respectively.[24]

On a well-positioned lateral view, a straight line drawn through the long axis of the radius should normally pass through the axis of the lunate and that of the capitate as well. Alteration of this relationship typically indicates lunate subluxation, dislocation, or instability.[18]

On the lateral view, the distal radius once again is seen to have a 20-degree angulation relative to the long axis of the radius, this time in a volar (palmar) direction. The range is 10 to 25 degrees.[18]

An angle may be drawn on the lateral view between the long axis of the scaphoid and the lunate. This angle is normally 30 to 60 degrees. An angle of 80 degrees or more indicates dorsal instability of the lunate, described as dorsal intercalated segmental instability (DISI). Similarly, if this scapholunate angle is less than 30 degrees, and if the capitolunate angle is 30 degrees or more, it indicates volar intercalated segmental instability (VISI).[18]

The carpometacarpal joint spaces normally have a "zig-zag" configuration. If this is lost, it may be a sign of disruption of the carpometacarpal joint region due to trauma or arthritis.

The pronator fat pad appears on the lateral view as a lucency between the pronator quadratus muscle and the flexor tendon sheaths.[18] The scaphoid fat pad appears as a thin lucency paralleling the scaphoid bone, lying between the radial collateral ligament, laterally, and the abductor pollices longus tendon, medially. Blurring of either the pronator or the scaphoid fat pads is a useful sign of swelling or edema of the wrist and may sometimes suggest occult pathology such as a scaphoid fracture.[7,53,54]

The thenar, hypothenar, pararadial, and paraulnar soft tissues may also be observed for evidence of swelling or edema, which appears as a blurring between the soft tissues and the subcutaneous fat. These soft tissues are more variable and less helpful than the pronator and scaphoid fat pads in the evaluation of milder to moderate abnormality.[18]

### Radiology of the lower extremities
GARY LINDQUIST
CYNTHIA BAUM

**Hip and pelvis.** The major part of the pelvis is typically visualized with a single A-P view. Both lower extremities are internally rotated approximately 20 degrees so as to elongate the femoral necks and take the trochanteric processes out of superimposition with the femoral necks. The basic hip study should employ three views. This includes an A-P pelvic view, an A-P spot hip view, and a lateral (frog leg) spot view of the side

of complaint (Case 23). The A-P pelvic view allows comparative assessment of the various paired structures of the pelvic girdle and hip regions while the spot A-P view brings the central ray to the area of interest allowing better projectional advantage. The lateral frog-leg spot offers a 90-degree or true lateral analysis of the proximal femur. Occasionally a bilateral frog projection can be performed as an expedient survey, particularly to rule out slipped capital femoral epiphyses.

The sacroiliac articulations lie on either side of the sacrum (see Case 15). They run in an oblique plane from posterior to anterior with the most anterior aspect of the joint visualized laterally. The iliac portions of the sacroiliac articulations are represented by the alae of the ilia. The sacroiliac articulation is ligamentous in nature along the superior one third of the joint while the lower one half to two thirds is synovial.

The femoral head is usualy hemispheric or slightly conical. It is interrupted along its axial border by the fovea centralis, which is the attachment of the ligamentous teres. The femoral neck progresses downward from the head. Any defects in the cortical or trabecular pattern would lend suspicion to an evolving stress fracture. There are some recognized lines of trabecular stress that are often seen in the femoral neck and proximal intertrochanteric region. These include the tensile and compression lines of stress. A relatively clear area or region of trabecular paucity is noted between these lines of stress which is called *Ward's triangle* (see Case 23).[18a] The greater and lesser trochanter are images with the lesser trochanter lying medial and the greater trochanter lateral and superior. A thin cortical line, called the intertrochanteric line, is noted connecting the two.

Various lines of mensuration have been employed for describing the anatomic relationships about the hip. In analysis of a slipped capital epiphysis, *Klein's line* tends to be the most sensitive measurement. This is a line drawn tangentially along the lateral aspect of the femoral neck extending superiorly to intersect the femoral epiphyses. This line should intersect the outer aspect of the epiphyses on both the A-P and frogleg views. If the line fails to intersect, it is probably caused by a slipped femoral epiphysis.[56a] Occasionally this line will appear normal on the A-P film, but will definitely show abnormality on the frog-leg view, which supports the necessity of employing this view in cases of suspected epiphysiolysis.

Another common line is *Shenton-Menard Arc* (Fig. 5-29). It is a curvilinear line extending up along the medial margin of the femur under the inferior surface of the superior pubic ramus. The line should be smooth and continuous. Any deviation may indicate a femoral dislocation, a slipped epiphysis, or even a fracture.[18a]

**AP spot hip**

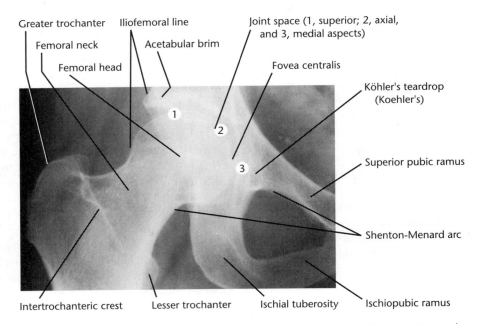

Greater trochanter   Iliofemoral line
Femoral neck   Acetabular brim
Femoral head
Joint space (1, superior; 2, axial, and 3, medial aspects)
Fovea centralis
Köhler's teardrop (Koehler's)
Superior pubic ramus
Shenton-Menard arc
Intertrochanteric crest   Lesser trochanter   Ischial tuberosity   Ischiopubic ramus

*Fig. 5-29*   A radiograph of the hip showing anatomical structures, Shenton-Menard arc, and the iliofemoral line.

The *iliofemoral line* is drawn along the lateral aspect of the ilium passing through a portion of the femoral head and extending along the tangential surface of the femoral neck (Fig. 5-29). This should be a smooth arcuate line. Any significant disruption in its course can be due to lateral displacement of the femur (dislocation or subluxation of the femur) in relation to the acetabular fossa such as in congenital hip dislocation.[43]

*Skinner's line* is drawn along the midshaft of the femur. A second line is constructed perpendicular to the first line along the top of the greater trochanter of the femur. The fovea centralis of the femur should extend above this line. Any deviation could indicate a subluxation, dislocation, epiphysiolysis, or even a fracture.[43]

*Waldenstrom's teardrop* distance is measured from the lateral aspect of Koehler's teardrop to the medial margin of the femoral head. If the distance is greater than 11 mm or if there is a difference greater than 2 mm when comparing the right and left sides then joint effusion should be suspected on the side of greater width.

The *femoral angle* is created by drawing an axis line along the shaft of the femur. A second line is formed along the axis of the femoral neck. The angle formed should measure between 120 to 130 degrees. A measurement less than 120 degrees is coxa varus and one more than 130 degrees is coxa vara.

**Knee.** Minimum examination of the knee should include projections at right angles to one another to visualize the region in two planes of view. The typical knee study consists of an A-P (or P-A) and a lateral view (Fig. 5-30). Many clinicians will include tangential, tunnel, or oblique views for further evaluation. The tangential view provides an axial depiction of the patella and its relationship with the femur (see Case 24). The tunnel allows excellent visualization of the intercondylar region of the femoraltibial articulation. The oblique view provides a different depiction of the knee to detect occult fractures and to provide another view of the joint space between the tibia and femur.

Typically an A-P knee radiograph is taken, but if the patella is the primary area of concern, a P-A view would be useful. The rationale is that there is less distortion or magnification of the part with the area of interest closest to the film. The collimated field should include the distal shaft of the femur to the proximal shafts of the tibia and fibula. In assessing alignment, the femur and tibia should be examined for varus or valgus deformity.

Various mensuration methods are available such as the *femoral and tibial angles* to determine the relationships about the knee (Fig. 5-30). The femoral angle can be measured by drawing one line along the margins of the femoral condyles and a second one through the midshaft of the femur (see Case 24). The angle formed is generally 75 to 85 degrees in both men and women. The tibia can be assessed in the same manner with a line along the plateau margins and a second through the tibial shaft. This angle is normally 85 to 100 degrees in men and 87 to 98 degrees in women.[23]

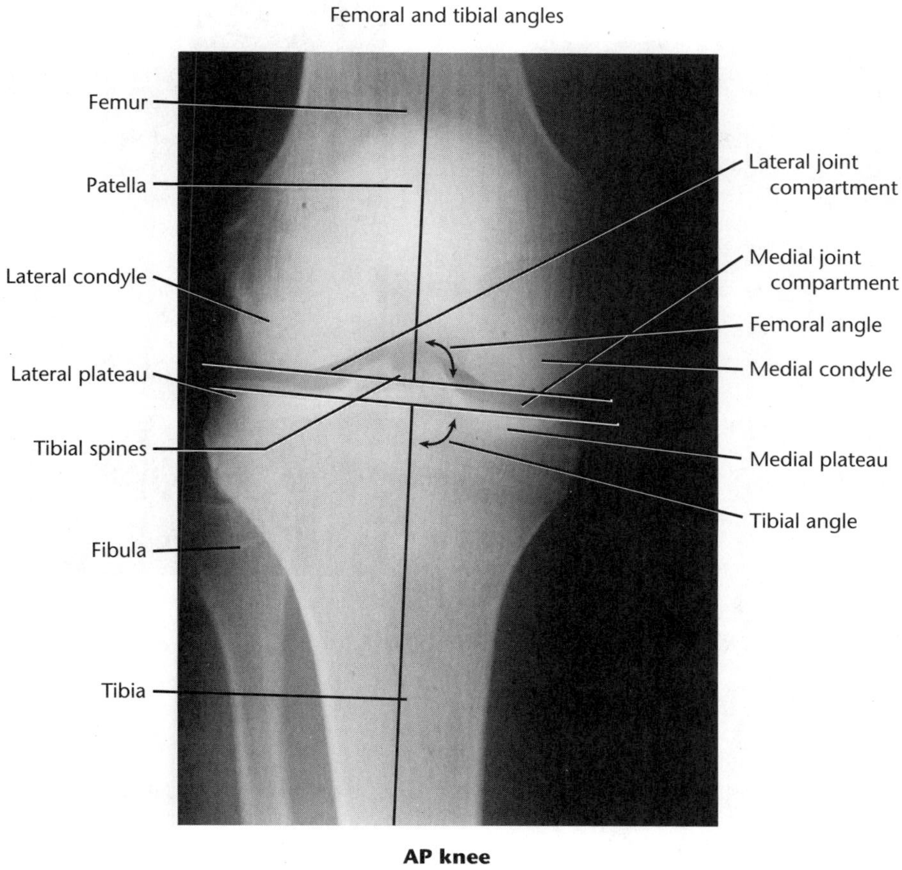

Femoral and tibial angles

Femur

Patella

Lateral condyle

Lateral plateau

Tibial spines

Fibula

Tibia

Lateral joint compartment

Medial joint compartment

Femoral angle

Medial condyle

Medial plateau

Tibial angle

**AP knee**

*Fig. 5-30*  An anterior-posterior radiograph of the knee with anatomical structures and the femoral and tibial angle.

Proper assessment of the lateral projection is based on good radiographic quality as well as positioning. Flexing the knee prevents rotation. The collimated field should include the area from distal femur to the proximal shafts of the tibia and fibula.

The medial femoral condyle extends lower than the lateral condyle so a 10- to 15-degree cephalic tube tilt will allow better visualization of the joint by superimposing the femoral condyles. If the point of clinical interest is the condylar surfaces, then the tube should not be tilted. This will allow better detection of defects along the femoral condyles. The relationship of the patella can be studied in this view by the *patellar position method.* The length of the patella and the distance from the inferior pole of the patella to the tibial tuberosity are compared. The lengths should be equal.[23] An increase in the patellar tendon length of more than 20% compared to the patellar length signals patella alta.

The patella-femoral joint is roughly equivalent in width to the tibiofemoral joint space. The anterior and superior aspect of the patella can show spurring from the attachment of the quadriceps tendon.

The lateral film is most sensitive for evaluating effusion of the joint. It is suggested that the lateral view be performed with the knee flexed at least 20 degrees, but not more than 45 degrees, to see the proper relationship of the suprapatellar bursa between the femoral and suprapatellar fat pads. The bursa is normally flat, measuring less than 5 mm in sagittal depth. A depth greater than 5 mm suggests joint effusion. The bursae are continuous with the joint capsule and are a sensitive indicator of joint effusion.[41a]

**Ankle.** The standard views of the ankle are the A-P, medial oblique (Mortise view), and lateral views (Fig. 5-31). The A-P ankle view includes the collimated field from the distal tibia and fibula through the talocalcaneal junction.

The primary purpose of the A-P ankle view is to illustrate the coronal relationship of the talocrural articulation and its surrounding bony elements of the tibia, fibula, and talus. The anatomic landmarks of the distal tibia include the medial malleolus and the lower tibial plafond that forms the lower articular surface of the tibia. Often in the adult, the physeal scar can be noted

**Mortise view of ankle**

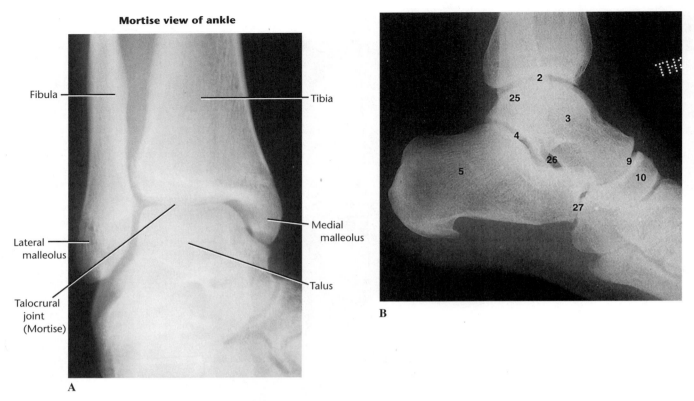

Fibula

Tibia

Lateral
malleolus

Medial
malleolus

Talocrural
joint
(Mortise)

Talus

A

B

*Fig. 5-31* **A,** Mortise and **B,** lateral radiographic views of the ankle, and its corresponding antomical structures. 2, Ankle joint; 3, talus; 4, talocalconeon joint; 5, calcaneus, forming the heel; 9, talonavicular of talocalcaneonavicular joint; 10, navicular bone; 25, shadow of lateral malleolus of fibula overlying tibia and talus; 26, tarsal sinus; 27, calcaneocuboid joint (on the lateral side). (**B** from: McMinn RM, Gaddum-Rosse P, Hutchings RT, Logan BM: *McMinn's functional and clinical anatomy,* St. Louis, 1995, Mosby, with permission.)

progressing transversely through the distal tibial metaphysis and is sometimes seen through the distal fibula. The distal tibia articulates with the fibula forming a fibrous type of joint. The lower aspect of the fibula forms the lateral malleolus. The dome or trochlea of the talus creates the talar portion of the talocrural joint. The joint space should be relatively symmetric in width along its medial, superior, and lateral margins. The lateral portion of the joint space is not visualized to full advantage on this view, which is the reason the medial oblique projection is performed.

The other term for the oblique view is the mortise view because it allows better visualization of this joint. The view brings the lateral malleolus out of superimposition with the talus allowing visualization of the lateral component of the talocrural articulation. It also allows visualization of the distal tibia-fibula articulation. The A-P and oblique projections of the ankle are sensitive for ruling out sites of injury along the lower tibia and fibula.

The lateral ankle view includes the lower tibia and fibula caudally through the talus and calcaneal structures. The medial and lateral malleoli tend to superim-

pose in this projection, with the lateral malleolus slightly more posterior. The talus however, is visualized much more thoroughly in profile, with the head, neck, and body areas demonstrated. The subtalar articulation is represented in profile, below which lies the calcaneus with the sustentaculum tali projecting from its medial aspect. The soft tissues superior to the calcaneus are represented most notably by the Achilles tendon. Anterior to that is the pre-Achilles tendon fat pad. The triangular intersection of the Achilles tendon with the calcaneus is the region of the retrocalcaneal bursa, a location that is sometimes swollen because of mechanical irritation (Achilles tendinitis) or inflammatory arthritis.[41a]

In cases of suspected ligamentous instability, eversion and inversion stress views can be performed. Inversion will test the lateral collateral ligament, whereas eversion will check the medial collateral (deltoid) ligament (see Case 25).

Two lines of measurement are helpful in assessing the ankle. *Boehler's angle* is formed by two intersecting lines connecting the three highest points on the upper surface of the calcaneus. This angle normally measures 20 to 40 degrees. An angle less than 20 degrees is abnormal and most likely suggests an intrinsic comminuted fracture.[43]

The *heel pad* measurement is the distance from the plantar surface of the calcaneus to the skin. A pad measuring more than 25 mm is considered abnormal.[56a]

**Foot.** There are three basic views of the foot. These include the A-P or dorsoplantar view, the oblique view, and the lateral view. In examining the foot the collimated field includes the entire region.

The A-P foot radiograph is taken with the plantar surface of the foot against the film (Fig. 5-32). The bases, shafts, and heads of the metatarsals and phalanges should be examined individually. The bases of the metatarsal structures are usually flat and the heads are convex. The first digit has two phalanges: the distal and proximal phalanges. The other digits have three phalanges: the proximal, middle, and distal phalanges.

Some of the tarsal bones can be visualized on the A-P view. The calcaneus and talus are difficult to see because of superimposition. The navicular bone is rectangular and articulates proximally with the talus. The cuboid bone as its name implies is rather square and articulates with the calcaneus proximally. The medial cuneiform is best visualized with very little overlap with the intermediate cuneiform.

The oblique view is performed with the foot rotated approximately 25 degrees medially. The medial aspect of the foot shoud be against the film. This allows the lateral aspect of the foot to be displayed better. The base of the fifth metatarsal is well demonstrated along with the lateral cuneiform. The oblique view may also be useful in displaying an occult fracture site.

The lateral projection is performed similarly to the lateral ankle view with the lateral aspect of the foot against the film. The entire foot should be included on the radiograph and the central ray should be the center of the foot. The calcaneus and talus are well visualized. The soft tissues can be evaluated for swelling and foreign bodies. Similarly to the ankle, the heel pad distance and Boehler's angles should be examined.

The individual toes can be studied as well. An A-P and a lateral view are considered mandatory and an oblique view may also be useful. Appliances can assist in positioning the toes. Innovation is a key factor for a successful toe radiograph.

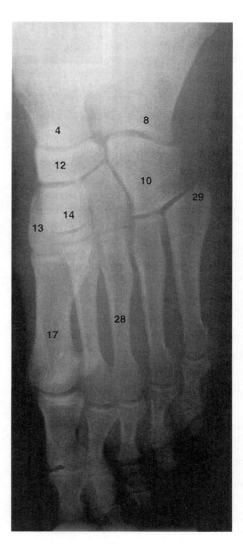

**Fig. 5-32**   A radiograph of the foot and its anatomical structures. 4, Talus; 8, calcaneus, the largest tarsal bone forming the heel at the back; 10, cuboid bone; 12, naviocular bone; 13, medial cuneiform bone; 14, intermediate cuneiform bone; 17, shaft of the first metatarsal bone; 28, third metatarsal bone. (From: McMinn RM, Gaddum-Rosse P, Hutchings RT, Logan BM: *McMinn's functional and clinical anatomy.* St. Louis, 1995, Mosby, with permission.)

**REFERENCES**

1. Alexander C: The acromiohumeral distance in health and disease, *Proc Coll Radiol Aust* 3:102, 1959.
2. Allman FL: Fractures and ligamentous injuries of the clavicle and its articulations, *J Bone Joint Surg.* 49A:774, 1963.
3. Basmajian JV, DeLuca CJ: *Muscles alive: Their functions revealed by electromyography,* ed 5, Baltimore, 1985, Williams & Wilkins.
4. Bejjani FJ, Landsmeer JMF: Biomechanics of the hand. In Nordin M, Frankel VH, editors: *Basic biomechanics of the musculoskeletal system,* Philadelphia, 1989, Lea & Febiger.
5. Bohrer SP: The fat pad sign following elbow trauma, *Clin Radiol* 21:90, 1970.
6. Borysenko M, Beringer T: *Functional Histology,* ed 3, Boston, 1989, Little, Brown & Co.
7. Carver RA, Barrington NA: Soft tissue changes accompanying recent scaphoid injuries, *Clin Radiol* 36:423, 1985.
8. Celli L, et al: Some new aspects of the functional anatomy of the shoulder, *Ital J Orthop Traumatol* 11:83, 1985.
9. Chansky HA, Iannotti JP: The vascularity of the rotator cuff, *Clinics in Sports Med* 10:807, 1991.
10. Cormack, DH: *Essential Histology,* ed 1, Philadelphia, 1993, Lippincott.

11. Dempster WT: Mechanisms of shoulder movement, *Arch Phys Med Rehabil* 46:49, 1965.

12. Evans EM: Rotational deformity in the treatment of fractures of both bones of the forearm, *J Bone Joint Surg* 27:373, 1945.

13. Evans RC: *Illustrated essentials in orthopedic physical assessment,* St. Louis, 1994, Mosby.

14. Fawcett DW: *Bloom and Fawcett: A textbook of histology,* ed 7, Philadelphia, 1986, Saunders.

15. Garth W: Evaluating and treating brachial plexus injuries, *J Muscuioskeletal Med* 55, 1994.

16. Geneser F: *Textbook of histology,* ed 1, Philadelphia, 1986, Lea & Febiger.

17. Gerard JA, Kleinfield SL: *Orthopaedic testing,* New York, 1993, Churchill Livingstone.

18. Gilula LA, editor: *The traumatized wrist and hand: Radiographic and anatomic correlation,* Philadelphia, 1992, Saunders.

18a. Greenspan A: *Orthopedic radiology: A practical approach,* Philadelphia, 1988, Lippincott.

19. Hammer WI: *Functional soft tissue examination and treatment by manual methods: The extremities,* Gaithersburg, 1991, Aspen.

20. Inman VT, et al: Observations on the function of the shoulder joint, *J Bone Joint Surg* 26A:1, 1966.

21. Johnson KE: *Histology and cell biology,* ed 2, Baltimore, 1991, Williams & Wilkins.

22. Junqueira LC, Carneiro J, Kelly RO: *Basic histology,* ed 7, Norwalk, 1992, Appleton & Lange.

23. Keats TE, Lusted LB: *Atlas of roentgenographic measurement,* ed 5, Chicago, 1985, Year Book Medical Publishers.

24. Keats TE, et al: Normal axial relationships of the major joints, *Radiology* 87:904, 1966.

25. Kelly DE, Wood RL, Enders AC. *Bailey's textbook of microscopic anatomy,* ed 8, Baltimore, 1984, Williams & Wilkins.

25a. Kessler RM, Hertling D: The Hip. In Hertling D, Kessler RM: *Management of common musculoskeletal disorders,* ed 2, Philadelphia, 1990, Lippincott.

26. Kettelkamp DB, Jacobs AW: Tibiofemoral contact area: determination and implications, *J Bone Joint Surg,* 54A:349, 1972.

27. Kopell HP, Thompson WAL: *Peripheral entrapment neuropathies.* Malabar, 1976, Robert E. Krieger Publ Co.

28. Kronberg M, Nemeth G, Brostrom LA: Muscle activity and coordination in the normal shoulder: An electromyographic study, *Clin Orthop Rel Rsch* 257:76, 1990.

29. Last RJ: *Anatomy, regional and applied: The upper limb,* section 2, Edinburgh, 1972, Churchill Livingstone.

30. Leeson TS, Leeson CR, Paparo AA: *Text/Atlas of Histology,* ed 1. Philadelphia, 1988, Saunders.

31. Lev-Toaff AS, Karasick D, Rao VM: Drooping shoulder: nontraumatic causes of glenohumeral subluxation, *Skel Radiol* 12:34, 1984.

32. Lippitt S, Matsen F: Mechanisms of glenohumeral joint stability, *Clin Orthop* 291:20, 1993.

33. London JT: Kinematics of the elbow, *J Bone Joint Surg* 63A:529, 1981.

34. Moore KL: *Clinically oriented anatomy,* ed 3, Baltimore, 1992, Williams & Wilkins.

35. Morrey BF, Chao EY: Passive motion of the elbow joint: A biomechanical analysis, *J Bone Joint Surg* 58A:501, 1976.

36. Nordin M, Frankel VH: Biomechanics of the hip. In Nordin M, Frankel VH, editors: *Basic biomechanics of the musculoskeletal system,* Philadelphia, 1989, Lea & Febiger.

37. Nordin M, Frankel VH: Biomechanics of the ankle. In Nordin M, Frankel VH, editors: *Basic biomechanics of the musculoskeletal system,* Philadelphia, 1989, Lea & Febiger.

38. Norrell HG: Roentgenologic visualization of the extracapsular fat. Its importance in the diagnosis of traumatic injuries to the elbow, *Acta Radiol* 43:205, 1954.

39. Perry J: Biomechanics of the shoulder. In Rowe CR editor: *The shoulder,* New York, 1988, Churchill Livingstone.

40. Petersson CJ, Redlund-Johnell I: Joint space in normal glenohumeral radiographs, *Acta Orthop Scand* 54:274, 1983.

41. Poppen NK, Walker PS: Normal and abnormal motion of the shoulder, *J Bone Joint Surg,* 58A:195, 1976.

41a. Resnick D, Niwayama G: *Diagnosis of bone and joint disorders,* ed 2, Philadelphia, 1988, Saunders.

42. Rockwood CA, Green DP: *Fractures,* Philadelphia, 1975, Lippincott.

43. Rogers LF: *Radiology of skeletal trauma,* New York, 1982, Churchill Livingstone.

44. Rogers SL, MacEwan DW: Changes due to trauma in fat plane overlying the supinator muscle: A radiographic sign, *Radiology* 92:954, 1969.

45. Ross MH, Romrell LJ: *Histology,* ed 2, Baltimore, 1989, Williams & Wilkins.

45a. Rowe LJ, Yochum TR: Radiographic positioning and normal anatomy. In Yochum, TR, Rowe LJ, editors; *Essentials of skeletal radiology,* vol 1, Baltimore, 1987, Williams & Wilkins.

46. Schwab GH, et al: Biomechanics of elbow stability: the role of the medial collateral ligament, *Clin Orthop* 146:42, 1980.

47. Deleted in galleys.

48. Silliman JF, Hawkins RJ: Classification and physical diagnosis of instability of the shoulder, *Clin Orthop* 291:7, 1993.

49. Smith DN, Lee JR: The radiological diagnosis of post-traumatic effusion of the elbow joint and its clinical significance: The displaced fat pad sign, *Injury* 10:115, 1978.

50. Stevens A, Lowe J: *Histology,* New York, 1992, Gower Medical Publishing.

51. Storen G: The radiocapitellar relationship, *Acta Chir Scand* 116:144, 1995.

52. Stuchin S: Biomechanics of the wrist. In Nordin M, Frankel VH: *Basic biomechanics of the musculoskeletal system,* ed 2, Philadelphia, 1989, Lea & Febiger.

53. Terry DW, Jr, Ramin JE: The navicular fat stripe: A useful Roentgen feature for evaluating wrist trauma, *Am J Roentgenol* 124:25, 1975.

54. Volz RG, Lieb M, Benjamin J: Biomechanics of the wrist, *Clin Orthop* 149:112, 1980.

55. Wheater PR, Burkitt HG, Daniels VG: *Functional Histology,* ed 2, New York, Churchill Livingstone.

56. Winter D: *Biomechanics and motor control of human movement,* ed 2, New York, 1990, Wiley-Interscience Publication.

56a. Yochum TR, Rowe LJ: Measurements in skeletal radiology. In Yochum TR, Rowe, LJ, editors. *Essentials of skeletal radiology,* vol 1, Baltimore, 1987, Williams & Wilkins.

57. Zuckerman JD, Matsen FA: Biomechanics of the shoulder. In Nordin M, Frankel VH: *Basic biomechanics of the musculoskeletal system,* ed 2, Philadelphia, 1989, Lea & Febiger.

## SUGGESTED READINGS

Bergmann TF, Peterson DH, Lawrence DJ: *Chiropractic technique,* New York, 1993, Churchill Livingstone.

Hammer WI: *Functional soft tissue examination and treatment by manual methods: The extremities,* Gaithersburg, 1991, Aspen.

Kendall HO, Kendall FP, Wadsworth GE: *Muscles: Testing and function,* ed 3, Baltimore, 1992, Williams & Wilkins.

Magee DJ: *Orthopedic physical assessment,* ed 2, Philadelphia, 1992, Saunders.

Moore KL. Clinically oriented anatomy, ed 3, Baltimore, 1992, Williams & Wilkins.

Nordin M, Frankel VH: *Basic biomechanics of the musculoskeletal system,* ed 2, Philadelphia, 1989, Lea & Febiger.

Perry J: Biomechanics of the shoulder. In Rowe CR editor: *The shoulder,* New York, 1988, Churchill Livingstone.

# CHAPTER 6    *Human locomotion (gait)*

**CASE**

*Connection*

1, 2, 4, 5, 23, 24, 25, 26

## KEY TERMS

*Child growth and development*
*Neonatal reflexes*
*Higher-order reflexes*
*Monosynaptic reflex arc*

*Motor unit*
*Lever system*
*Kinematics and kinetics*
*of human walking*

## NEUROSCIENCE OF HUMAN LOCOMOTION
### Reflexes pertinent to human locomotion

CHARLES N. R. HENDERSON

Human locomotion (gait) is a learned phenomenon that requires the development of neuronal synapses for reflexes as well as intentional motor actions. Intentional motor actions are a complex composite of cortically initiated actions, reflexes at the spinal cord and brain stem levels, and modulatory influences from the cerebellum and the basal ganglia. None of these components act alone.[5] Alteration in the character or magnitude of a reflex is often the earliest and most subtle sign of neurologic dysfunction. The patient's reflexes may be the most objective evidence of neurologic function obtained during an examination. Although patients can voluntarily influence their reflexes to some degree, reflexes are less readily controlled than are muscle strength, sensory testing, coordination, or range of motion. This section will focus on the reflexes needed for "normal" human locomotion.

**Postural and righting reflexes.** A normal adult can stand erect and rise from a recumbent position without any difficulty. Maintaining an upright posture and righting are essential reflex actions accomplished by interaction of spinal, visual, and vestibular reflexes. Although almost the entire central nervous system is involved, the reflex centers for posture and righting are thought to be located in the brain stem.[8] Reflexes related to the postural and righting reflexes can be demonstrated in neonates and infants. Some of these reflexes are the Moro (startle) reflex, neck righting reflexes, tonic neck reflexes, and stepping reactions.

*Moro reflex* (startle reflex) is present during the first 3 months of life. A sudden loud noise, light, or movement causes an infant to reflexively extend and abduct and flex and adduct the extremities and spine. Typically this reflex disappears over the next few months. However, children with cerebral damage and associated motor deficits may continue to demonstrate this reflex for years.

The *Landau reflex* (righting reflex) is present during the first 1 to 2 years of life. A normal infant held prone in the examiner's hand will extend the head and spine. When the infant is held supine, the head and spine flex. Passive flexion of the infant's head will also cause the spine to flex. This response is caused by labyrinthine (mostly utricle and saccule) and neck righting reflexes.

*Tonic neck reflexes* are present in the first 4 to 6 months of life. They are the combined result of labyrinthine and neck-righting reflexes and are the first reflexes to illustrate the development of the neuronal circuitry of gait. These reflexes are produced by the examiner moving the subject's head relative to the rest of the body (Fig. 6-1). When the head is turned or tilted to the side, the ipsilateral limbs will extend, supinate, and become rigid; the contralateral limbs will flex and pronate. The muscle tone of the flexed limb is always less than that of the extended limb. Similarly, if the head is flexed, the upper limbs flex and the lower limbs extend; and, if the head is extended, the upper limbs extend and the lower limbs flex. Also firm pressure over C7 results in relaxation of all four limbs.

**Neck righting response.** This response is thought to represent a maturation of components of the tonic neck reflex. It is seen in the infant at 4 to 6 months of age, after the disappearance of the tonic neck reflexes. When the infant is held supine, the examiner turns the head to the side. The shoulder, trunk, and pelvis rotate toward the side to which the head faces. This reflex disappears at about the time the child can arise without first rotating to its abdomen.

It will be noted in this section that antigravity support of the body is principally a reflex act. But, contraction of antigravity muscles to maintain upright posture must not be rigid. Walking and running both require slight, but precise, shifts in the position of the head and trunk in harmony with placement of the feet. Therefore, maintaining an upright posture (equilibrium) during normal activity requires rapid and ongoing adjustment of the postural reflexes.

## Maintenance of equilibrium

Equilibrium, or balance, is the body's exact and almost instantaneous counteraction to the forces of gravity. This is accomplished by cerebellar modulation of the vestibular nucleus in response to a constantly changing barrage of proprioceptive information.[6] Proprioceptive information arises from deep tissues (mechanoreceptors in ligaments and joint capsules, muscle spindles, and golgi tendon organs), skin, the labyrinthine apparatus (especially the utricle, but also the saccule and semicircular canals), and the retina.[6] Therefore, even the standing posture is not a static condition. The body is constantly swaying to and fro in readjustment to maintain the center of gravity. This sway is not simply a pivot from the ankles, but from the hips as well.[5]

All voluntary movements are conducted at the risk of losing postural equilibrium and so are accompanied by strategies to regain this equilibrium. There are essentially three strategies for the control of upright stance:

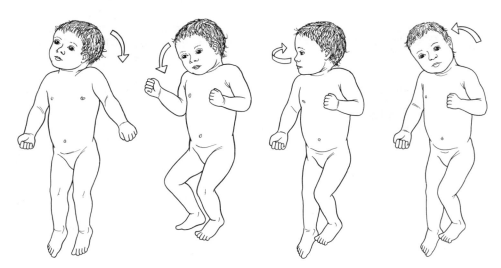

*Fig. 6-1*   The tonic neck reflexes normally present in an infant. The extremities respond by reflexive positioning, depending on the position of the neonate's head and neck.

(1) *Postural preparations* that are initiated prior to a voluntary movement (for example, widening the stance, bending the knees, and arching the low back prior to lifting something heavy). (2) *Postural accompaniments* (*feedforward control*) that occur simultaneously with each voluntary movement. This involves unconsciously anticipating the effect of a movement of posture and making compensatory adjustments during the motion. (3) *Postural reactions* (*sensory-based feedback*) strategies that trigger automatic postural adjustments. They usually occur within 100 milliseconds (for example, regaining balance after slipping on an icy spot).[11,20]

Normal gait requires a highly coordinated shift of body weight from side to side along with counterrotation of the trunk and swinging of the upper limbs. Postural reflexes constantly modulate the antigravity muscles to maintain upright posture while standing, walking, or running. These activities require ongoing integration of both extracranial (from muscle, joint, and skin) and cranial (visual and labyrinthine) proprioceptive information. These inputs converge and are integrated in the brain stem and cerebellum.[7,13] The labyrinthine input arises from the otoliths (saccule and utricle) and the three semicircular canals and is conducted by the vestibular nerve to the vestibular nucleus in the brain stem and directly to the cerebellum.[13] Most of the neurons in the vestibular nucleus also receive cervical proprioceptive input. From the vestibular nucleus, neurons project to the cerebellum carrying both labyrinthine and cervical proprioceptive information. Vestibulospinal projections are important for reflex adjustments of posture and gait. Visual proprioceptive information is routed to the inferior olive in the rostral medulla. Inferior olive neurons project to the cerebellum where they converge with the labyrinthine projections.[1,16]

Extracranial proprioceptive inputs provide information concerning the position and motion of the head, trunk, and extremities. The cervical muscles are particularly important in this regard. They contain an unusually large number of proprioceptive receptors, having six to eight times more muscle spindles than do other muscles.[3] The critical nature of cervical input to the maintenance of normal equilibrium is demonstrated in a study by De Jong.[9] In this study, local anesthetics injected into the neck induced vertigo, ataxia, and nystagmus in animals and man. An interruption anywhere along the major pathway for extracranial proprioceptive information may produce ataxia.

The integration of cervical proprioceptive input with visual information is also essential for accurate location of an object in visual space. This was demonstrated in an elegant experiment reported by Biguer.[3] The tip of a physiotherapy vibrator (100 Hz) was applied to the posterior neck muscles in the depression below the left lateral occiput of human subjects. This produced an illusion in which a visual target appeared to move to the right of its actual position. Muscle spindles in the suboccipital muscles sent inappropriate signals to the cerebellum (as if the head had been turned to the right to maintain visual fixation). Increasing the amplitude of the vibration increased the magnitude of the illusion. Thus, extracranial proprioceptive input may be critical to other special sensory functions.

Cranial proprioceptive input provides information with regard to gravity and head position or movement. The labyrinthine receptors in the inner ear also allow the eyes to focus on a stable image (visual fixation) during head movement (vestibuloocular reflexes), as well as allow postural adjustment (vestibulospinal reflexes). As noted in the subjects above, visual proprioceptive input can compensate to a substantial degree for both labyrinthine and extracranial proprioceptive loss. This is why tests for station and gait are done with the eyes open and closed (for example, Romberg's test).[6]

Visual information alone can provide strong simulation of movement. A common example is the brief, but uncomfortable sensation of falling or moving backward that is experienced when a car parked next to you unexpectedly moves forward. This sensation is brief because it is rapidly suppressed. The mismatch between extracranial and cranial proprioceptive inputs within integrative centers of the brain stem and cerebellum produces short-term suppression of the incongruent proprioceptive information. Continued mismatch of these inputs produces a "sensory conflict" which may be experienced as motion sickness, imbalance, or vertigo.

**Stepping.** During normal gait, the head and trunk are held erect, the feet are slightly everted, and the steps are bilaterally symmetric. Each individual develops a highly characteristic postural rhythm that opposes displacement of the body's center of gravity with each step. As an individual steps forward, the advancing lower limb flexes at the hip and knee and dorsiflexes at the ankle. The pelvis moves almost imperceptibly, elevating and rotating forward on the side of the advancing limb. Meanwhile, the contralateral shoulder and upper limb swing forward as a counterbalance. The heel of the advancing foot strikes the ground first and the individual's full weight shifts to that foot. Supportive forces are progressively distributed from the heel to the outside of the sole, across the metatarsal arch, and finally, at the "push off," to the first metatarsal and great toe.

Stepping is largely a reflex that is present at birth. Prior to the development of voluntary stepping (within the first year), infants display a *placing reaction*. If the infant is held vertically, and the dorsum of the feet touch the underside of the examining table, the infant will reflexly place each foot on the top of the table. Similarly, if the same infant is held vertically with its feet placed firmly on the top of the examining table, the flexors and extensors of the lower limbs will contract, locking the joints of the lower limbs. In addition, the infant will usually make reflex stepping motions. In lower mammals, but not in primates, a stepping response can be induced in some animals that have the spinal cord surgically separated from higher centers (for example, spinal cats). This suggests that the basic circuitry for stepping is present in the spinal cord of these animals. In primates, however, stepping requires participation of higher reflex centers (such as the posture center in the rostral mesencephalon).

### Higher order reflexive mechanisms

Understanding the role of reflex function in normal health and disease is essential to the clinician. Much of the patient's response to treatment will be mediated through reflex mechanisms. Even voluntary movement has a reflex component. Intentional motor actions are a complex composite of cortically initiated actions, reflexes at the spinal cord and brain stem levels, and modulatory influences from the cerebellum and the basal ganglia. None of these components act alone.[5] Alteration in the character or magnitude of a reflex is often the earliest and most subtle sign of neurologic dysfunction. The patient's reflexes may be the most objective evidence of neurologic function obtained during the examination. Although patients can voluntarily influence their reflexes to some degree, reflexes are less readily controlled than are muscle strength, sensory testing, coordination, or range of motion. Moreover, abnormal reflexes are quite difficult to simulate. It is stressed that interpretation of reflexive responses must not be made in the absence of a complete examination (including history, inspection, spinal examination, and indicated ancillary studies [for example, diagnostic imaging, paraspinal instrumentation, and clinical laboratory tests]). The basic reflex circuitry and reflex development are discussed here.

### Basic reflex circuitry

A reflex is simply a stereotyped, involuntary response to a sensory stimulus. Each reflex has a sensory (afferent) limb that carries information into the central nervous system and a motor (efferent) limb that carries the response signal away from the central nervous system. One or more interneurons may be interposed between the afferent and efferent limbs, the whole complex constituting the *reflex arc*. All elements of the reflex arc must be intact to obtain a normal response. The neural circuit shown in Figure 6-2 is the simplest reflex arc—the *muscle stretch reflex*. In this reflex there is no interneuron interposed between the afferent and efferent limbs. Reflex arcs increase in complexity from this simple, monosynaptic circuit to those with multiple interneurons that synapse bilaterally and involve several levels along the rostrocaudal extent of the central nervous system.

The neural circuitry of the simple muscle stretch reflex, the withdrawal reflex, and the refinement of reciprocal and crossed effects demonstrate the essential concepts of somatic reflex function.

**Muscle stretch reflexes.** Indirect stimulation of sensory receptors within a striated muscle, by striking a tendon or bone with a reflex hammer, or direct stimula-

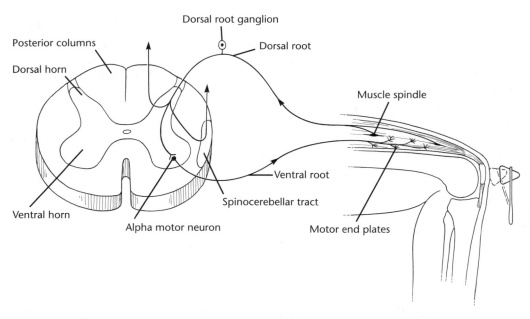

*Fig. 6-2*   Monosynaptic reflex arc initiated by the deep tendon reflex.

tion (striking the muscle itself) produces a brief lengthening of the muscle followed immediately by a reflex contraction. Similar reflex arcs exist for the cranial nerves, but involve brain stem nuclei. The afferent limb of the arc is formed by Ia fibers arising from muscle spindles within the belly of the muscle. These fibers terminate directly (without interneurons) on a motor neuron in the ventral horn of the spinal cord. The efferent limb of the reflex arc is formed by the axons (alpha motor fibers) arising from these motor neurons. These fibers terminate as motor end plates on the muscle fibers. Brief lengthening of the muscle produces a signal that travels rapidly through the afferent and efferent limbs of the arc with only one synapse (*monosynaptic reflex*). This signal is excitatory. It causes the quadriceps muscle to contract, producing the visible and palpable response sought by the examiner.

Normal muscles do not all give the same response to a tendon tap. The extensor muscles of the upper limbs respond more rapidly and forcibly than do the flexor muscles. This is because flexor muscle excitation is rapidly inhibited by impulses from higher (supraspinal) centers within the normal central nervous system. This relationship can be readily observed in most individuals by comparing the biceps (flexor) reflex to the triceps (extensor) reflex.

As noted above, directly stimulating muscle spindles by striking the muscle belly will produce a contraction. This contraction usually persists for only a short time after the stimulation. After muscle denervation, direct stimulation produces a prolonged contraction response (myotatic irritability) while indirect stimulation (for example, tendon percussion) fails to produce a contraction.

**Withdrawal reflex.** While the biceps reflex illustrates a deep somatic reflex, the withdrawal reflex is an example of a superficial somatic reflex. In the withdrawal reflex, the afferent limb arises from cutaneous or mucosal receptors that respond to noxious stimuli (nociceptors). The muscle stretch reflex involves only the muscle that is stretched, whereas the withdrawal reflex involves a whole region of the body. A typical response is a rapid withdrawal of the upper limb when the fingertip touches a hot burner. This is a fortuitous reflex action, occurring before the subject has time to think about it. Withdrawing the limb requires participation of motor nuclei at multiple segmental levels of the spinal cord. In the withdrawal reflex, nerve fibers arise from cutaneous nociceptors in the fingertip and, upon entering the spinal cord, bifurcate into branches that project to cord segments above and below the point of entry. These ascending and descending branches give off collateral branches that terminate on interneurons, some of which also project to other spinal levels. The interneurons terminate on alpha motor neurons that form the efferent limbs of

the reflex. The end result is the rostrocaudal spread of sensory information–producing contraction of the many muscles (with varying spinal innervation levels) required to withdraw the finger from the hot burner.

**Reciprocal and crossed effect of a reflex.** The two reflexes discussed above are very simple, involving only prime movers, and only one side of the body. Clearly, this is a great simplification of our daily experiences. Additional refinements permit smooth and effective movements that characterize our normal reflex actions. To understand these refinements it is useful to consider the two basic reflexes introduced above.

The muscle stretch reflex involves only the muscle that was stretched (the primary muscle). This is certainly the strongest response. However, other muscles (synergists) that assist the action of the primary muscle are also recruited. Their contractions are much weaker, but they assist in relaxing the primary muscle by producing movements that bring its origin and insertion together. In a similar fashion, muscles that oppose the motion of the primary muscle, and therefore oppose its shortening, are inhibited (for example, Renshaw cells). These refinements of the basic muscle stretch are known as reciprocal effects (reciprocal excitation and reciprocal inhibition).

The withdrawal reflex introduced another degree of complexity, involvement of multiple longitudinal levels of the central nervous system. The reader may have already realized that withdrawing a threatened body part requires stabilization of the other parts of the body. This is the final refinement introduced here. For the finger to have been effectively withdrawn from the burner the shoulder girdle would also have to be stabilized. In addition, the trunk and lower limbs would be extended rapidly. These actions involve not only the longitudinal extent of the nervous system, but contralateral regions as well. These "crossed effects" are nicely demonstrated by a person stepping on a tack. Rapid withdrawal of the foot must be accompanied by an equally rapid extension of the contralateral lower limb. Involvement of this extended limb is accomplished by excitatory and inhibitory interneurons that cross the cord.

The reflex mechanisms discussed above are quite basic but they help in the understanding of much more complex somatic activities such as posture and gait.

### Postural and gait reflexes

Maintaining a standing posture, walking, or running requires a complex interaction of virtually the entire central nervous system. To simplify the task of reviewing the reflexes involved, we will examine three major components that are common to both walking and running: (1) antigravity support of the body, (2) maintenance of equilibrium, and (3) stepping. There are voluntary and reflex motor interactions in each of these components.

**Antigravity support of the body.** A neurologically intact individual arises from a prone position by the interaction of a family of postural reflexes called the *righting reflexes.* Upright posture is then maintained by reflex extension of the lower extremities, neck, and trunk by means of the antigravity muscles.[4] The smooth sequence of actions that accompany the act of arising (look up, sit up, and stand up) requires communication between a postural center (or centers) in the midbrain reticular formation and more caudal brain stem areas (the pontine and medullary reticular formation and the vestibular nuclear complex). Descending fibers from the lateral reticular area (especially from the pontomedullary reticular formation), as well as from the vestibular area (especially from the lateral vestibular [Dieters'] nucleus) provide ongoing excitation of spinal reflexes. In this way, tone is maintained in the antigravity muscles. There is also a localized area within the medial reticular formation of the caudal medulla that, when stimulated by descending fibers from the mesencephalic postural center, inhibits spinal reflexes. This arrangement permits upright posture without conscious effort through tonic output of the lateral reticular and vestibular areas. However, upright posture must be modified to perform locomotion. Postural tone is modified by the mesencephalic postural center sending excitatory impulses to the medial reticular area of the caudal medulla, which inhibits spinal reflexes, or by the postural center inhibiting the lateral reticular and vestibular areas.

Transecting the neuroaxis provides instructive effects on muscle tone and spinal reflexes. A transverse cut that isolates the spinal cord from the brain stem produces flaccid paralysis, but spinal reflexes remain intact. If the neuraxis is cut transversely at the middle of the mesencephalon, or at the midpons, the pontomedullary reticular formation and the vestibular area are isolated from the descending modulatory influences of the posture center. Lacking this control, the lateral reticular and vestibular areas send unchecked excitatory stimuli to the spinal cord reflexes. This produces tonic spasticity in the antigravity muscles and hyperreflexia. In quadrapeds this means rigid extension of all four limbs, but in primates there is rigid extension of the lower limbs and rigid flexion of the upper limbs.

There are four righting reflexes: *optical, labyrinthine, neck,* and *body righting* reflexes. Although optical righting reflexes require cortical integration, the midbrain (superior colliculus and the reticular formation) provides essential mediation with the pontomedulary reticular formation and vestibular nuclear complex. When the eyes are turned, the head and body are also turned toward the object viewed. Normally, vision does not play an essential role in posture or equilibrium. However, when proprioceptive information from other sources (labyrinth or deep tissues) is sufficiently compromised, visual information becomes essential. This is readily demonstrated by patients with tabes dorsalis. These patients have lost proprioceptive input from deep tissues primarily due to degeneration of the posterior columns and dorsal roots of the spinal cord. They become very dependent on visual information to walk or even maintain standing posture.

Labyrinthine righting reflexes respond to changes in position of the head and act upon the muscles of the entire body. Of specific interest is the effect these reflexes have upon the neck and other antigravity muscles of the body. When the body is tilted, the labyrinthine reflex (mostly through the utricle) increases the tone of antigravity muscles bilaterally, but the muscles of the neck are contracted such that the head is returned to an upright position. Similarly, when the head is rotated, the labyrinthine reflex (through the semicircular canals) increases the tone of the neck muscles on the side toward which the face is rotated.

The neck righting reflex is a spinal cord reflex located in the upper two or three cervical segments. The afferent limb arises from the deep tissues of the neck. The efferent limb acts upon the muscles. When the head is rotated, the pelvis tilts slightly toward the contralatral side, while the shoulders and hips rotate toward the ipsilateral side.

The body righting reflex is centered in the medulla. Proprioceptive information from the deep tissues of the trunk and limbs ascend to the medulla. The efferent limb of the reflex is mediated through the vestibular nuclear complex.

Gait is highly individual. The general build, or even the identity of individuals can be guessed by the unique sound pattern of their gait. In addition, masculine and feminine characteristics can be differentiated in a gait. Finally, there are highly characteristic modifications of gait associated with various disease conditions (for example, cerebellar gait, sensory ataxia, festinating gait, hysterical gait, and spastic gaits) (see Cases 2, 4, and 5).

## Muscle mechanics

Muscle contraction is an extremely complicated and chemically balanced phenomenon that occurs many times daily. The scientific understanding of muscle contraction and strength production is limited. This section will focus on striated muscle and its physiologic function.

### Physiology of muscle contraction
GENE TOBIAS

The ability of the neuromusculoskeletal (NMS) system to perform movement and control posture depends on skeletal muscle contraction. Skeletal muscle contraction occurs by the *sliding filament mechanism.* This mechanism utilizes the contractile proteins that make up the *thick* and *thin filaments* of the sarcomeres within muscle. The thick filament is composed of *myosin* molecules arranged with their "tail" portions pointing toward the center of the thick filament with the "head" portions found at the ends of the thick filament. Each myosin "head" is normally oriented at about a 90-degree angle with respect to its "tail." The thin filament is composed of three proteins: *actin, troponin,* and *tropomyosin.* Actin has a binding site for the myosin head and troponin has three binding sites referred to as the C-site, T-site, and I-site.

When skeletal muscle is relaxed, the following conditions exist:

1. The muscle cell membrane potential equals the resting membrane potential.
2. The $Ca^{2+}$ ion concentration inside the muscle cell is low.
3. The C-site on troponin is unoccupied; tropomyosin is binding to troponin at the T-site (T refers to tropomyosin).
4. Actin binds to troponin at the I-site (I refers to inhibition of contraction).
5. Tropomyosin covers the actin-binding site of the myosin head.
6. Muscle tension is low indicating that only a few actin and myosin proteins are binding.

During skeletal muscle contraction, the following sequence of events occurs:

1. The neruon action potential triggers acetylcholine release at the synapse, between the alpha motor neuron and skeletal muscle fiber. A muscle end plate potential results creating a muscle action potential immediately outside the end-plate region by depolarizing the muscle cell to the threshold potential.
2. The muscle action potential travels along the cell membrane, through the T-tubular membrane that depolarizes the membrane of the sarcoplasmic reticulum (SR) inside the cell.
3. Voltage-dependent gates on SR membrane protein $Ca^{2+}$ channels open, increasing the membrane permeability to $Ca^{2+}$.
4. $Ca^{2+}$ enters the muscle cytoplasm from the SR and binds to troponin at the C-site (C refers to $Ca^{2+}$).
5. The bond breaks between actin and troponin at the I-site.
6. Tropomyosin moves with respect to actin to uncover the actin-binding site for the myosin head.
7. The myosin head binds to the actin binding site creating a crossbridge between the thick and thin filament increasing muscle tension.
8. The myosin head releases energy rapidly (like a gun

firing) and moves to a more acute angle of about 45 degrees.
9. The thick filament slides along the thin filaments toward both z lines resulting in shortening of the sarcomere and the muscle (Fig. 6-3).

Muscle relaxation occurs by the following sequence of events:

1. The muscle action potential ends.
2. The SR membrane repolarizes and the membrane $Ca^{2+}$ channel gates close.
3. $Ca^{2+}$ is removed from the C-site on troponin and pumped back into the SR by a SR membrane $Ca^{2+}$ ion pump (requiring ATP).
4. Actin binds to troponin at the I-site.
5. ATP binds to the myosin head causing the crossbridge to break.
6. Tropomyosin covers up the binding site on actin for the myosin head.
7. The myosin head enzyme (ATPase) converts the bound ATP to free ADP plus phosphate and energy and uses the energy to change the myosin head position back to 90 degrees with respect to the tail and the long axis of the thick filament (recock the gun).
8. The muscle tension decreases.

These mechanisms for skeletal muscle contraction and relaxation are the same for all muscles of the body. The basis for the NMS system's ability to perform the two functions of movement and posture control in part is due to two different types of muscle: fast twitch glycolytic (FG, type II) muscle and slow twitch oxidative (SO, type I) muscle. Exercise physiologists argue that there are other muscle types: FG, SO, and an intermediate type, fast twitch oxidative glycolytic (FOG or type IIb). Fast twitch muscles contract and relax quickly; slow twitch muscle fibers contract and relax slowly. Table 6-1 lists the other differences in anatomic, biochemical, and physiologic characteristics between the muscle types. The fast twitch muscle fibers generally are designed for quick, fine movements (phasic), whereas, slow twitch muscle fibers are designed for gross, sustained contractions (tetanus, tonic) for prolonged control of posture. The selection of the muscle type among the muscles of the body appears to be determined by the alpha motor neurons through synaptic transmission and through neurotrophic factors.

The sliding filament theory explains concentric muscle activity; however, the theory is limited in its explanation of eccentric muscle activity. How a muscle produces tension during a lengthening action is a physiologic mystery. Recent literature on the subject describes the action of actin and myosin as a screw. When contraction occurs, the myosin head torques around the longitudinal axis of the myosin molecule. This finding can possibly

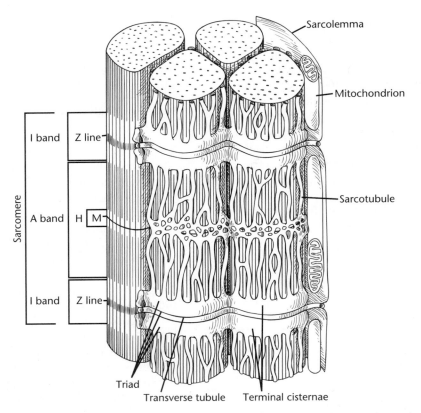

**Fig. 6-3** Histologic appearance of the actin and myosin filaments of striated muscle. *ATP,* adenosine triphosphate; *Ca,* calcium.

spread more light on the physiologic events that occur during eccentric muscle action.

**Muscle biomechanics.** Striated muscle (skeletal muscle) has many biomechanical properties that make it an exceptional organ. Its ability to volitionally contract and relax and cause human motion make it an essential organ. Striated muscle is composed of active and passive components. Its active components consist of actin and myosin fibrils that create changes in muscle length depending on the neurologic and tonic demands. The passive components do not contract and consist of *epimysium, perimysium,* and *endomysium* fibrous coverings that wrap around different layers of the muscle. The endomysium wraps each fibril, the perimysium wraps each muscle bundle, and the epimysium wraps the complete muscle. The passive components also consist of the tendon that attaches muscle to bone.

The active components produce a certain amount of force (tension) at the insertion of the muscle that causes joint motion to occur. The passive components are elastic and participate in the total tension produced by the muscle. The passive components act similarly to a rubber band. When they are lengthened (stretched) a potential energy is produced. When the stretch is released, the tissue returns to its original shape and the stored potential energy is changed to kinetic energy, adding to the total force the muscle can achieve. The elastic

**Table 6-1** Characteristic differences between fast and slow twitch skeletal muscle fibers

| Characteristics | Fast twitch | Slow twitch |
|---|---|---|
| Twitch duration | Short | Long |
| Mitochondria | Few | Many |
| Myoglobin concentration | Low | High |
| Color | White | Red |
| Blood supply | Low | High |
| Energy substrate | Glucose | Glucose and fatty acids |
| Energy metabolism | Aerobic glycolysis | Oxidative phophorylation |
| Time to fatigue | Rapid | Slow |
| Motor unit size | Small | Large |
| Action potential frequency to produce tetanus | High | Low |
| Biomechanical role | Flexor | Extensor |
| Function | Movement | Postural control |

components are divided into two categories: (1) parallel elastic components (epimysium, perimysium, and endomysium) and (2) the series elastic (tendon) components. The parallel elastic components are in parallel with the active muscle components. When the muscle is at a resting length, or shortened, these components are slack and produce no tension. As the muscle lengthens past its resting length, tension is produced in the parallel elastic components in a nonlinear fashion.[21] A length-tension curve describes the interaction of the active and elastic components (Fig. 6-4). First described by Hill in 1941, the maximum amount of active component tension occurs at the resting length of a muscle. The passive components contribute potential energy to muscle tension as the muscle is lengthened beyond its resting length. As is seen from the length-tension curve, production of tension by the active components decreases after the resting length is reached, this action being caused by a decrease in the number of cross-bridges that are formed. The passive components, however, now begin to display a steep increase in tension. This illustrates the stiffness properties of these components. The slope is steep enough to add to the total tension produced within the muscle. The maximum that a muscle can be stretched before its tension curve decreases is 20% beyond its resting length.[21]

During human motion the passive components are used by stretching muscle. A typical example of this muscle activity are basketball players. While performing a jump shot, they will quickly flex the knees and then jump by forcefully extending their knees.

The series elastic components (tendons) do not respond in the same manner as do the parallel elastic components.[21] When the active components of muscle produces tension, the series elastic components stretch and add to the total energy being produced by the muscle. The most frequent mechanical description of the relationship between active and passive muscle components is described by a dash-pot spring diagram. The active components of the muscle are presented as the dash-pot and the passive components are described by the spring (Fig. 6-5).

**Motor unit and muscle activity.** The motor unit consists of one motor neuron and the muscle fibers it innervates. When a motor nerve impulse is received by a muscle, many motor units are activated and a muscle contraction (activity) is produced. There are three different types of contraction that a skeletal muscle can produce: concentric, eccentric, and static muscle actions (See Glossary).

**Force-velocity relationships.** Another important variable of striated muscle is its *force-velocity relationship*. During a concentric muscle action the load produced by the muscle is inversely proportional to the velocity at which it can produce that load (Fig. 6-6). In an eccentric muscle action, force and velocity of contraction can be increased beyond that produced by a concentric muscle action of the same muscle. At the end point, built-in muscle mechanisms (for example, the Golgi tendon organ [GTO]) will prevent the muscle from producing any further force to protect it from injury.

Variables that affect the force-velocity relationship are as follows:

1. The length and angle of the fiber of the individual muscle at the time of contraction (pennate versus longitudinal).
2. Muscle temperature. At temperatures outside the 82.5° to 107.6° F (28° to 42° C) range actin-myosin filaments do not respond to a stimulus in the same manner, and the muscle loses the ability to contract.
3. Order of muscle recruitment and muscle fiber composition. Recruitment order is dependent on the rate and temporal properties of a muscle contraction. Some of the variables of the rate of muscle contrac-

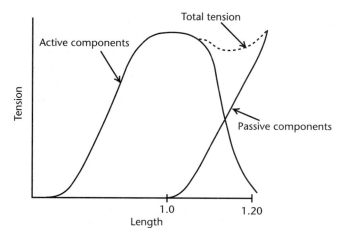

**Fig. 6-4** The length-tension curve of striated muscle. Muscle produces maximum force at approximately 20% beyond its resting length ($L_0$).

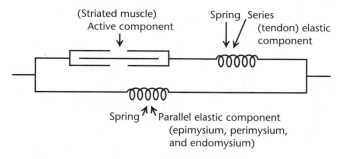

**Fig. 6-5** A dash-pot diagram representing the active component, passive-parallel, and passive-serial components of muscle.

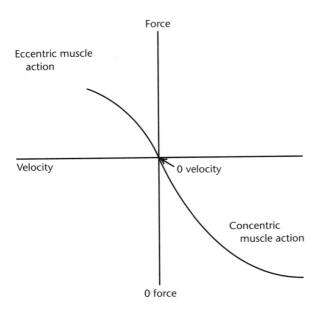

**Fig. 6-6** Force-velocity relationship of striated muscle. Note that an eccentric action can produce more force and velocity than a concentric action.

tion are: oxygen supply to the muscle (the amount of myoglobin in the muscle); fiber type—slow oxidative, fast oxidative glycolytic, or fast glycolytic; source of ATP; and the size of the motor nerve innervating the muscle (a large nerve innervates fast glycolytic muscle)

4. Number of joints traversed by the muscle. Muscles that traverse one joint are used for strength. Muscles that traverse two or more joints are for joint range of motion

5. Muscle origin and insertion in relation to the axis of rotation of a joint. The closer the origin and insertion of a muscle is to the axis of rotation, the less moment can be produced by that muscle on that joint (for example, the supraspinatus and deltoid muscles)

6. The lever system. The lever system is the final determinant of the force-velocity curve[15] and is described in the paragraphs that follow. Figure 6-7 exemplifies the principle of the lever system within the human body.

There are three different types of lever systems: A *first-class lever* is described as a seesaw. In a first-class lever, the resistance force and effort force are located on opposite sides of the axis. The motion of the head upon the cervical spine in flexion and extension is described as a first-class lever. Flexion of the neck at a slow rate, against gravity, occurs by an eccentric action of the posterior cervical musculature (effort force). The resistance force is the head, its center of mass is located at the zygomatic arch, and the axis of rotation is located

at the occiput-C1 joint. Another example of a first-class lever system is flexion at the waist. The erector spinae muscle (effort force) allows the trunk to flex forward against gravity. The center of rotation is the lumbar spine and the center of mass is located at the approximate level of the umbilicus (resistance force).

A *second-class lever* system is exemplified by a wheelbarrel. In this type of lever system, the resistive force is less than the effort force. A person standing on their toes is an example of a second-class lever. The effort force of the triceps surae muscle group is greater than the resistance force of gravity located at the midfoot. The second-class lever system is used by the body when a great amount of force (strength) is needed to lift or move a large resistive force (such as the weight of the human body).

In a *third-class lever* system the effort force is located between the resistive force and the axis of rotation. This is the most common lever system in the human body and is used to produce high joint velocities. Elbow flexion is an example of a third-class lever system. The resistive force is located at the center of mass of the forearm, the effort force is the insertion of the brachialis, and the axis of rotation is the elbow.

## THE BIOMECHANICS OF HUMAN LOCOMOTION (GAIT)
GARY M. GREENSTEIN

The focus will now shift to the basics of normal biomechanics of gait and its appearance during human walking. As is presented in Cases 1, 2, 4, and 23 there are obvious variations in the presence of gait in patients who have suffered from upper and lower motor neuron lesions and injury inflicted on joints (hip, knee, ankle or foot). These gait variations are studied by the clinician so that the lesion can be located.

As presented above, ability to walk develops through a sequence of events that are learned through a child's growth and development. The purpose of locomotion is to accelerate and decelerate the center of gravity in a given direction using the least amount of energy (high efficiency). In this section, terminology and kinematics of gait will be discussed first, followed by the sequencing of muscle activity (kinetics).

### Terminology

The terminology of gait defines the position of the joints and appendages of the lower extremities in relation to their position to the center of gravity. Terms such as stride, step, gait cycle, heel contact, midstance, and other descriptors of gait are used to describe the position of the lower extremity in its attempt to move the center of gravity in a given direction. These terms are discussed in this section and in the Glossary.

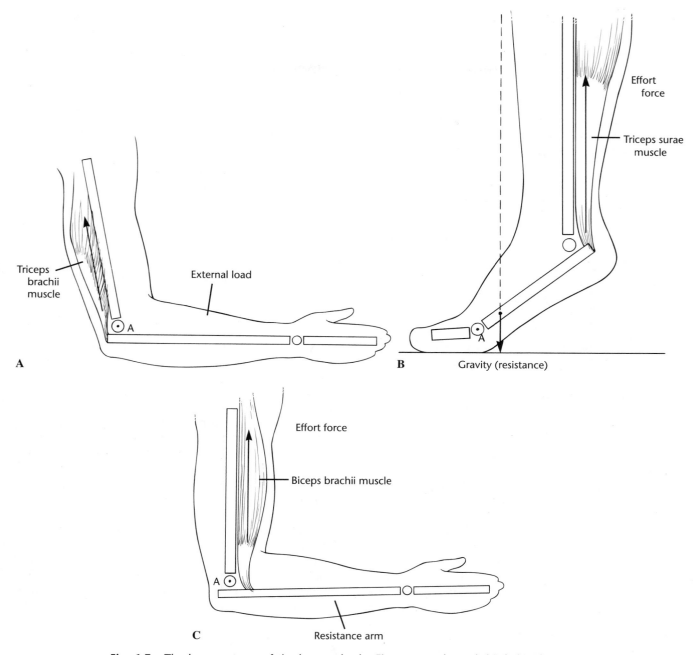

*Fig. 6-7*   The lever systems of the human body. First-, second-, and third-class levers. In a first-class lever system (**A**) the effort arm may be farther, closer, or equidistant from the axis of rotation as is the resistance arm. In a second-class lever (**B**) the effort arm is always farther from the axis of rotation than is the resistance arm and the axis. In a third-class lever (**C**) the effort arm is always closer to the axis of rotation than is the resistance arm.

The most common terms used in gait are: stride, stance phase, and swing phase. A *stride* is defined as ipsilateral heel contact to ipsilateral heel contact and includes all the subcategories of the gait cycle (Fig. 6-

8). The two subphases of a stride are the *stance* and the *swing phase.* In stance phase the foot is in contact with the ground whereas during swing phase the foot is not on the ground.

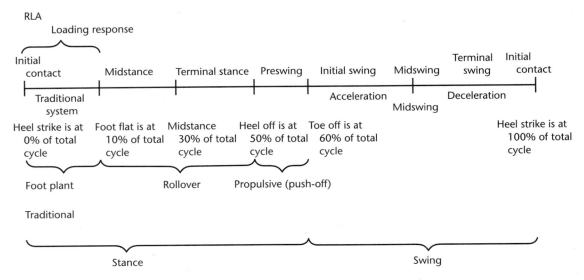

**Fig. 6-8** A gait stride and its subphases. Comparison of the terminology used in the Rancho Los Amigos System (RLA) and the traditional system.

**Stance and swing phases of the gait cycle.** The stance phase during "normal" human walking comprises 60% of the stride, with the swing phase constituting the other 40% of the total stride. A commonly used descriptor of gait (traditional terminology) defines five subcategories in the stance phase of gait: heel contact (strike), foot-flat, midstance, heel-off, and toe-off. Heel contact initiates the stance phase of gait, when the foot first makes contact with the ground. Toe-off occurs at the end of the stance phase, when the toes push off from the ground and the lower extremity proceeds into swing phase (see Glossary). The first 10% of the stance phase occurs when the foot makes complete contact with the ground (heel contact to foot-flat). From foot-flat to heel-off the center of gravity rolls over the foot and prepares the lower extremity for the propulsive phase of gait (heel-off to toe-off), the last 10% of the stance phase. The swing phase consists of three subdivisions: (1) toe-off to acceleration; (2) acceleration to midswing; and (3) midswing to deceleration.

**The Rancho Los Amigos system.** The Gait Laboratory at Rancho Los Amigos (RLA) has revised gait cycle terminology to a functional categorization (Fig. 6-8 and Table 6-2). Heel contact (strike) in the traditional classification is described as *initial contact* in the RLA system. Initial contact occurs when the heel makes contact with the ground. The *loading response* phase occurs immediately following initial contact and continues until the contralateral extremity lifts off the ground at the end of double support phase.[15] The midstance phase in the traditional system is the point at which the center of gravity is located directly over the supporting foot. In the RLA system *midstance* begins when the contralat-

eral foot lifts off the ground and the center of gravity has progressed over and ahead of the supporting foot. In the traditional system, heel-off occurs when the heel leaves the ground. In the RLA system *terminal stance* begins at the end of midstance and proceeds to the point just prior to initial contact of the contralateral foot or following heel-off of the same foot.[15] In the traditional system, toe-off is the point at which the toe is the only part of the foot on the ground and is being lifted off the ground. In the RLA system, this is the *preswing phase* which encompasses the period from heel-off to toe-off.

A comparison of the RLA system during the swing phase of gait to the traditional categorization shows that the acceleration phase of the traditional system is classified as the *initial swing* in the RLA system. Initial swing begins at the same point as the acceleration phase and continues until maximum knee flexion occurs. The

**Table 6-2** Comparison of the traditional and Rancho Los Amigos (RLA) terminology

| Traditional | RLA |
| --- | --- |
| Heel contact (strike) | Initial contact |
| Heel contact to foot-flat | Loading response |
| Foot-flat to midstance | Midstance |
| Midstance to heel-off | Terminal stance |
| Heel-off to toe-off | Preswing |
| Toe-off to acceleration | Initial swing |
| Acceleration to midswing | Midswing |
| Midswing to deceleration | Terminal swing |

*Modified from Norkin CC, Levaugie PK: Joint-structure and function: a comprehensive analysis, ed 2, Philadelphia, 1989, Lea & Febiger.*

*midswing* of the RLA classification occurs immediately following maximum knee flexion and continues to the point where the tibia is in a vertical position, when acceleration of the lower extremity occurs. *Terminal swing phase* of the RLA system includes the point at which the tibia is in a vertical position to a point just prior to initial contact, when deceleration of the lower extremity occurs. In this text a combination of the two systems will be used to exemplify the gait cycle better.

**Support phases of gait.** During the gait cycle there are two locations when both feet are on the ground (double-support phase), and one location where one foot is on the ground (single-support phase). At no time during walking are both feet off the ground (this differentiates walking from running). The double support phase is defined as initial contact (heel-strike to flat foot [traditional]) of the lower extremity and preswing (heel-off to toe-off [traditional]) of the contralateral lower extremity. Further progression of the gait cycle causes one foot to lift off the ground and proceed through the swing phase. The other lower extremity continues through the stance phase and is in the single-support phase of gait where one foot is on the ground.

## Kinematics of the gait cycle

Kinematically, there is a sequence of closed-chain and opened-chain events that occur in the lower extremity during the gait cycle. Closed chain events are synonymous with the events that occur during the stance phase of gait, and opened-chain events occur during the swing phase of gait.

**The rules of gait.** Some simple rules need to be observed when studying the kinematics of the lower extremities during gait. First, motions of the thigh and leg are produced by synchronous motions of the hip and knee. Secondly, external and internal motions of the talus are synchronous with the external and internal rotation of the lower extremities (hips and knees). Thirdly, when the talus rotates internally, the calcaneous, at the subtalar joint, everts; and, when the talus rotates externally, the calcaneous inverts. Lastly, when the calcaneous inverts, the foot adducts, and when the calcaneous everts, the foot abducts. The motions of the hip, knee, ankle, and foot during the gait cycle are presented in Tables 6-3 and 6-4. The following discussion will focus briefly on the anatomy of the joints of the lower extremities and the response of these joints to loads during gait. The kinetics of the muscles of the lower extremities during the stance phase of the gait cycle will also be discussed.

**Joint anatomy and its response to load during gait.** The hip, like all other joint articulations, is specifically designed to withstand maximum loads during certain phases of motion. The ball-and-socket shape of the hip joint allows for freedom of motion and maintains stabil-

**Table 6-3**  A summary of the motions of the joints of the lower extremities during one stride

Stance Phase:

1. Initial contact (heel contact [strike])
   Hip: flexed and slightly rotated externally
   Knee: slightly flexed, slightly rotated externally, varus
   Ankle: slightly dorsiflexed
   Foot: slightly supinated
2. Just past heel contact
   Hip: flexed and along the sagittal plane, no rotation
   Knee: slightly flexed, no rotation, no varus or valgus
   Ankle: neutral
   Foot: neutral
3. Foot flat
   Hip: flexed and maximally rotated internally
   Knee: slightly flexed, maximally rotated internally, valgus
   Ankle: plantar flexed
   Foot: pronated
4. Just before heel-off
   Hip: extended and no rotation
   Knee: slightly flexed, no rotation, no varus or valgus
   Ankle: dorsiflexed
   Foot: neutral
5. Heel-off
   Hip: extended and slightly rotated externally
   Knee: slightly flexed, slightly rotated externally, varus
   Ankle: dorsiflexed
   Foot: slightly supinated
6. Toe-off
   Hip: extended and externally rotated
   Knee: Increased flexion, externally rotated, varus
   Ankle: plantar flexed
   Foot: supinated

Swing Phase:

   Hip: moving from extension to flexion, moving from external rotation to slight external rotation at heel contact
   Knee: flexed, externally rotated, varus moving toward slight external rotation, and slight varus at heel contact
   Ankle: dorsiflexed moving toward slight dorsiflexion at heel contact
   Foot: supinated moving toward slight supination at heel contact

ity throughout all phases of the gait cycle. Femoral head anteversion and acetabular anterior projection help increase the stability of the hip joint when the lower extremity is internally rotated (foot-flat to just before heel-off, loading response to terminal-stance phases). This anatomic development is in response to the maximum torques that are generated through the hip during this period of the stance phase of gait.[19]

The knee also has built-in anatomic nuances. The joint is not well supported by bone. It depends on soft tissue structures to maintain stability and allow motion. Internal and external rotation of the knee is supported by the size and surface area of the femoral condyles and tibial plateaus. The medial femoral condyle and tibial plateau have a larger surface area than do the lateral structures. This increases the surface area contact

*Table 6-4* Joint motion of the lower extremities in the sagittal plane during one stride

| Joints | Stance phase | | |
| --- | --- | --- | --- |
| | Heel contact | Midstance | Toe-off |
| Hip | 20 degrees flexion | 0 degrees | 10 degrees extension |
| Knee | 5 degrees flexion | 15 degrees flexion | 25 to 30 degrees flexion |
| Ankle | 1 to 2 degrees dorsiflexion | neutral | 120° plantar flexion |
| Foot | slight supination | resupination | supination |
| Toes | 0 degrees | 0 degrees | 50 to 60 degrees extension |

| Joints | Swing phase | | |
| --- | --- | --- | --- |
| | Initial swing | Midswing | Terminal swing |
| Hip | 40 degrees extension | 0 degrees | 30 degrees flexion |
| Knee | 60 degrees flexion | 30 degrees flexion | 5 degrees flexion |
| Ankle | 10 degrees plantar flexion | 0 degrees | 1 to 2 degrees dorsiflexion |

*Modified from Perry J: Gait analysis: normal and pathological function, Thorofare, NJ, 1992, Slack Inc.*

(closed pack position) that occurs at foot-flat when the torques are the highest in the knee.[19] At this position, the ligaments and capsule of the knee are taut, adding additional support, and assist in the dissipation of forces to prevent stress risers at any one point in the knee.

The synovial fluid in each joint articulation also acts as a buffer preventing stress risers and keeps friction to a minimum. The synovial fluid is behaving as a *viscoelastohydrodynamic* structure during joint motion. As pressures within the joints change dynamically, the synovial fluid dissipates the forces by causing hyaline cartilage displacement (wave action) and fluid motion effects.[14,21]

In the ankle joint, the body shape of the talus allows forces to be dissipated at heel strike and at toe-off. The frustrum shape allows the ankle to be in a closed packed position. This allows forces to be generated through the ankle, permits the absorption of shock and generates the necessary muscle contraction at the preswing phase.

As in the hand, many joints are involved in the structure and function of the foot. Joint number alone decreases the stresses occurring in any one area of the foot. The flexibility of the joints and muscles allows for a large range of motion to occur (for example, the toes during the preswing phase of gait). Any deviation from normal foot mechanics may lead to pain and changes anywhere along the kinematic chain (see Case 26). The

kinematics of the ankle and foot will be discussed in more detail.

**Ankle and foot relationship during gait.** The ankle joint, as described in Chapter 5, is a hinge joint that produces two motions: plantar flexion and dorsiflexion. Of interest is the closed-chain motion that occurs between the ankle (mortise) joint and the subtalar joint. The bones that articulate and form the subtalar joint are the talus and the calcaneous. The talus is part of the mortise joint and the subtalar joint. Kinematically, calcaneal motion causes a response of the talus that, in turn, causes internal and external lower extremity rotation (that is, calcaneal eversion causes internal rotation of the calus and lower extremity.[12,17]

Calcaneal eversion results in the midfoot being internally rotated and the forefoot becoming slightly varus relative to the midfoot. This foot position is described as *supination*. Calcaneal inversion causes the midfoot to rotate externally and the forefoot to become valgus relative to the midfoot (*pronation*) (Fig. 6-9).

During gait, the ankle travels through four arcs of motion.[17] Twice during each gait cycle the ankle alternately plantar flexes and dorsiflexes. During the swing phase of gait the ankle dorsiflexes only. The other three phases occur during the stance phase of gait. The entire range of motion of the ankle during walking is from 20 to 40 degrees and averages 30 degrees.

The closed-chain response of the ankle and foot is as follows: At heel contact the ankle is dorsiflexed and moving toward plantar flexion, and the foot is slightly supinated. At foot flat the mortise joint is plantar flexed and the foot is at its maximal pronated position. From foot-flat to just before heel-off the mortise joint is changing from plantar flexion to dorsiflexion. The foot, in turn, is coming out of maximal pronation and is moving toward its neutral position (resupinating). From heel-off to toe-off the mortise joint is plantar flexing and the foot is supinated. Foot pronation unlocks the joints and allows the foot to adapt to any terrain. Foot supination locks the joints and produces a rigid lever for the propulsive phase of gait. The pressures that occur in the "normal" foot during the stance phase of the gait cycle are presented in Figure 6-10. Pressure location is determined by supination and pronation and the location of the center of gravity.[12,18] Clinically, if the foot does not function properly by staying pronated for too long a period of the gait cycle, the propulsive phase of gait may be altered leading to injury (see Case 26). In Case 26 the plantar fascia is being overstretched because the foot is not locking during the propulsive phase. This leads to a poor push-off phase during gait.

### Kinetics of gait

The purpose of locomotion is to use as little energy as possible to propel the body in a specific direction. The

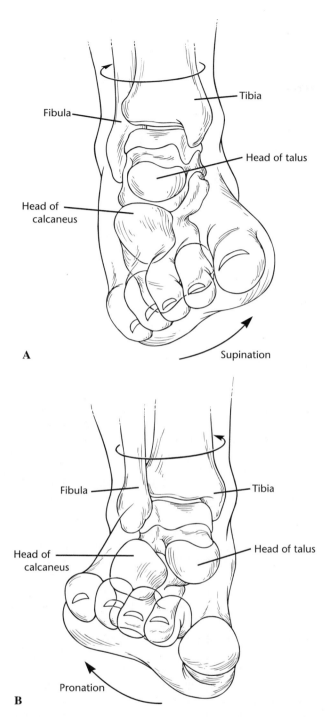

**A**

Supination

**B**

Pronation

*Fig. 6-9*   Foot pronation and supination and its relationship to the subtalar joint.

three mechanisms are used, but eccentric muscle action is predominant. The goal of eccentric muscle activity is to decelerate a limb so that it can be positioned properly.

The kinetics of gait is a complicated topic. As techniques of evaluation become more sophisticated research is unraveling more of the intricacies of locomotion. Inman and coworkers[10] were the first to describe and quantify the kinematics and kinetics of human gait. Since that time several laboratories have looked at the kinetics of human locomotion. The most common technique used to evaluate human kinetics is electromyography (EMG). Electromyography, as does any tool, gives limited information about the muscles being evaluated. EMG cannot determine how the muscle is actually functioning during motion (for example, whether the muscle is producing an eccentric, concentric, or static action), nor can it determine muscle strength. It only records the active components of the muscle.[2] High-speed cinematography helpes solve some of these problems. With the use of a high-speed camera (computer-driven cameras) and EMG it is easier to determine when muscle is producing a force eccentrically, statically, or concentrically. Today, cinematography and EMG are far more sophisticated. Fine-wire needle electrodes are inserted into individual muscles and electronically driven cameras collect and transmit information to a computer that interprets the information with greater accuracy. To evaluate motion in three dimensions requires two high-speed cameras that view the same limb simultaneously. Markers attached to the subject are recorded by the cameras and information is interpreted by the computer, giving a more detailed picture of the kinetics and kinematics of human motion.

The following discussion is a combination of the findings of several authors.[10,12,17] Figure 6-11 illustrates the muscle activity of major muscle groups involved with human locomotion. The purpose of muscle activity during gait is to provide joint stability, stability to retain balance during motion, and mobility necessary for locomotion. Many of the muscle groups necessary for proper locomotion will be discussed. It is impossible to cover all the muscles of the lower extremities; however, this section will provide a good understanding of the kinetics of gait.

### Vectorial components of locomotion

A clearer picture of muscle activity during locomotion can be presented through the understanding of ground reaction force vectors. From the vectors, joint moments can be determined and evaluated. These evaluations provide the reader with a more acurate picture of muscle activity during gait. This section will present the kinetics of the stance phase of gait.

**Vectorial components at initial ground contact.** At initial ground contact, the ground reaction force vec-

forces that are applied to the body to cause motion at the joints are the muscles. Striated muscle can produce a force by three different types of contractions: eccentric, concentric, and static actions. During locomotion all

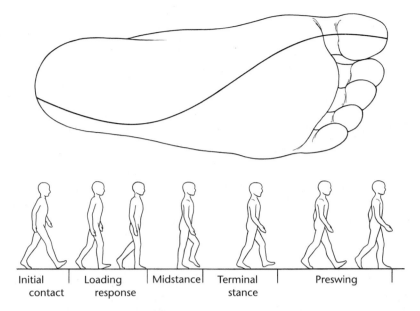

**Fig. 6-10** Pressure distributions of the foot during the stance phase of gait.

tor is located at the heel (point of attachment). The direction of the vector is vertical and the force is minimal when compared to a loading response (Fig. 6-12). The type of moments that are produced at initial ground contact are (1) a small flexor moment at the ankle, (2) a large extensor moment at the knee, and (3) an even larger flexor moment at the hip. The musculature surrounding the joints would need to produce forces at the hip, knee, and ankle that would control the momentum and give stability to the joint. Any divergence of these muscles from their normal activity could possibly cause joint injury.

At initial contact the hamstring muscles produce an eccentric action to prevent the momentum of the hip and knee from causing hip hyperflexion and knee hyperextension. Since large forces are needed to prevent hyperflexion of the hip by the hamstrings, this would cause the forces produced at the knee to be great and cause knee hyperflexion. To counterbalance the knee forces produced by the hamstrings, the quadriceps become active and produce a counterforce (static action) to control knee position, thereby, increasing stability and increasing shock absorption at the knee.

At the ankle, since the moment arm is small, the anterior compartment of the leg produces an eccentric action that controls the flexor moment of the ankle. The amount of force produced by each muscle group during the different phases of gait depends on the total moment needed to cause the desired motion (moment = force × perpendicular distance). If the moment arm is large then the amount of force needed to control joint motion

will be large and the moment will be large. If the moment arm is short then less force is needed to produce the motion necessary at the joint and the moment is less.

**Vectorial components during the loading response.** At this phase in the gait cycle the main focus is to restrain knee flexion and ankle plantar flexion and to stabilize the hip.[17] This is the phase in which the greatest muscular activity occurs. The knee now flexes to 18 degrees, and 10 degrees of ankle plantar flexion and subtalar valgus also occur.[17] There is negligible knee motion from initial contact to the end of the loading response.

The ground reaction force during the loading response phase of gait is primarily located at the heel but the vector has now shifted, relative to its location at initial contact, slightly posterior to the ankle and knee and slightly anterior to the hip (Fig. 6-12). An interesting mechanism now exists between the anterior compartment muscles of the leg and ankle and knee. The ankle plantar flexion proceeds to 10 degrees. This motion is controlled by eccentric action of the anterior compartment muscles. The origin of these muscles is the anterior aspect of the tibia. The location of the ground reaction force vector and the action of the muscles of the anterior compartment of the leg pull the tibia forward relative to the femur, producing knee flexion. When the forefoot makes contact with the ground the anterior leg muscles discontinue their activity and the anterior forces applied to the tibia decrease. The limiting factor of knee flexion at the end of the loading response is the rapid increase in eccentric activity (30% of manual muscle test [MMT])

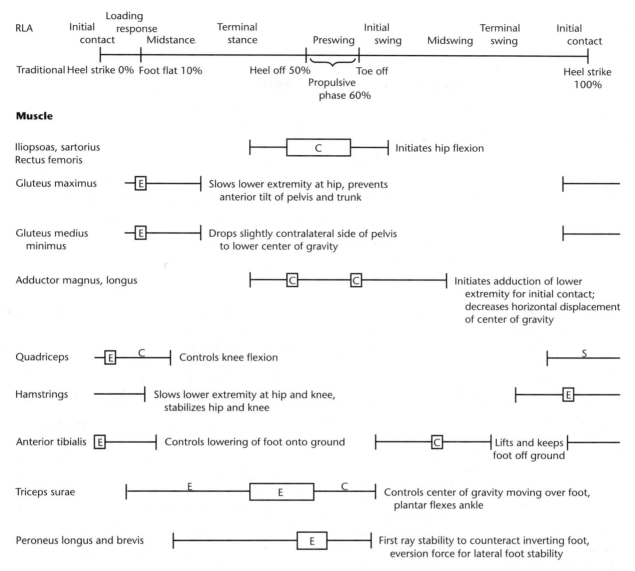

**Fig. 6-11** Muscle activity and its affect during gait. Presented is the Rancho Los Amigos system (RLA) and traditional system. The muscles listed are the major muscles involved in gait. Note that agonist and antagonist muscles may be active during the same gait phase. These muscles act as a group to control motion about a joint (i.e., quadriceps and hamstrings). Also note that muscles are not continually active during the gait cycle. *E,* Eccentric muscle activity; *C,* concentric muscle activity. Lines represent area in which muscle activity occurs. Rectangles represent areas of greatest activity for the designated muscle or muscle group.

of the three vasti of the quadriceps muscle group. The rectus femoris muscle does not participate because it would produce a force on the hip causing the hamstring and gluteus maximus muscles to contract more forcefully. The combination of the anterior leg muscles and the quadriceps results in a shearing force at the knee joint. The anterior cruciate ligament and the hamstring muscles resist the shearing forces produced by these muscle groups and both play a major role in knee stability during the loading response phase.

At loading response, the origin of the hamstrings contributes to pelvic stability. Because the ground reaction vector is slightly anterior to the hip, and the hip is flexed 30 degrees, a flexion moment is present. To counterbalance this moment the gluteus maximus and adductor magnus muscles produce an eccentric action to prevent further hip flexion.

A flexion moment is produced at the trunk at the end of the loading response. This moment is present because the ground reaction force vector is anterior to the trunk.

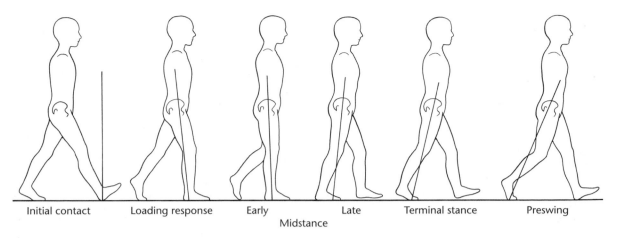

| Initial contact | Loading response | Early | Late | Terminal stance | Preswing |

Midstance

*Fig. 6-12* Example of the torque vectors during the gait cycle.

A quick eccentric action of the erector spinae and other extensor muscles counterbalances this moment.

Pelvic motion in the coronal plane at loading response helps facilitate lower extremity adduction and lower the peak of vertical displacement of the center of mass.[10,17] The pelvis, during this phase, drops 5 degrees on the unsupported side. Pelvic unleveling is produced by an eccentric action of the hip abductors (gluteus medius, gluteus minimus, upper gluteus maximus, and tensor fascia lata muscles) of the supported extremity.[17]

Coronal plane motion of the foot at the end of the loading response phase is subtalar valgus (calcaneal eversion and talus medial rotation and lowering of its head). This hindfoot motion allows the lower extremity to absorb the shock of the ground by unlocking the joints of the foot to adapt to any type of ground contour (the foot pronates). The muscles that control subtalar valgus are the tibialis anterior and tibialis posterior.

During the loading response phase the lower extremity rotates medially (transverse plane motion). This rotation is exemplified at the ankle by the talus rotating internally on the calcaneous at the subtalar joint. The tibia rotates internally but is limited by the amount of medial rotation that occurs at the talus. Further medial rotation occurs at the knee because there is more surface area on the medial condyle of the femur and the medial tibial plateau than on the lateral condyle and tibial plateau. This difference in surface area allows the lateral aspect of the knee to lock first, causing medial rotation of the femur on the tibia. The muscles that control femoral internal rotation are the hamstring muscles. The semimembranosis muscle is active into the midstance phase of gait. The biceps femoris ceases during the load-ing response. The persistent activity of the semimem-branosis causes medial rotation of the tibia and supports the response of internal rotation of the talus.[17] However, overall the femor rotates more, internally, than the tibia, causing internal knee rotation.

**Vectorial components during midstance.** At early midstance the ground reaction force vector has shifted forward to project from the midfoot. The lower extremity is now in an almost vertical position, with the center of mass almost directly over the ground reaction force vector. The muscle activity generated at the hip and knee has terminated and now switches to the triceps surae muscle group (especially the soleus) located at the posterior compartment of the tibia. The activity of the soleus controls ankle dorsiflexion by restraining the rate of tibial forward advancement.[17] The knee continues to extend (almost to 0 degrees) and is controlled by the activity of the gastrocnemius. The hip abductors are also active in providing pelvic stability and supporting erect posture. This provides a base for an upright alignment of the trunk.

At late midstance the ground reaction force vector has now progressed to the metatarsal heads and is vertical. It is anterior to the ankle and knee and slightly posterior to the hip. This produces moments that cause the ankle to dorsiflex and the knee and hip to extend. Momentum produced by the contralateral swinging limb and the heel rocker are the major factors that bring the ankle into dorsiflexion during this phase of gait.[17] The triceps surae muscle group controls the motion of the tibia and therefore retains ankle dorsiflexion. The ankle goes from 7 degrees of plantar flexion at the beginning of the midstance phase to 4 degrees of dorsiflexion at the end of the midstance phase.

Muscle sequencing of the triceps muscles during the midstance phase of gait reveals that the soleus contracts eccentrically just before the gastrocnemius. Because the origin of the soleus is on the tibia and the origin of the gastrocnemius is on the femur, the earlier action of the soleus allows ankle dorsiflexion to occur earlier. This allows knee flexion to progress to 18 degrees at the onset of midstance, when the vector is posterior to the knee joint, to 10 degrees when the vector is anterior to the joint at the end of midstance. As the femur advances over the tibia, the knee extends because the tibia is being held in place by the contracting soleus. The quadriceps continues to show activity until the ground reaction force vector is anterior to the knee. Quadriceps activity is considered to pull the femur forward.

During early midstance the semimembranosus muscles minimally help control hip extension from 30 degrees to 10 degrees. At the end of midstance the thigh is in a vertical posture. The action of the quadriceps and gluteus medius is to cause an anterior pelvic tilt, which increase lumbar lordosis and helps the pelvis support an upright posture.

**Vectorial components during terminal stance.** The major component of progression of the body is free forward fall. Its effects on body balance cause a temporary instability in the sagittal plane. As the body rolls forward over the forefoot, the ankle dorsiflexes to 20 degrees and the heel simultaneously rises. The knee at this phase has completed its extension. The ground reaction force vector is located at the metatarsal heads (most of the force is over the large toe). The moment at the ankle is large, with the vector located anterior to the joint. The result is a large ankle dorsiflexion moment produced by the gastrocnemius and soleus muscle group. The action of these muscles not only causes ankle dorsiflexion but also produces tibial stability.

The ground reaction force vector now moves posterior to the knee. This unlocks the knee and causes it to begin flexion. The unlocking is supported by the action of the gastrocnemius.

### Other components of gait

During gait the human body attempts to propel itself in a straight line without horizontal body sway or vertical displacement. The anatomic mechanisms that keep horizontal sway to a minimum are the femoral neck-shaft angle and adduction of the lower extremity during the stance phase of gait. The femoral neck-shaft angle is normally in the range of 120 to 130 degrees.

Vertical displacement of the center of gravity during gait is controlled by many determinants. Vertical displacement is described as a sagittal plane sinusoidal wave. The greatest vertical displacement occurs during the double and single support phases of the stance phase of gait. At double support the center of mass is located

at its lowest point—it is in the trough of the sinusoidal wave. At single support phase (midstance) the vertical displacement is at its highest point, located at the peak of the sinusoidal wave.

The major determinant of vertical displacement of the center of gravity is the motion that occurs at the pelvis. The center of gravity is elevated to decrease the vertical displacement that occurs in the trough by pelvic rotation in the horizontal (transverse) plane. This rotation will produce 8 to 10 degrees of ipsilateral rotation (a total of approximately 20 degrees rotation) and elevate the center of gravity. At its highest point (peak of the sinusoidal wave) the center of gravity is lowered by pelvic rotation in the coronal (frontal) plane. During the single support phase the eccentric action of the gluteus medius slightly drops the contralateral pelvis allowing the center of gravity to correspondingly lower (Fig. 6-13).

Inman[10] describes the knee-ankle-foot relationship as another determinant to vertical displacement. At foot contact, the foot is slightly supinated, the ankle is moving from dorsiflexion to plantar flexion and the knee is slightly flexed, externally rotated, and in varus. The positioning of these joints at heel contact cause the center of gravity to be slightly elevated, therefore lifting it from the bottom of the trough. During human walking the joints of the lower extremities move in harmony. As the foot is preparing to make ground contact the joints and muscles of the lower extremity are reacting in synchrony. The foot is in a certain position that is supported by the position of the ankle, knee, and hip. This synchronous motion of joints and muscles is a closed chain. The action of one muscle group causes

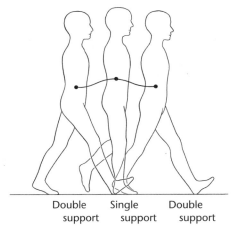

Double        Single        Double
support      support      support

*Fig. 6-13*  The vertical displacement of the center of gravity during the different phases of the gait cycle. At the double-support phase, the center of gravity is in the trough and at the single-support phase, it is at the peak of the sinusoidal wave.

other muscle groups to act certain ways, causing joints to be moved into certain positions. On the other hand, when a clinician examines an individual joint (for example, testing the knee through active and passive ranges of motion) the motion of the knee is not affecting the motion of other surrounding joints (hip, ankle, and foot). The examination of individual joints is considered an open-chain evaluation.

In summary, the basics of neurologic growth and development, muscle physiology and biomechanics of human locomotion are presented in this chapter. This topic is very complicated but provides imperative information to the clinician who is treating neuromusculoskeletal disease. The human body is a dynamic, adapting structure that cannot be examined by individual evaluation of a joint. The surrounding structures and their interrelationships with the joint undergoing examination must be considered.

## REFERENCES

1. Adams RD, Victor M: Disorders of stance and gait. In *Principles of neurology*, ed 5, New York, 1993, McGraw-Hill.
2. Basmajian JV, DeLuca CJ: *Muscles alive: Their functions revealed by electromyography*, ed 5, Baltimore, 1985, Williams & Wilkins.
3. Biguer B, et al: Neck muscle vibration modifies the representation of visual motion and direction in man, *Brain* 111:1405, 1988.
4. Brown JJ: A systematic approach to the dizzy patient, *Neurol Clin* 8:209, 1990.
5. Burt AM: *Textbook of neuroanatomy*, Philadelphia, 1993, Saunders.
6. DeMyer WE: *Technique of the neurologic examination: A programmed text*, ed 4, New York, 1994, McGraw-Hill.
7. Frank JS, Ear M: Coordination of posture and movement, *Phys Ther* 70:855, 1990.
8. Ghez C: Posture. In Kandel ER, Schwartz JH, Jessell TM: *Principles of neural science*, ed 3, New York, 1991, Elsevier.
9. Haerer AF, editor: *De Jong's The neurologic examination*, ed 5, Philadelphia, 1992, Lippincott.
10. Inman VT, Ralston HJ, Todd F: *Human walking*, Baltimore, 1981, Williams & Wilkins.
11. Lacquaniti F: Automatic control of limb movement and posture, *Curr Op Neurobiol* 2:807, 1992.
12. Michaud TC: *Foot orthoses and other forms of conservative foot care*, Baltimore, 1993, Williams & Wilkins.
13. Nolte J: *The Human Brain: an introduction to its functional anatomy*, ed 3, St. Louis, 1993, Mosby.
14. Nordin M, Frankel VH: *Basic biomechanics of the musculoskeletal system*, ed 2, Philadelphia, 1989, Lea & Febiger.
15. Norkin CC, Levangie PK: *Joint structure and function: a comprehensive analysis*, ed 2, Philadelphia, 1992, F.A. Davis Co.
16. Nutt JG, Marsden CD, Thompson PD: Human walking and higher-level gait disorders, particularly in the elderly, *Neurology* 43:268, 1993.
17. Perry J: *Gait analysis: normal and pathological function*, Thorofare, NJ, 1992, Slack Inc.
18. Root ML, Orien WP, Weed JH: *Normal and abnormal function of the foot: clinical biomechanics*, vol 2, Los Angeles, 1977, Clinical Biomechanics Corporations.
19. Skinner SR, et al: Functional demands on the stance limb in walking, *Orthopedics* 8:355, 1985.
20. Stein RB: Locomotion control. In Adelman G, editor: *Encyclopedia of neurosciences*, vol 1, Boston, 1987, Birkhauser.
21. Winter DA: *Biomechanics and motor control of human movement*, ed 2, New York, 1990, Wiley-Interscience Publication.

## SUGGESTED READINGS

Michaud TC: *Foot orthoses and other forms of conservative foot care*, Baltimore, 1993, Williams & Wilkins.
Perry J: *Gait analysis: normal and pathological function*, Thorofare, NJ, 1992, Slack Inc.
Winter DA: *Biomechanics and motor control of human movement*, ed 2, New York, 1990, Wiley-Interscience Publication.

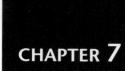

# CHAPTER 7

# *Treatment/management*

EDWARD ROTHMAN
GARY M. GREENSTEIN

**CASE**
*Connection*

1, 2, 3, 4, 5, 6, 7, 8, 9, 10,
11, 12, 13, 14, 15, 16, 17,
18, 19, 20, 21, 22, 23, 24,
25, 26

■

### Definitions

**Musculoskeletal and neuromuscular injury: treatment and management relationships**

**Tissue response to mechanical injury**
  Inflammatory (acute) stage
  Circulatory response
    Cellular events
    Chemical mediators of inflammation
  Arachidonic acid cascade
  Effect of ischemia on soft tissues
  Clinical signs of acute inflammation
  Chronic inflammation
  Tissue healing: repair and regeneration stage
    Remodeling or maturation phase
  Specific tissue response to injury
    Long bone healing
    Striated muscle healing
    Tendon injuries
    Ligament injuries

**Treatment and management protocols**
  Immediate treatment protocols
  Intermediate treatment protocols
  Long-term treatment protocols
  Integration of somatosensory and motor cortices

■

### KEY TERMS

Inflammation and tissue
  response
Healing response
Conservative care
Medications
Definitions
Passive/active care
Immediate, intermediate,
  and long-term goals

Mobilization
Manipulation/adjustment
Active/resistive exercise
Janda
Sensory integration
Proprioceptive
  neuromuscular facilitation
Plyometrics

Recent efforts by managed care organizations and state boards to produce protocols of treatment for physi-cal medicine problems[38] have resulted in a number of recently published treatment guidelines.[17,39] These pro-tocols are usually based on consensus opinions of groups of "expert" clinicians. This textbook is a problem-oriented approach to case management in which the reader is challenged to develop a plan to manage each clinical presentation. The goal is to formulate a manage-ment plan that will positively affect the patient's prob-lem and health quickly and at the lowest possible cost.

Considering that 90% of the population will have a musculoskeletal or neuromuscular injury or problem, it is surprising that only a few treatment/management protocols are established beyond anecdotal routines. There is little consensus among clinicians regarding the management of most musculoskeletal and neuromuscu-lar injuries and conditions.

This chapter presents the basic science infrastructure to support treatment and management decisions for musculoskeletal and neuromuscular injuries. The chap-ter consists of three parts. A discussion of the response of the body to injury is followed by discussion of thera-peutic modalities and procedures. This discussion is un-dertaken as the clinical approach of the basic sciences. Finally, an overview of management decisions and goals is presented as a way of organizing conservative man-agement of body injury.

The management and treatment are not rigid guide-lines but are instead based on evolving approaches cen-tered on reproducible outcomes. This chapter is not a cookbook of treatment but rather an attempt to suggest protocols that can be thoughtfully evaluated and con-sidered.

### DEFINITIONS

The lack of a standardized vocabulary in physical medi-cine leads to problems in communication. Chiropractic alone has over 40 different therapeutic approaches or techniques,[3] with adherents to specific schools of thought often having their own specialized vocabulary.

The following definitions are offered for the purpose of clear communication and understanding.

Management and treatment, though similar, have several differences. *Management* is a global term involving the clinical decision process. It includes diagnostic and therapeutic procedures. It involves treatment methods that are given in the office and those that are prescribed. For the purpose of our discussion, *treatment* is defined as the therapeutic care given to the patient in the office.

*Treatment modalities* include electric, mechanical, and chemical methods of passive therapy that are applied, in some way, to the patient. They do not include manual procedures.

Several terms are often used interchangeably in manual medicine. However, the following definitions are offered for continuity. An *adjustment* is any chiropractic therapeutic procedure that utilizes controlled force, leverage, direction, amplitude, and velocity and that is directed at specific joints or anatomic regions.[15,16] A *manipulation* is similar to an adjustment but defined more broadly. It is a manual procedure that involves a directed thrust to move a joint past the physiologic range of motion, without exceeding the anatomic limit.[15] *Mobilization* is the movement applied singularly or repetitively within the physiologic range of motion of a joint without imparting a thrust or impulse. The therapeutic purpose is to restore joint mobility.[16]

Sandoz's chart is used to define the difference between manipulation and mobilization more clearly (Fig. 7-1). There are four stages involved in the normal range of motion of a synovial diarthrodial joint. The first stage is the active range of motion of the joint accomplished by muscle contraction. The second stage is a slightly greater range of motion produced passively. This stage is called *joint play*. It is defined by the elastic barrier of joint resistance. The elastic barrier is a clinical term. There is no implication, by definition, that further forced motion produced by manipulation will cause permanent deformation. Any technique, performed properly, should not injure a joint or the surrounding tissues.

The third stage is defined as motion beyond the elastic barrier. The area beyond the elastic barrier is the *paraphysiologic* space. It does not go beyond the anatomic integrity of the joint and this is where manipulation occurs. A "crack" may or may not be heard during manipulation. This sound depends on the gapping or shearing forces applied to articulating surfaces and is caused by the formation and release of nitrogen bubbles as the joint capsule area expands.[15]

The fourth stage is pathologic. The paraphysiologic space is exceeded and the joint capsule is damaged. The degree of damage depends on the amount of injury to the bone and surrounding soft tissue structures. The damage may result in hypermobility leading to joint instability.

*Reactivation* is the measured capacity of therapeutic management to eliminate the clinical problem. The goal is to return the patient to the level of health and activity enjoyed prior to the injury. The patient has the potential for complete recovery.

*Rehabilitation* is defined as the process required to bring a patient to a maximum functioning point after injury or a poor therapeutic outcome. This may not be at a level the patient enjoyed prior to being injured or struck with an illness. For example, individuals with severe head trauma will not be able to function at their previous level, whereas those suffering from a mild-to-moderate lumbar sprain should be able to return to full function.

There are several definitions of *conservative treatment*. Some define it as any procedure other than surgery. Other schools of thought consider conservative treatment as being limited to manipulation and lifestyle counseling. In this text, conservative procedures are those that do not include surgery or prescription medications.

## MUSCULOSKELETAL AND NEUROMUSCULAR INJURY: TREATMENT AND MANAGEMENT RELATIONSHIPS

Several factors influence healing and repair of a joint and the contiguous tissues. The degree of inflammation, circulation, congenital anomalies, neurologic disease, and systemic disease must be considered when developing a management plan.

The most common problems treated by manual medicine physicians are those arising from trauma. The trauma may be severe or mild and may be caused by a single overwhelming force or by repetitive actions.

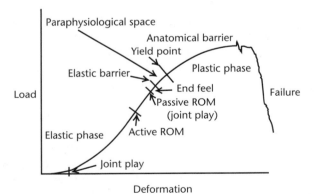

*Fig. 7-1* Clinical motion palpation analogy (Sandoz's pie chart) on a typical load-deformation curve of a viscoelastic material. Clinical joint testing takes place within the elastic phase of viscoelastic tissues not in the plastic phase; therefore injury does not occur to tissues during motion palpation evaluation or the application of an adjustment or manipulation. Tissue stiffness (i.e., joint stiffness) is exemplified by the slope of the curve.

*Macrotruama* is caused by a sudden change in the relationship of joint surfaces and surrounding tissues. The cause is a quick, often unsuspected force that cannot be dissipated by the supporting structures. *Microtrauma* is most often caused by repetitive mild forces. These forces do not exceed the elastic limit of tissue, but because of temporal relationships, tissue fatigue and failure occur. Improper management of macro- and microtrauma leads to joint degeneration. Part of the clinician's role is to slow down the process of degeneration.

Kirkaldy-Willis[24] proposed a model to explain the spinal degenerative process, which, theoretically, could be extended to include all other synovial diarthrodial joints. In this model, the process begins with joint dysfunction in which hypomobility and muscle splinting are present. Other clinicians, such as Janda, describe the "functional hypermobility" model[20,21] in which the joint does not have an increased global range of motion. The motion within the normal range is altered. This is a significant motion palpation finding. The chiropractor interprets this as a movement change between articulating surfaces found between joint play and end feel.

Joint dysfunction may result in degeneration. In the spine, joint degeneration is characterized by loss of hyaline cartilage, disc disruption, and capsular laxity. This could result in degenerative changes seen on x-ray examination.

Panjabi[34] describes this phenomenon as a change in the "neutral zone." As joint degeneration progresses, the neutral zone increases, accompanied by laxity in the capsule and other surrounding tissues. The hypothesis suggests that aging tissues lose elasticity and therefore greater joint motion is required to produce tissue tension and stiffness. This may be a reason why joints become slack or hypermobile.[24]

The second stage of degeneration of Kirkaldy-Willis's paradigm is instability, which results in increased global range of motion. The stabilization phase is the result of the joint degenerative process[24] and is characterized by the body's attempt to reduce excessive motion. An example of this process is osteophyte formation as a result of excessive stresses placed on the disc and the surrounding soft tissue structures.

Sensory disturbance, resulting in symptoms ranging from discomfort to pain, can occur in any of the stages. Since pain is the driving force for patients seeking care, it is imperative to determine whether the involved joint is in a dysfunction, instability or stability stage. The choice of treatment may depend on this information.

A traumatic event may begin the degenerative process or may accelerate a process that has already started. The injury may cause instability immediately, ranging from hypermobility to dislocation. The body will attempt to stabilize the joint but the attempt is not always successful.

The Kirkaldy-Willis model leads to a discussion of management and treatment. What different therapeutic actions can be employed at the different stages to influence proper healing? One goal of treatment is to prevent dysfunction from cascading to instability and then to degenerative stability.

## TISSUE RESPONSE TO MECHANICAL INJURY

Acute injury to the neuromusculoskeletal system can be caused by two mechanical methods: sudden severe loads that cause macrotrauma and temporal repetitive loads that produce microtrauma.[25,26]

Macrotrauma results in immediate tissue damage. Common causes of such injury are sudden severe overloads (compression, tension, shear, or laceration).[26] Once a tissue is injured the process of healing begins immediately and consists of the inflammatory response phase, the fibroblastic-repair phase, and the maturation-remodeling phase.[26]

The scope of this chapter does not permit or warrant an in-depth discussion of the intricacies of these stages. The focus will be on basic mechanisms and those aspects that are relevant to clinical management justified by scientific evidence for intervention.

### Inflammatory (acute) stage

Inflammatory response mediators are precipitated by tissue injury. The signs of inflammation are redness (rubor), swelling (tumor), pain (dolor), heat (calor), and altered function.[9] Acute inflammation is of relatively short duration, lasting a few hours to a few days and consists of hemodynamic events, cellular events, and inflammatory mediators.

### Circulatory response

Hemodynamics is defined as the changes in vascular flow caused by injury. The fluids of inflammation consist of transudates, exudates, and pus. The circulatory response in acute inflammation is a typical response to tissue injury and it consists of edema (the hallmark of acute inflammation) caused by initial vasoconstriction followed by vasodilatation of the local blood vessels (precapillary arterioles). This causes a concomitant increase in blood flow into the arterioles and opening of new microvascular beds in the area leading to the objective findings of heat and redness.

The capillary vasodilatation is accompanied by increased hydrostatic pressure in the dilated vessels, initially resulting in transudation into the extravascular space. The flow of transudate is short-lived. An increase in intravascular hydrostatic pressure or a decrease in intravascular osmotic pressure will result in an overall increase in the movement of fluid out of the capillary. This leads to the initial flow of transudate. The abundant flow of exudate (that is, serum high in protein) is the result of the increase in capillary permeability caused by chemical factors (such as, bradykinin) that reduce the intravascular osmotic pressure and increase the osmotic pressure of the interstitial tissues. The increase in osmotic pressure in the interstitial tissues leads to an impairment of the return of fluid to the blood on the venous end of the capillary causing a net outflow of fluid, thereby also producing edema (Starling's hypothesis).

The extravasation of exudate causes increased pressure on the capillaries that leads to a slowing of the circulation and results in red cell concentration in small vessels with increased viscosity of the blood (blood stasis). The accumulation of red cells, stasis of blood, and chemotaxis of platelets to the area help develop a blood clot.

**Cellular events.** *Neutrophils* and *leukocytes* are drawn to the injured area because of chemotactic agents. Leukocytes play an important role in the cellular response.[9] They engulf and degrade foreign material through phagocytosis and lysosomal enzyme activity. The leukocytes adhere to the endothelium because of inflammatory agents such as interleukin-1 and other chemical mediators. Neutrophils predominate in the first 24 hours postinjury, during the next 48 hours they are replaced by leukocytes.

Phagocytosis and degranulation destroy foreign material in the injured area. Phagocytosis consists of four distinct steps. The material is first recognized as foreign by the leukocyte. This is followed by movement of the leukocyte toward the foreign material, which is engulfed by the leukocyte and surrounded by a phagocytic vacuole. Lastly, the vacuole discharges its contents and the material is degraded. The system is not intact and leakage of proteolytic enzymes into healthy tissue surrounding the area can increase tissue necrosis. Necrotic tissue produces chemical reactants that stimulate further cellular movement through chemotaxis and, thus, the cycle is perpetuated.

**Chemical mediators of inflammation.** The chemical mediators originate from plasma cells and damaged tissues (Table 7-1). Included in the chemical mediator arsenal is the complement system. Activation of the complement system results in increased vascular perme-ability, chemotaxis, opsonization prior to phagocytosis, and lysis of target microorganisms. This system is initiated by either the classic pathway or the alternate pathway. Although a detailed explanation of the complement system will not be provided, its importance is emphasized.

The system plays a major role in cleaning the injured area. C5a is chemotactic to neutrophils, eosinophils, basophils, and leukocytes. The system also activates the lipoxygenase pathway, which increases chemotaxis. C3b and C3bi are opsonins that recognize receptors on neutrophils, macrophages, and eosinophils. These mechanisms attract the cells that clear the injured area of foreign material. C5b to C9 is the membrane attack complex (MAC) and is the final lytic component of the complement pathway.[9]

The complement system assists in vascular permeability to promote edema. The chemotactic events and production of opsonins are essential in attracting cells that clear the injured area of foreign material.

### Arachidonic acid cascade

Arachidonic acid is important in inflammation and hemostasis (Fig. 7-2). It is a 20-carbon polyunsaturated fatty acid derived from the conversion of linoleic acid. The two pathways by which arachidonic acid is metabolized are the cyclooxygenase pathway and the lipoxygenase pathway.

The cyclooxygenase pathway produces prostaglandins that cause vasodilatation, pain by irritating free nerve endings, edema, and fever. Another product of this pathway is throboxane, which is found in platelets. It is a potent platelet aggregator and blood vessel constrictor. Prostacyclin is found in the vessel wall and is a potent platelet inhibitor and vasodilator.

Clinically, this is important to understand because the cyclooxgenase pathway can be inhibited by anti-inflammatory medications. These include nonsteroidal anti-inflammatory medication such as aspirin and indomethacin, as well as prednisone, a steroidal anti-inflammatory drug.

The lipoxygenase pathway generates leukotriens. These are potent chemotactic agents that facilitate leukocyte aggregation and increase vascular permeability.[9]

There are many acute inflammation mediators. These systems are intimately intertwined with no single system working alone. This ensures a system with checks and balances. All the chemical mediators have a short half-life. Some mediators destroy others, (for example, kinase destroys bradykinin). Antioxidants absorb oxygen-derived free radicals. Some mediators damage surrounding tissue. For example, proteolytic enzymes in the leukocytes cause damage to endothelium and other tissues. Mediators such as bradykinin and the prostaglandins irritate nerve endings and produce pain.

*Table 7-1* Chemical mediators of inflammation within blood

| Cell-derived mediators | | Plasma-derived mediator |
|---|---|---|
| Preformed | Newly synthesized | |
| Serotonin | Cytokines | Clotting/fibrinolytic system |
| Histamine | Leukotrienes | Complement system |
| Lysosomal enzymes | Platelet activating factor | Kinin system |
| | Prostaglandins | |

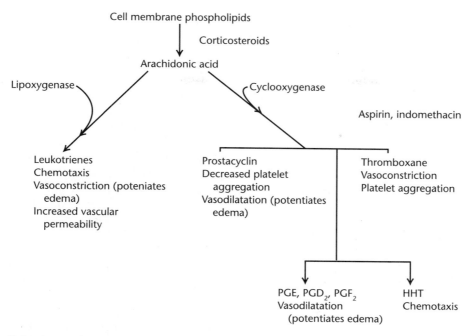

*Fig. 7-2*  Formation of arachidonic acid metabolites during the inflammatory process.

## Effect of ischemia on soft tissues

All cells are affected by ischemia. Mitochondria are extremely sensitive to ischemic changes and will swell in response to ischemia. This causes the collapse of the cytochrome oxidase and electron transport enzyme systems and results in the release of intracellular calcium ion stores that act as signals for increased phospholipase and calcium-dependent protease enzyme activity.[26] Phospholipid degeneration causes a loss of the cell membrane. An interesting theoretical speculation is that this may be one of the changes or pathways of aging.[35] The release of oxygen free radicals by neutrophils and other phagocytes produces further cell damage. The clinical importance of these events is clear. The question is, should inflammation be controlled?

## Clinical signs of acute inflammation

The classic signs of inflammation were described by Celsus and Virchow[9] and are swelling, redness, heat, pain, and loss of function. The chiropractor most often addresses muscle and joint-complex injuries in which the inflammatory process is a response to necrotic tissue resulting from injury and degeneration and is rarely caused by systemic disease, such as infection, cancer, or immunologic disease.

Inflammation should be controlled to reduce the pathologic effects. However, inflammation should not be stopped because of the positive effects of the process. Knowing when to intervene and to what extent is essential for appropriate case management.

Understanding the process of inflammation provides a blueprint for control. Rest, ice, compression, and elevation (RICE) are simple basic methods to influence the inflammatory process without shutting it down. Rest and ice decrease pain, swelling, and blood flow. Ice or cryotherapy offers brief tissue analgesia. It decreases capillary permeability and dampens the effects of circulatory histamines. Compression decreases edema. Elevation reduces blood stasis and improves venous return.

Nonsteroidal anti-inflammatory drugs such as aspirin, ibuprofen, and naproxen offer a relatively safe way to control inflammation and pain. Nutritional pharmacology and botanical medicine play similar roles. Vitamin C and bioflavanoids, such as Quercitin, have anti-inflammatory effects. Bromalain, derived mainly from pineapple, has a long history as an anti-inflammatory agent. Salicylate-containing botanicals such as *Bryonia* and *Spirea ulmaria* have been used for centuries to control inflammation and pain.

In contemplating methods to control inflammation a question arises. Does changing the natural course of the inflammatory process hamper tissue healing? This is a risk-versus-benefit question. Inflammation, if left uncontrolled, can cause tissue damage. Is there a greater exogenous risk from controlling inflammation or from letting the inflammation follow a natural course? Another issue is function. How important is it to return a joint complex to full function?

Movement is an important aspect of joint health. For example, allowing and encouraging motion after knee surgery decreases the chance of degenerative joint changes.[36,37] Soft tissues require stress and strain to direct collagen fiber healing. Without stress and strain the body tends to lay collagen down in a haphazard pattern causing scar formation.[44] Collagen fibrils are aligned in the direction of stress and strain forces. This promotes healing and a return to normal function. This is true whether a joint complex is injured or whether the injury is limited to a muscle.[26,44]

A problem may arise if forces are applied too early in the healing process, and tissue damage may result. There are a number of considerations in deciding what force or exercise to apply, how much to apply, and when to apply it.

Unfortunately, these issues are neither defined nor adequately addressed in the scientific literature. Clinical decisions have more to do with the clinical acumen and experience of the treating clinician than with standardized methodology.

The clinician must take into consideration the healing rate of the individual, the amount of tissue damage, and the vascularity of the injured area. Understanding these issues allows the clinician to tailor a program for the specific problem and, more importantly, to a specific patient.

### Chronic inflammation

The most challenging condition to treat in physical medicine is the chronic musculoskeletal problem. The person with a chronic problem often experiences acute exacerbations and the persistent pain becomes problematic. Not only do the physical findings have to be addressed but emotional and psychologic issues must also be dealt with. The results of treatment may be frustrating for both the clinician and patient.

There are a number of parameters that define chronic problems. A common time period, noted by several authors, designating a problem as chronic is 3 months.[39] This definition is limiting in that no consideration is given to the level or consistency of pain. The effects on activities of daily living are not considered. However, the clinician managing the case must consider these aspects when developing a reasonable therapeutic approach.

The definition of a chronic pain syndrome needs to be revised. It is suggested that the definition of persistent pain that affects a person's daily activities for more than 3 months or pain identified in the same area for 6 months that remisses and exacerbates and affects normal daily activities may clarify the definition.

What occurs with chronic pain? Is a nonimmunologic chronic condition really inflammatory? Histologic examination of tissues that have been injured and in which chronic pain is located shows signs of inflammation.[9] However, chronic inflammation differs from acute in-

flammation in the cell types found in the involved area. The monocytes and leukocytes found during the acute inflammatory response are replaced by macrophages, plasma cells, and lymphocytes.[9] Macrophages predominate, especially in highly vascularized areas. Monocytes, once they project through the vascular wall, change into macrophages. In acute inflammation the precipitating stimuli are generally short lived. Therefore, the macrophages are usually not activated and die or are cleared through the lymphatic system. In chronic inflammation macrophages are activated.

Tissue destruction and fibrosis are evident in these histologic samples. Macrophages produce biologically active substances, many of which are toxic to healthy and damaged tissue. Some of these substances have chemotactic properties, whereas others promote fibroblastic proliferation and collagen deposition. In turn, tissue is damaged and function impaired.

Chronic inflammation may occur because of a number of different insults. Two examples are persistence of any injury-causing stimulus and interference with the normal healing process.

Injuries resulting from overuse are seen very frequently in worker's compensation cases. A repetitive task performed improperly or for a long period of time without a break produces microtraumatic events. Slow, sometimes imperceptible, acute inflammatory tissue reactions progress to chronic ones causing pain and tissue dysfunction.

The mechanism of chronic inflammation following repetitive trauma is poorly understood. One speculation is that continued abuse stimulates the local release of cytokines. This results in autocrine and paracrine modulation leading to cell activity and scar tissue formation.[1]

### Tissue healing: repair and regeneraton stage

Tissue repair with regeneration begins about 48 hours after a traumatic event. The process usually lasts for 6 to 8 weeks. It is controlled by macrophages, which release chemotactants and proteolytic enzymes that activate fibroblasts and growth factors.

The reparative cells consist of modified chondroblasts, fibroblasts, and myofibroblasts. These cells are found in dense, linear-oriented collagenous matrix that lays down type III collagen. Type III collagen consists of small fibrils that are not cross linked. Repair is characterized by a shift from type III to type I collagen. Type I collagen is typically found in skin, bone, tendons, and organs. Cartilage and blood vessels contain types II, III, and IX collagen.[9,26] The driving force of the reparative process is relative tissue hypoxia and large amounts of lactate. The lactate is produced by macrophages and causes vascular proliferation, or angiogenses.[25]

**Remodeling or maturation phase.** The remodeling phase is characterized by an increase in extracellular matrix organization, a return to a normal biomechanical response to loads (within 80%), and a normal biochemical profile. Collagen maturation with realignment in the direction of stresses and strains is usually present by the second month postinjury in tendons and ligaments.[12,44] However, the biomechanical properties at this time are only about 30% of the initial tendon or ligament strength. A complete return to normal strength depends on the severity of the injury, preexisting condition of the area, and treatment. Ligaments and tendons may never regain their initial strength.[44]

## Specific tissue response to injury
### Long bone healing
EMILE GOUBRAN

Case 23 presents a patient who has fractured a long bone. The events that occur in a simple fracture of a long bone in which the two segments of the broken bone have been brought together and aligned will be discussed.

In the area of the fracture, bleeding occurs from ruptured capillaries and blood fills the spaces between the broken ends. Osteogenic cells from the periosteum and endosteum migrate to this area and around the fractured site. Those at the site differentiate to osteoblasts and begin to lay down trabeculae of cancellous bone at the fracture site to form the internal callus.[4] The osteogenic cells at the periphery of the fracture differentiate to chondroblasts that develop the hyaline cartilage collar,

the external callus around the fracture, which provides a support to the fracture site (Fig. 7-3). The cartilage then will ossify in the same manner described for endochrondral ossification. The original bone formed by the cartilage collar and at the site of fracture through activity of osteoblasts is cancellous. In areas of the bone where compact bone is to develop in the shaft, the cancellous bone turns to compact bone through laying down of concentric lamellae in the cavities between bone trabeculae to convert them to Haversian systems. Excess bone tissue at the periphery of the healing site will be removed through the activity of osteoclasts. Subsequent remodeling occurs to bring the bone to its orginal condition, especially in young individuals.[8]

**Striated muscle healing.** Muscle injuries are commonly classified by the degree of strain. The injury usually involves the muscle-tendon unit. Common injuries include the acute strain, avulsions, contusions, fatigue- and exercise-induced muscle injury, and delayed onset muscle soreness syndrome (DOMS).[26] DOMS usually appears in 12 to 48 hours. The lactic acid build-up theory is not supported by current research. The biochemical response is actually similar to the acute inflammatory response.[26]

The common forces applied to muscle that cause injury are direct blows resulting in contusions and sudden voluntary concentric or eccentric overload contractions.[14] Muscle fatigue is often caused by repetitive use over long periods of time and contributes to the risk of

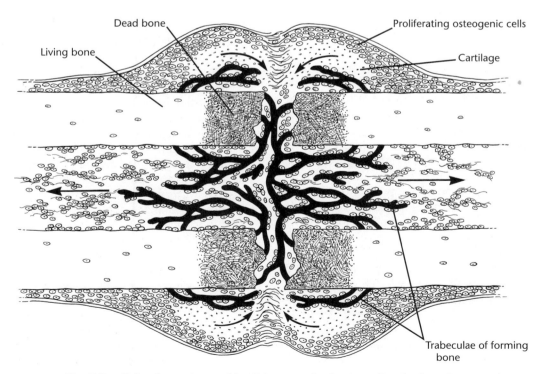

***Fig. 7-3***   Callus formation and healing around a fracture site of a long bone.

injury by decreasing the load-to-failure capacity of the muscle-tendon unit and diminishing the ability of the unit to absorb energy. This can lead to muscle failure.[7]

Strain injuries are categorized according to macroscopic and microscopic tissue changes. A mild strain, or first-degree strain, causes some pain, minimal structural damage, minimal hemorrhage, and early resolution; and, mild strain injuries are self-limiting. Moderate, or second-degree, strain injuries occur when there are incomplete or partial thickness tears at the myotendon junction. This is accompanied by pain, significant local hemorrhage, and inflammation. Some functional loss of the muscle unit occurs in second-degree strains. Severe, or third-degree, strain injury may result in rupture of the muscle or myotendon junction. The injury displays stunning pain, inflammation, obvious swelling, and hemorrhage.

It was not clear, until recently, whether striated muscle could regenerate and proliferate. The general opinion was that all injured muscle are replaced by fibrous tissue. However, it is now known that striated muscle can go through the degeneration-regeneration cycle as long as the basement membrane and blood supply are intact.[44] If the basement membrane is not disturbed, reserve cells are able to differentiate and proliferate to form new skeletal muscle. After injury, recovery of strength may begin in 48 hours because of fibrous components in the clot. If the basement membrane is disturbed, scar tissue forms. Scar tissue creates soft tissue adhesions that restrict contractile and joint function. This can result in a loss of 10% to 20% of muscle contractile strength.[33]

Striated muscle is bathed in blood because of a well-developed blood supply. If blood supply is compromised, ischemia occurs resulting in degneration. The first phase of degeneration is characterized by membrane damage, disruption of sarcomeres at the z bands, mitochondrial swelling, and nuclear pyknosis.[44] This is followed by cell-mediated fragmentation of the damaged muscle fiber. Macrophages are attracted into the area via chemotactic agents and fragment the necrotic muscle fibers. The speed of macrophages entry into the area depends on the extent of ischemia. If blood vessels are not seriously damaged, phagocytosis may occur in 12 hours. However, if there is substantial blood vessel damage, phagocytosis may not take place for several weeks.

**Tendon injuries.** Biomechanically, tendons are strong, flexible viscoelastic structures. They are strong enough to sustain high tensile muscle forces, yet flexible enough to angulate around bony surfaces and deflect beneath retinacula to change the final direction of muscle pull.[6] Failure occurs when the tendon is stretched more than 5% beyond its original length.[13] Normal elastic stresses are 3% to 5%.

Fatigue or over-stress tendon injury requires long periods of time to heal because of minimal blood supply. This can be contrasted to direct muscle injury and healing. During tendon healing, collagen fibers realign according to applied loads. Unique to the tendon is the paratendon, which is loose areolar connective tissue that covers the tendon. It protects the tendon during motion and enhances gliding. If damage occurs to the paratendon, friction develops during motion, causing inflammation and pain. During healing, a lack of stress and strain promotes scar tissue formation, resulting in limited joint motion caused by limited muscle contraction (see p. 191, section on muscle length-tension relationships).

**Ligament injuries.** Sprain is the term commonly used to describe injuries to ligaments. Ligaments heal as do other vascularized tissues, despite a limited blood supply, and have similar biomechanical properties similar to those of tendons.[6] Injury is followed by blood clot formation, hematoma, and soft tissue inflammatory repair.[26] However, once a ligament is injured, it does not retain its original biomechanical properties.

Ligaments reinforce joint capsules supporting bone-to-bone structures. Ligaments are excellent force buffers and shock absorbers because of their ability to crimp. Crimping allows applied stresses without corresponding increases in strain. This permits protection of excessive joint motion. Scar tissue limits this ability, causing greater strain to be applied to the ligament during joint motion. When ligaments fail, muscles crossing the joint are the only structures supporting the joint.

## TREATMENT/MANAGEMENT PROTOCOLS

Treatment and management are divided into three stages: immediate, intermediate, and long-term care. Treatment time periods for each of these categories are not well defined. Clinical acumen defines treatment periods. Pain contributes to treatment-time decisions but is not the only deciding factor. Joint assessment plays a greater role as a determining factor of treatment and management protocols and time determinants.

Immediate care and management is associated with the acute inflammatory response. Usually, this phase lasts 3 to 4 days when the pain is most severe. Intermediate care and management begins at the end of the inflammatory phase. It lasts until there is sufficient healing to avoid compromise. The most aggressive passive-therapies are applied during this period. Pain dissipates and activity levels increase during this time period. Long-term care is a relative term. Management of the patient moves toward active exercise therapy. Therapeutic goals are evaluated at the end of the intermediate phase and the beginning of long-term management.

Individual response to therapy and time after injury are the most important indicators in directing these treatment phases. Immediate procedures relying on acute-phase modalities may be skipped or limited. Patients with chronic pain or dysfunction usually bypass this phase. Even patients with a fresh injury may be able to move directly into an intermediate treatment protocol. Clinical decisions are based on presentation and objective data. The doctor needs to treat the patient, not the injury. There is a strong caveat here. Treatment guidelines are, literally, just guidelines. Clinical thought guided by experience is the determining factor in management decisions. Patients should not be forced into categories simply because of time.

## Immediate treatment protocols

The immediate goal is *controlling* inflammation and pain. There are multiple treatment modalities that can influence inflammation. Cryotherapy is inexpensive and simple. Applications of cold affect the circulatory response of inflammation. The length of time for cold therapy is governed by the *Hunting reflex*. Simply stated, vasoconstriction is followed by vasodilatation. If ice is applied for no longer than 10 minutes at a time, vasoconstriction occurs without reflex vasodilatation. This controls circulation and produces an anesthetic effect. The muscle spindle is desensitized to length changes and nociceptive fibers are inhibited.

Anti-inflammatory medication also assists during this treatment phase. Nonsteroidal anti-inflammatory drugs (NSAIDs) are most commonly used. Aspirin traditionally has been the most frequently used NSAID but ibuprofen has now taken the place of aspirin. These medications chemically inhibit arachidonic acid metabolism.[41] Steroid or sympathomimetic anti-inflammatory drugs are the most potent medications. They are rarely used in musculoskeletal injuries because the risks outweigh the benefits. They are beneficial in treating systemic inflammatory diseases.

Locally, substances such as salicylates, cortisone, lidocaine, and potassium iodide control inflammation and pain with relatively few side effects. If iontophoresis is used to deliver the drug, burning with the low-voltage direct electric current necessary for iontophoresis is of great concern, and the procedure must be closely monitored.

These substances can be delivered transcutaneously through iontophoresis and phonophoresis. These transdermal drug delivery systems are produced by unfacilitated diffusional transport resulting from concentration gradients. Diffusional flux can be induced by electric currents (iontophoresis) or mechanical vibration (phonophoresis).[18]

Different electric modalities may be used to block pain. The modalities do not control inflammation. In fact, with some electric therapy modalities vasodilatation can occur, increasing the inflammatory response.

Each electric therapy modality has a mode of action to accomplish a specific goal. However, any type of stimulation at a sensory level stimulus (SLS) and a high frequency, 80 to 120 Hz, initially changes or blocks pain perception. The *pain-gait* theory describes this phenomenon. Fast conducting afferent axons are stimulated, thereby blocking slower conducting nociceptor fibers.

All electric units, whether transcutaneous electric stimulation (TENS), direct (DC), alternating (AC), or high voltage (HVG) stimulate high velocity (large diameter) sensory axons.[2,32] This blocks or changes nociceptive reception of the anterolateral system at Rexed level II (substantia gelatinosa).[10,32] Many of the neurons in Rexed level II use enkephalins as neurotransmitters and their stimulation inhibits the projection (tract) neurons and blocks the projected nociceptive stimulus.[10] Pain inhibition, however, may be temporary because sensory fibers adapt to continual stimulus. All nociceptive pathways are affected by the sensory stimulation generated by electric stimulation therapy (see Chapter 2).

Pain relief in these first few days posttrauma is of primary concern to the patient. However, manipulation and mobilization, used judiciously, play an important role in producing a quicker recovery. The general rule for these modalities is to treat only as much as the patient can tolerate. If manipulation increases pain the force should be reduced, the adjustment changed, or the procedure discontinued.

Mobilization techniques aid the clinician or therapist in determining the amount of tolerable motion in the injured area. Grade 1 mobilization is less invasive than is grade 4. Grade 5 constitutes joint manipulation.

The decision of whether to manipulate is based on experience. Even though backing off from painful manipulation techniques is suggested, some clinicians, relying on experience, recommend moving through pain. Mobilization techniques outlined by Maigne and Keltonborn help determine levels of tolerance. If a patient can tolerate grade 4 mobilization, manipulation can usually be performed. In experienced hands, adjusting and manipulation may be undertaken in the immediate phase. The usual method to determine whether a thrust should be applied is to monitor the patient's response during "set-up." If pain increases, a different approach or procedure should be attempted. In spinal manipulation, adjusting the contralateral joints may be indicated if the attempt at adjusting the involved side elicits too much pain (assisted versus resisted procedures).[3] Some motion is evoked in the involved joint but without using direct force.[3]

Exercise is not usually prescribed during the first 2 or 3 days postinjury. Basic self-care includes rest, ice applications for 10 minutes at a time, compression if mechanically possible and necessary, and elevation if possible (RICE). This program is followed by gentle progressive activities to increase ranges of motion.

Patient education is paramount throughout all phases. Instruction in proper self-care techniques and nutritional aids to healing improve compliance and outcome. Advice such as lying supine with knees bent supported by two pillows and a rolled towel placed under the neck offers comfort to the patient. Depending on the severity of the injury, instruction about proper movement and lifting can avoid reinjury or exacerbation of symptoms. Education is integral to management.

## Intermediate treatment protocols

In the intermediate phase both treatment and management become aggressive and active. Mobilization, manipulation, and adjusting may be vigorously applied. Passive therapeutic modality goals switch from controlling inflammation and pain to increasing circulation, joint motion, and muscle contraction. Procedures to affect motor level stimulus and joint mobility are now considered.[19,23]

Electric stimulation is directed toward muscle stimulation by causing contraction and relaxation of fibers through lower frequency and higher intensity stimulation. This, in turn, increases blood supply and, hence, metabolite exchange, promoting healing.

Cold applications can be increased from 10 minutes to 20 minutes. Alternating hot and cold is extremely effective in increasing circulation and can replace the 20-minute cold applications.

Intermittent mechanical traction and massage are excellent ways to increase circulation, joint mobility, and soften tissues. Passive movement of tissues, taking into account patient tolerance, can be less painful than active movement and affords early tissue warmth, activity, circulation, and mobility. These techniques may allow transition to early active therapy.

Ultrasound may be employed to heat deep tissues that are not reached by application of hot packs. Deep muscles and joint capsules can be reached with ultrasound. Caution must be taken in ultrasound application since heat tends to build up at dissimilar tissue interfaces such as at the periosteum-bone interface. Ultrasound has been shown to increase local cortisol levels.[40] It increases the temperature of deep structures enough to cause tissue relaxation. This deep heat is produced with continuous ultrasound. When heat is contraindicated, such as during the acute inflammatory phase, pulsed ultrasound can be used with good result. The mechanical disruption assists in tissue healing.

Exercise during the intermediate stage plays an essential role in increasing healing and restoring function. The effects of stresses and strains on healing tissue and collagen realignment has already been discussed. This can be accomplished with stretch and exercise. Early mobility decreases healing time and improves therapeutic outcome.

Specific exercise protocols come into play with certain conditions. For example, William's flexion exercises and other similar programs apply tensile forces to the posterior annular disc fibers and the posterior longitudinal ligament. The theory for these types of exercise suggests that bulging nuclear material can be forced to the disc center.

McKenzie offers a different approach but similar outcome.[31] Centralization of the pain to the low back and out of the leg in a lumbar radiculopathy is the goal. This is accomplished by finding an extension position while prone that reduces or eliminates the leg pain. The McKenzie protocol also attempts to decrease the antalgic position.

Stretching maneuvers increase muscle flexibility by readjusting the muscle spindle.[42] Common procedures involve muscle contraction followed by an instantaneous muscle stretch (that is, postisometric relaxation and postcontraction stretch).

## Long-term treatment protocols

Increasing passive and active range of motion by manipulation, stretch and exercises, and incorporating uniplanar and multiplanar exercise protocols are the goals of the long-term treatment protocol. Muscle strengthening, synergy, and patterned motion with proprioception are evaluated and initiated. In this phase, patients must take an active role in their treatment.

Exercise protocols begin with active and resistive exercises that are uniplanar motions (that is, isotonic, isokinetic, and isometric exercises). Active and resistive exercises consist of the patient moving the affected joint through a range of motion with an applied resistive force or weight. The force may be applied by the clinician resisting the patient's motion; a weight applied to the extremity would also provide resistance during the motion.

Multiplanar exercises consist of resistance being applied along many different motion directions. These type of exercises can be performed in a non–weight-bearing or weight-bearing apparatus. The patient walking on an injured ankle is applying multiplanar motions to the ankle with the resistance of body weight.

Janda[20,21] prescribes to the belief that proprioceptive feedback mechanisms are affected by musculoskeletal injury. He proposes that proprioceptive neuromuscular facilitation (PNF) exercises be introduced to improve function and coordination of the injured area. By the use of the wobble board and Swiss ball, the activity of sensory, conscious, and unconscious proprioception is incorporated in the reactivation process, thereby decreasing time of disability, improving function, and improving long-term effects in a shorter period of time.

## Integration of somatosensory and motor cortices

The effect of proprioceptive retraining on neuromusculoskeletal injury is a subject that has been appearing in the recent rehabilitative and reactivation literature in the chiropractic profession. Janda and Lewit, both major contributors to this literature, have hypothesized that neuromusculoskeletal injury interrupts normal proprioceptive feedback mechanisms that inhibit an expedient return to normal function of the injured patient.[21,28] It has been difficult for the clinician, who treats neuromusculoskeletal problems, to develop protocols that prevent an acute injury from becoming a chronic problem. Janda[20,21] suggests that chronicity is caused by the inadequate retraining of the proprioceptive mechanisms and cortical programs that are changed because of pain and dysfunction. His hypotheses originate from the disciplines of neurology, physical therapy, and occupational therapy beginning with the studies of Sister Kinney, Brunnstrum,[27] and leading to A. Jean Ayres.[2a]

Janda and Lewit explain the clinician's inability to treat chronic pain as directly related to the change in the programming of the proprioceptive mechanisms and state that musculoskeletal injury is partially caused by an ineffective reaction time of muscle contraction in response to proprioceptive stimuli. This reaction time needs to be corrected so that further injury can be prevented. Proper muscle sequencing during motion is also essential to proper musculoskeletal function.[20,21] Injury occurs because of the inability of muscles to reflexively react to a change in posture. In the patient with musculoskeletal injury, the neuromusculoskeletal system must be retrained to respond to a change in external loads by reflexive muscle responses that result in a change of posture.[20,21]

Janda's treatment of chronic musculoskeletal problems are similar to the therapies used on the "clumsy" child. The clumsy child is defined as a youngster who has no neuroanatomic anomaly but has sensory, proprioceptive, and/or motor problems. These problems can include learning deficits. The child has problems integrating information from the surrounding environment and selecting or coordinating proper motor responses. Something is amiss in the sensorimotor networking of this child's neurologic system. The problem can be located in the motor learning program, the sensory interpretation program, or the postural or balance program located in the different neuroanatomic structures of the spinal cord and brain. Each area plays an integrative role in proper sensory interpretation with motor function and learning behavior.

The major anatomic areas of concern have been presented in this chapter and in Chapter 2. The vestibular system, with the cerebellum and the postcentral gyrus of the cerebral cortex, determines sensory input and its integrative role with balance, conscious (that is, joint position sense and motion position sense during voluntary motion), and unconscious proprioception (for example, posture).

In turn, postural and balance correction, joint position changes, and sensory responses are interpreted by the motor system of the precentral gyrus, the supplementary motor and premotor gyrus of the cerebral cortex, the basal ganglia, and the cerebellum.

Integration of these systems produces active movement. Active movement provides the basis for developing neuronal models that are used to plan more complex movements that develop motor control.[11] Treatment of patients with sensory, proprioceptive, or movement disorders requires active participation of the patients to move their bodies in planned coordinated activities. Passive motion does not have the same effect as does active motion on the sensory, proprioceptive, and vestibular pathways, which in turn do not produce proper motor response and ultimately, motor control.[22]

Three theories attempt to explain motor control: closed-loop, open-loop, and schema theory. In the closed-loop theory active joint motion is compared to a "reference of correctness" located in the sensory centers. A neuronal model of "how it feels" to move is then compared to the actual motion, and subtle changes are made that correct any discrepancies.[5,30] The open-loop view proposes that muscle commands are preprogrammed and, once triggered, run their course without correction from sensory feedback. A combination of these theories (schema theory) proposes that there are three types of response-produced feedback: feedback arising from the muscles as they contract (that is, spindle and Golgi tendon organ); feedback from body movement in space (that is, proprioception); and feedback from the environment (that is, sensory information, light touch, and pressure). These feedback mechanisms are then compared to the schema of the closed-loop comparison of how the movement is supposed to occur. The preprogram of the muscle command (open-loop) is then fed forward to the muscles with correction (feedforward mechanism).

Janda suggests that chronic injury to the neuromusculoskeletal system, if not corrected, allows the patient to develop compensatory networks in the proprioceptive and motor plans. The clinician trains this system through exercises that will direct the proprioceptive, sensory, and motor systems to the correct neuronal model (that is, the neuronal model before the injury). Janda proposes that treatment of the chronic back pain patient be directed at the achievement of good function of all peripheral structures, the development of reasonably good muscle balance, and the activation of the spinocerebellovestibular circuits for sensory motor stimulation.[20]

Treatment consists of retraining proper muscle firing sequences and proprioceptive feedback mechanisms that lead to the correction of motor control. The use of the wobble board, balance board, and large balance balls attempts to achieve the common goal of improving muscle sequencing and proprioceptive control. Proper foot position (that is, the foot flexed and narrowed) and the use of a specific standing surface produces specific proprioceptive and light touch stimuli that promote proper feedback stimulus. By certain exercises, an attempt is made to use subcortical reflexive muscle mechanisms to help the patient respond to sudden changes in posture. These authors feel that proper training improves proprioception and motor function to prevent further injury, decrease chronic pain, and return the patient to the activities of daily living.

The use of eccentric and concentric exercise machines (such as Cybex and Kin-com) and plyometrics takes functional exercise protocols to a new level. Biomechanically, striated muscle will produce more active contractile tension during an eccentric muscle action and it will produce greater concentric action if the concentric action is preempted by a fast eccentric action. Hill's length-tension curve illustrates the tension that can be produced in a muscle that is lengthened beyond its resting point (Fig. 6-4). The contractile components in muscle (the actin-myosin fibrils) produce their maximum force at the muscle's resting length. At this length, the distance between each z band is approximately 2.5 $\mu$m, and there is a maximum number of cross-bridges between the actin and myosin filaments. When the length of the z band is changed, the number of cross-bridges are affected and a decrease in force occurs. At full length (approximately 4 $\mu$m) the filaments are pulled apart and there are no more cross-bridges, reducing the tension produced to zero. As the z-band length shortens from the resting length there is an overlap of the cross-bridges and an interference occurs causing a reduction in muscle tension. A full overlap of the actin-myosin filaments

occurs at 1.5 $\mu$m and the muscle tension approaches zero.[43] The parallel elastic components (the epimysium, perimysium, and endomysium) and the series elastic components (the tendon) will produce tension when stretched beyond the muscle's resting point. The series elastic component does not produce significant tension during most human movement, but during high-performance movements in which the demand upon the muscle is to produce a great amount of force, the series elastic component is responsible for a high amount of elastic storage (for example, when a muscle lengthens just prior to rapid shortening).[43] In plyometric exercises the principle of rapid eccentric activity (muscle lengthening) preceding rapid shortening (concentric action) is exemplified. Exercises such as jumping to the floor and then springing forward causes the quadriceps of the knee to lengthen and rapidly shorten; catching and throwing a medicine ball by torquing the trunk are examples of muscles lengthening prior to shortening (Fig. 7-4). The purpose of these exercise protocols is to more precisely copy what a muscle does during normal human motion.

In summary, the literature pertaining to management of musculoskeletal and neuromuscular injury is limited. This chapter has summarized the scientific basis of the tissue-healing process. Patient management strategy is to correlate immediate, intermediate, and long-term goals with the healing process. A protocol has been developed to link science with management. That protocol consists of (1) initial control of inflammation, (2) passive treatment (that is, modalities, mobilization, adjustment, and manipulation), (3) passive and active range of motion improvement through active resistive

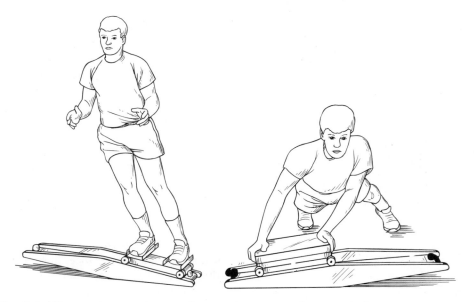

***Fig. 7-4*** Plyometrics exercises used to produce eccentric action before concentric muscle action.

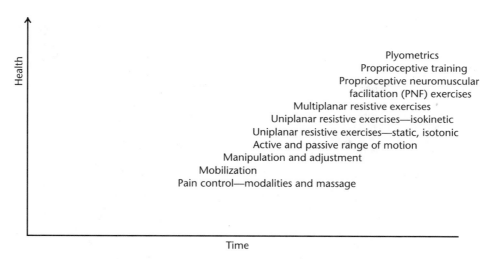

**Fig. 7-5**   Goals of patient management. A patient may begin and end at any part of the management plan.

exercises along one plane, (4) proprioceptive exercises along multiplanes, and (5) plyometrics (Fig. 7-5). The working diagnosis determines where along this protocol the patient will begin treatment. The ultimate goal of patient management may not require that the patient go through all the steps mentioned in this protocol. The goals of the patient may be achieved without needing many of the listed steps. This protocol is an attempt to give organization to the treatment of musculoskeletal and neuromuscular problems and to improve communication between the clinicians treating patients with these problems so that better and more effective care can be given.

## REFERENCES

1. Almekinders LC, Banes AJ, Ballinger CA: Inflammatory responses to fibroblasts to repetitive motion, *Trans Ortho Res Soc* 17: 678, 1992.
2. Alon G: Principles of electrical stimulation. In: Nelson RM, Currier DP, editors: *Clinical electrotherapy*. Norwalk, 1987, Appleton & Lange.
2a. Ayres AJ: Sensory integration and learning disorders, Los Angeles, 1972, Western Psychological Services.
3. Bergmann TF, Peterson DH, Lawrence DJ: *Chiropractic technique*. New York, 1993, Churchill Livingstone.
4. Borysenko M, Beringer T: *Functional histology*, ed 3, Boston, 1989, Little, Brown & Company.
5. Brooks VB: *The neural basis of motor control*, New York, 1986, Oxford University.
6. Carlstedt CA, Nordin M: Biomechanics of tendons and ligaments. In Nordin M, Frankel VH, editors: *Basic biomechanics of the musculoskeletal system*, ed 2, Philadelphia, 1989, Lea & Febiger.
7. Chow GR, et al: The effect of fatigue in muscle strain injury, *Trans Orth Res Soc* 15:148, 1990.
8. Cormack, DH: *Essential histology*, ed 1, Philadelphia, 1993, J.B. Lippincott.
9. Cotran et al, editors: *Robbins: pathological basis of disease*, Philadelphia, 1994, Saunders Co.
10. Cramer GD, Darby SA; Pain of spinal origin. In Cramer GD, Darby SA: *Basic and clinical anatomy of the spine, spinal cord, and ANS*, St. Louis, 1995, Mosby.

11. Fisher A, Murray E, Bundy A: *Sensory integration: Theory and practice*, Philadelphia, 1991, F.A. Davis Co.
12. Frank C, et al: Normal ligament properties and ligament healing, *Clin Orthop* 196:15, 1985.
13. Fung YCB: *Biomechanics: mechanical properties of living tissues*, New York, 1981, Springer Verlag.
14. Garrett WE: Muscle strain injuries: Clinical and basic aspects, *Med Sci Sports Exerc* 22: 436, 1990.
15. Gatterman MI: *Chiropractic management of spine related disorders*. Baltimore, 1990, Williams & Wilkins.
16. Gatterman MI: *Foundations of chiropractic: subluxation*, St. Louis, 1995, Mosby.
17. Haldeman S, Chapman-Smith D, Petersen DM: *Guidelines for chiropractic quality assurance and practice parameters: Proceedings of the Mercy Center consensus conference*, Gaithersburg, 1993, Aspen Publications.
18. Henley EJ. *Transcutaneous drug delivery: iontophoresis, phonophoresis. Critical Reviews in Physical Medicine and Rehabilitation*, vol 2, Issue 3, Boca Raton, 1991, CRC Press Inc.
19. Herzog W, et al: Forces exerted during spinal manipulative therapy, *Spine* 18:1206, 1993.
20. Janda V: Treatment of chronic back pain, *J Manual Med* 6: 166, 1992.
21. Janda V: Muscles, central nervous motor regulation and back problems. In Korr IM, editor: *Neurobiologic mechanisms in manipulative therapy*, New York, 1978, Plenum Press.
22. Kalaska JF: The representation of arm movements in postcentral and parietal cortex, *Canadian J Physiol Pharmacol* 66:455, 1988.
23. Kawchuk GN, Herzog W: Biomechanical characterization (Fingerprinting) of five novel methods of cervical spine manipulation, *J Manip Physiol Therap* 16:573, 1993.
24. Kirkaldy-Willis, WH: The three phases of the spectrum of degenerative disease. In Kirkaldy-Willis WH, editor: *Managing low back pain*, ed 2, New York, 1988, Churchill Livingstone.
25. Leadbetter WB: An introduction to sports-induced soft-tissue inflammation. In Leadbetter WB, Buckwalter JA, Gordon SL: *Sports-induced inflammation*. Park Ridge, 1990, American Academy of Orthopaedic Surgeons.
26. Leadbetter WB: Management and treatment of systemic and regional injuries. In Fu F, Stone D, editors: *Sports injuries: mechanisms, prevention, treatment*, Baltimore, 1994, Williams & Wilkins.
27. Lehmkuhl LD, Smith LK: *Brunnstrom's clinical kinesiology*, ed 4, Philadelphia, 1983, F.A. Davis Co.
28. Lewit K: Functional pathology of the motor system. In *Proceedings of the fourth congress of the international federation of manual medicine*, Prague, 1974.

29. Lewit K: *Manipulative therapy,* Avicenum, 1974, Prague.

30. Matthews PBC: Proprioceptors and their contribution to somatosensory mapping: Complex messages require complex processing, *Canadian J Physiol Pharmacol,* 66:430, 1988.

31. McKenzie RA: *The lumbar spine: mechanical diagnosis and therapy,* Waikanae, 1981, Spinal Publications Limited.

32. Nelson RM, Currier DP: *Clinical electrotherapy,* Norwalk, 1987, Appleton & Lange.

33. Nikolaou PK, et al: Biochemical and histological evaluation of muscle after controled strain injury, *Am J Sports Med* 15:9, 1987.

34. Panjabi MM: The stabilizing system of the spine. Part I. Function, dysfunction, adaptation, and enhancement, *J Spinal Discord* 5:383, 1992.

35. Rubin E, Farber JL, editors: *Pathology,* Philadelphia, 1988, Lippincott.

36. Salter RB, et al: Continuous passive motion and the repair of full-thickness articular cartilage defects: A one-year follow-up, *Trans Orthop Res Soc* 7:167, 1982.

37. Salter RB, et al: The biological effect of continuous passive motion on the healing of full-thickness defects in articular cartilage: An experimental investigation in the rabbit, *J Bone Joint Surg* 62A:1232, 1980.

38. Scholten JHG, Van Weel C: *Function status assessment in family practice: The Dartmouth COOP functional health assessment charts/WONCA,* Lelystad, 1992, MediTekst.

39. Shekelle PG, et al: *The appropriateness of spinal manipulation for low-back pain: indication and ratings by an all-chiropractic expert panel,* Santa Monica, 1992, Research and Development.

40. Touchstone JC, Griffin JE, Kasparon M: Cortisol in human nerve, *Science* 142:1275, 1963.

41. Vane JR: Inhibition of prostaglandin synthese as a mechanism of action for aspirin-like drugs, *Nature* 232:231, 1971.

42. Voss DE, Ionta MK, Myers BJ: *Proprioceptive neuromuscular facilitation: Patterns and techniques,* ed 3, Philadelphia, 1985, Harper & Row.

43. Winter DA: *Biomechanics and motor control of human movement,* ed 2, New York, 1990, Wiley-Interscience Publication.

44. Woo SLY, Buckwalter JA, editors: *Injury and repair of the musculoskeletal soft tissues,* Park Ridge, 1988, American Academy of Orthopaedic Surgeons.

## SUGGESTED READINGS

Albert M: *Eccentric muscle training in sports and orthopaedics,* New York, 1991, Churchill Livingstone.

Bergmann TF, Peterson DH, Lawrence DJ: *Chiropractic technique,* New York, 1993, Churchill Livingstone.

Fu F, Stone D, editors: *Sports injuries: mechanisms, prevention, treatment,* Baltimore, 1994, Williams & Wilkins.

Hertling D, Kessler RM: Management of common musculoskeletal disorders: physical therapy principles and methods, ed 3, Philadelphia, 1996, Lippincott.

Kirkaldy-Willis WH: The three phases of the spectrum of degenerative disease. In Kirkaldy-Willis WH, editor: *Managing low back pain,* ed 2, New York, 1988, Churchill Livingstone.

Tyldesley B, Grieve JI: *Muscles, nerves and movement: kinesiology in daily living,* Boston, 1989, Blackwell Scientific.

Voss DE, Ionta MK, Myers BJ: *Proprioceptive neuromuscular facilitation: patterns and techniques,* ed 3, Philadelphia, 1985, Harper & Row.

Woo SLY, Buckwalter JA, editors: *Injury and repair of the musculoskeletal soft tissues,* Park Ridge, 1988, American Academy of Orthopaedic Surgeons.

# Glossary

*acceleration* The rate of change of velocity. Acceleration occurs in a linear direction or in an angular direction. An example of linear acceleration is applying a thrust to the spine. The force applied by an adjustment accelerates the spine in a certain direction. Acceleration is a vectorial quantity with a beginning point before the adjustment is applied and a distance it will travel (the end of its range). $a = \frac{1}{2}mv^2$, where a = acceleration, m = mass of body, and v = velocity of body.

*all-or-nothing phenomenon* If a cell depolarizes to the threshold potential, then an action potential will be produced.

*anesthesia* A complete loss of cutaneous sensation

*antagonist* A muscle that opposes the direct action of the agonist muscle

*ataxia* A failure to produce normal motor acts or jerky and uncoordinated motions during walking. Ataxia can be caused by sensory or motor deprivation. Sensory ataxia can be improved on by visual feedback mechanisms to guide limb positioning, whereas motor ataxia is not compensated by vision.

*axon hillock* The point of origination of an axon on the cell body and is located at the Nissl free origin.

*bradykinesia* Abnormal slowness of movement

*Cartesian coordinate system* In biomechanics this system is used to identify motion that is being studied in research. There is a right-handed and a left-handed system. The right-handed system is most commonly used in biomechanical research. In a Cartesian system there are three axes connected at their tails in a perpendicular fashion. Any object in motion can be described by this system. Any movement can be described by placing the coordinate system at a fixed position in the structure being studied. The motions that occur are (1) rotation around an axis and (2) motion along an axis.

*cartilaginous joint* A classification of a joint according to its structure. The bones of this joint are held together by cartilage and the joint is slightly moveable. These are of two types; (1) synchondrosis (synarthrosis)—the bones that make up this joint are united by hyaline cartilage. This is often a temporary joint because it fuses as human development progresses. An example is the epiphyseal plate of bone (growth plate) and the ischiopubic synchondrosis of the inferior ramus of the pubis and the ramus of the ischium. (2) symphysis (amphiarthrosis)—the bones in this joint are united by fibrocartilage and have limited motion (for example, intervertebral disc and pubic symphysis).

*center of gravity* A point at which the body mass is centered. In kinesiology, the center of gravity of the human body is located 55% from the floor of the total body height. The center of gravity moves according to related body structures. For example, when a person wants to initiate walking, the center of gravity is displaced anteriorly to begin the body in motion.

*center of mass* A point at which the body mass is centered. The center of mass of the human body is located 55% from the floor of the total body height. The difference between center of mass and the center of gravity is that the center of mass does not change in location; it is a fixed point. Each anatomic structure has a center of mass and a center of gravity. The center of mass is typically measured by taking the object of concern and hanging it from a wire. The point-at-which the object is balanced is the center of mass.

*chorea* Brief, jerky, and abrupt movements of any part of the body caused by an overactivity of dopaminergic neurons. The movements are random and continuous.

*closed chain* The motions that occur within a joint when the hand or foot are fixed in position. The joints of the lower extremities are closed chain during the stance phase of gait. The foot is fixed on the ground. During a push-up the joints of the upper extremity are performing closed-chain events.

*concave-convex rule* When a concave object moves on a fixed convex object the rotation and translation of the concave object is in the same direction. If a convex object moves on a fixed concave object the rotation and translation of the convex object is in opposite directions. When a patient is asked to extend the knee while seated, the tibia (concave object) will translate and rotate in the same direction relative to the fixed femur (convex femoral condyles).

*concentric muscle activity* The shortening of a muscle while it is producing a force (Fig. G-1).

*creep* A viscoelastic property that is a measurement of deformation of a material as the load remains constant. The intervertebral disc is a good example of creep. After arising in the morning a person is approximately 1.25 cm taller than when going to bed at night. This is caused by the constant loads applied to the intervertebral disc during the day that cause the disc to lose height over time (Fig. G-2).

*damping* A viscoelastic property of a material that constitutes resistance to the speed of the application of a load. The intervertebral disc exemplifies this principle well. During a slow (time) application of a load the water content in the disc can redistribute itself causing the disc to lose height with time (that is, creep occurs). However, if a load is applied quickly the water within the disc does not have the time to redistribute and the disc increases in its stiffness properties (that is, damping occurs). Both properties allow the disc to protect itself and the surrounding structures from the application of external loads that might cause internal fracture.

*deformation* A change in length or shape of an object. There are three types of deformation: compression, tension, and shear (Fig. G-3).

*degeneration* A change in tissue from a higher to a lower or less functionally active form. These structures are more vulnerable to either dynamic or cyclic overload that leads to mechanical fatigue and failure.[9]

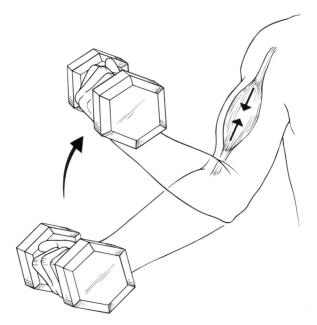

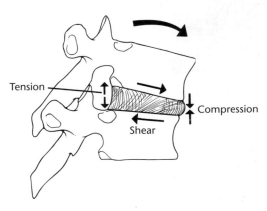

**Fig. G-3** Deformation in tension compression and shear.

**Fig. G-1** Concentric muscle activity. Muscle shortens during tension production.

**dermatome** The area of skin supplied by afferent nerve fibers by a single posterior nerve root.[5] A dermatome is an area of skin that receives sensory innervation from a specific spinal nerve root.

**diarthrosis (synovial)** A classification of a joint according to its function. This is an anatomic joint that is freely moveable. It incorporates a capsule that surrounds two bones that are covered with hyaline cartilage and is bathed in synovial fluid produced by synovium. The majority of joints in the human body are of this type (shoulder, elbow, wrist, and hand; hip, knee, ankle, and foot; spine).

**diencephalon** The diencephalon is considered the primitive brain and consists of all the thalamic structures: the thalamus, hypothalamus, epithalamus, and subthalamus. It encircles the third ventricle and is surrounded by the cerebral hemispheres. The cavity of the diencephalon is the narrow third ventricle lying between the right and left thalami.[11]

**dynamic stabilizer** A muscle that has constant unchanging muscle activity throughout a joint's range of motion. For example, the supraspinatus muscle shows a constant level of muscle activity (measured on electromyogram) throughout the range of motion during shoulder abduction.

**dysesthesia** An altered or perverted interpretation of sensation such as burning, tingling, or painful feelings in response to touch.[15]

**eccentric muscle activity** Lengthening of the muscle fibers while the muscle is producing a force. This type of muscle activity usually occurs when an anatomic structure motion is resisting gravity (for example, bending slowly at the waist) (Fig. G-4).

**elasticity** The property of a material or structure to return to its original form following the removal of a deforming load. In comparison, an elastic material is best illustrated by a rubber (or elastic) band. When a load is applied to the rubber band it deforms (flexible properties). When the load is removed from the rubber band, it returns to its original shape. A material that is not elastic is exemplified by chewing gum. When a load is applied to the chewing gum, it will deform, but when the load is removed the chewing gum

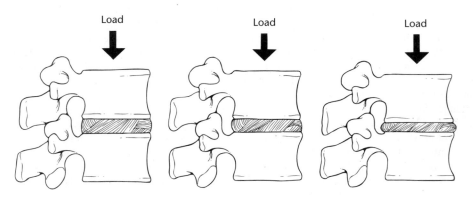

**Fig. G-2** Biomechanical creep.

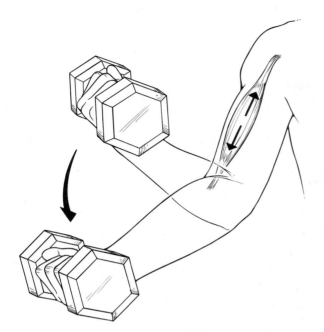

**Fig. G-4** Eccentric muscle activity. Muscle lengthens during tension production.

stays deformed and does not return to its original length (Fig. G-5).

**emigration** The process by which motile white cells escape from the blood vessels to the perivascular tissues.[4]

**exocytosis** The discharge from a cell of enclosed particles that are too large to diffuse through a cell membrane.[5]

**exudate** An inflammatory extravascular fluid that has a high protein concentration, much cellular debris, and a specific gravity greater than 1.020.[4]

**failure** fracture of an object caused by the presence of excessive loads (for example, bond fracture).

**fatigue** A viscoelastic property that is the process of formation and propagation of cracks in a structure subjected to repetitive load cycles. The applied load is generally below the failure load of the material. Repetitive cycle injury is a major cause of musculoskeletal problems in the athlete. Athletes who double their running distance in a very short period of time display fatigue type of injuries because of the increase in repetitive loads applied to the anatomic structures.

**fibrous joint** A classification of an anatomic joint according to its structure. There is almost no motion within a fibrous joint and it is held together by dense connective tissue or ligaments. There are three types of fibrous joints: (1) suture joint (synarthrosis)—found between the bones of the skull. These bones have a small amount of periosteum between them. (2) Gomphosis (synarthrosis)—similar to a suture joint in that it almost has no movement, but the shape of the joint is different. The joint is in the form of a peg fitting into a hole ("gomphos" means nail) and is held in place by dense connective tissue (for example, teeth). (3) Syndesmosis (amphiarthroidal)—the most moveable of the three types of fibrous joints. The bones are held together by ligaments ("syndesmo" means connective tissue) and are separated from each other by a considerable space that is bridged by an interosseous ligament (for example, distal radioulnar or distal tibiofibular joints).

**fixation** An object stuck in a certain direction (for example, C3 is stuck in right lateral bending relative to C4). This joint will move further into right lateral bending but will not be able to move in the other direction (left lateral bending).[2]

**flexibility** A measure of compliance to external loads by a material as it deforms. Flexibility is best described as a coefficient and is defined as the ratio of the amount of displacement produced to the load applied (meters/new-

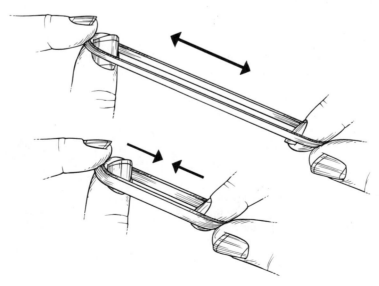

**Fig. G-5** Biomechanical elasticity.

ton). A flexible material is exemplified by three principles; (1) a flexible material needs less stress to deform; (2) flexibility = strain/stress; and (3) the less the slope of the stress/strain curve (or load/deformation) the more flexible the material.

**foot-flat** (flat-foot) Period of time when the foot is flat on the ground during the stance phase of gait.

**force** Any action that tends to change the state of rest or of motion of a body to which it is applied. Any influence that causes a change in position or alters the direction or speed of motion.[12]

**healing** A complex process that results in the restoration of anatomic continuity as a result of an orderly biologic repair process. There are four different qualities of soft wound healing: ideal, acceptable, minimal, and failed. An ideally healed wound is a soft tissue that has returned to normal anatomic structure, function, and appearance. An acceptably healed wound has restored anatomic continuity and sustained function, whereas a minimally healed wound has restoration of anatomic continuity but without a sustained functional result and the wound may therefore recur. In failed wound healing no anatomic restoration or sustained function is present.[9]

**heel-off** Period at which the heel comes off the ground during the stance phase of gait.

**heel rocker** Progression of the limb and body while the heel is the pivotal area of support.[12]

**Heuter-Volkmann rule** Abnormal bone growth (that is, lack of bone growth) caused by too much or not enough force (compression, tension or shear). Stresses being applied to an anatomic structure that are outside the normal range for normal response of that tissue (see Wolff's Law).

**hierarchical organization of neurons** This organization exists in the brain and is an explanation of how one descending tract can have influence on a parallel descending tract. Hierarchical order exists between the lateral corticospinal tract and the rubrospinal tract. The neurons of the lateral corticospinal tract are located in the cerebral cortex (higher level). They send axons to the red nucleus located in the midbrain (lower level). The red nucleus axons descend in the rubrospinal tract.

**hyperalgesia** Enhancement of the sensation of pain in response to other stimuli when peripheral tissues are damaged.

**hyperesthesia** Sensory stimuli that are more keenly felt than normal.[15]

**hypesthesia** Reduced sensation to touch.

**hypokinesia** A reduction in mobility caused by an increase in muscle tone. Movements are slow and stiff and are often caused by disease in the substantia nigra of the basal ganglia.

**inertia** The resistance of a body to any change in its state of rest or uniform motion. The property of all material bodies to resist change in the state of rest or motion under the action of an applied load.[16] This is an important concept when interpreting an automobile whiplash injury (acceleration-deceleration injury).

**isokinetic (isoinertia)** A form of exercise that causes muscles to contract and joints to move at a constant velocity because of a change in the external load. Cybex or Kincom are examples of these types of weight machines. They control the velocity of contraction by changing the external force the muscle is resisting by affecting the moment arm distance between the weight being lifted and the center of rotation. The most common technique used to produce this change in distance is a cam (Fig. G-6).

**isometric** A form of exercise that applies a constant external force and causes a static muscle contraction. Muscle activity is present but there is no change in the joint angle or muscle length. Grasping your hands and pushing them together causes the pectoralis major to produce a force but there is no change in the length of the muscle (Fig. G-7).

**isotonic** A form of exercise that applies a constant external force and produces a change in the velocity of muscle and joint motion (for example, flexing the elbow while holding a 20-lb dumbbell in the hand will allow the elbow to flex at a change in velocity during the action) (Fig. G-8).

**kinematic chain** Joints of the human body that are linked in such a way that motion of one joint affects the motion of others. During gait the motion of the foot affects the motion of the ankle as it affects the motion at the knee, and it, in turn, affects the motion at the hip. This describes a closed kinematic chain. An open kinematic chain exists when one joint moves without affecting the motion of other joints.

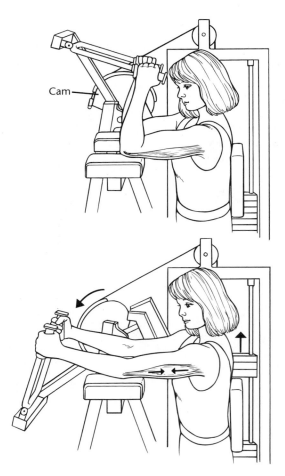

Cam

**Fig. G-6** Isokinetic exercise. The cam changes the moment arm.

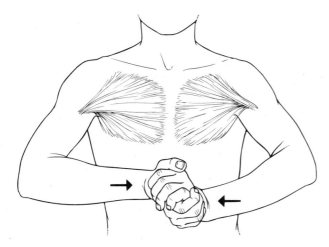

**Fig. G-7** Isometric exercise. Muscle activity with no change in length. No work is performed.

When the clinician examines the knee independently of other joints this is a closed kinematic chain.

**kinematics** The study of the motion of a body without considering the forces causing that motion. In biomechanics we consider how an object moves (for example, the spine) without considering the forces causing that motion (for example, striated muscle).

**labeled line code** individual receptors responding selectively to one type of stimulus.[8]

**lever arm** (see Moment Arm)

**load** A general term describing the application of a force or moment (torque) to a structure. An external quantity that is applied to an object. There are three types of loads: compression, tension, and shear.

**locomotion** The translation of the center of gravity through space along a path requiring the least expenditure of energy.[1]

**locomotor unit** The two lower limbs and the pelvis that provide the mechanics of walking.[12]

**manipulation** (1) A passive maneuver in which specifically directed manual forces are applied to vertebral and extra-vertebral articulations of the body, with the objective of restoring mobility to restricted areas.[6] (2) A manual procedure that involves a directed thrust to move a joint past the physiologic range of motion without exceeding the anatomic limit.[7]

**mesencephalon** Middle brain

**metencephalon** Hind brain

**microtrauma** Damage at the microscopic or molecular level of a tissue that can be produced by either a tension, compression, or a shear load that, most often, is well within the physiologic range (elastic range).

**midstance** Period of time when the center of mass is directly over the foot during the stance phase of gait (traditional system).

**moment** The product of force times the lever arm. Moment is a measurement of forces being applied to an object that cause that object to rotate about a point.

**moment (lever) arm** The perpendicular distance from the point of application of force to the axis of rotational motion. A moment arm changes length during motion. A simple example of this phenomenon is elbow flexion. The muscle that produces the force during elbow flexion is the brachialis. At 30 degrees of elbow flexion the moment arm is short, at 90 degrees of elbow flexion the moment arm increases, and at 145 degrees of elbow flexion the lever arm again decreases in length. If the force being applied by the brachialis is constant the moment produced would increase and decrease according to the moment arm length.

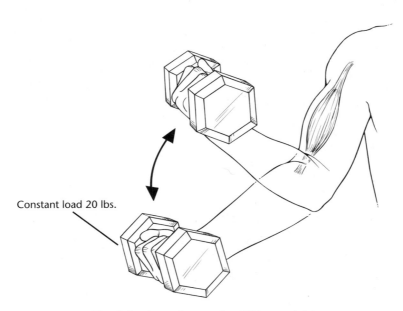

Constant load 20 lbs.

**Fig. G-8** Isotonic exercise. Lifting weights.

*momentum (p)* The measurement of the tendency of a body to continue in motion at a constant velocity. If the object being studied travels in a straight line linear momentum is being measured. If the moving body is spinning then angular momentum is measured.

*movement (involuntary)* A movement of a part of the body that cannot be started or stopped on a command.

*movement (voluntary)* A motion of any part of the body that can be started or stopped on command.

*myelencephalon* hind brain

*myotomal pain* Pain originating from muscle or tendon. This pain is described by the patient as a dull-diffuse ache.

*myotome* A group of muscles innervated from a single spinal segment.[5]

*necrosis* The structural changes that occur in living cells just prior to death. Necrosis occurs from the release of intracellular proteolytic enzymes or extracellular enzymes in response to a decrease in pH (increase in acid pH) from hypoxic or anoxic metabolism.[9]

*negative work* An expression used when an athlete trains the eccentric action of a muscle. An eccentric action, in this context, defines a muscle producing a force in the direction opposite to that the joint is moving (for example, during resisted flexion of the knee the quadriceps is producing an eccentric action to resist knee flexion).

*neuralgia* nerve pain similar to neuritis but displays objective motor weakness.

*neuritis* inflammation of a peripheral nerve or its surrounding structures that does not display any objective motor weakness (differentiating from neuralgia).

*neurogenic pain* Includes deafferentation pain, neuropathic pain, and sympathetically maintained pain. This pain occurs from a direct affect upon a nociceptive axon. Examples are nerve compression or a neuroma.

*neutral zone* A part of the total range of motion of a body in an anatomic plane that begins at its neutral position and ends when deformation of that object is initiated.

*open chain* The motions that occur within a joint when the most distal joint is not fixed. The motion of the upper extremity when grabbing for an object is an example of open-chain events of all the joints of the upper extremity. The swing phase of gait and the actions of the joints of the lower extremities are examples of an open chain.

*overuse* Broadly defined, a level of repetitive microtrauma sufficient to overwhelm the ability of tissues to adapt.[13]

*pain referral* Pain felt in a region much larger than the area immediately surrounding the damaged tissue. This area is most often a distance from the damaged tissue.

*paracrine* A cell that stimulates adjacent cells.

*paresthesia* Spontaneous sensation of prickling or tingling.[15] This word is often used instead of dysesthesia to mean a change in sensation.

*pattern code* Different temporal patterns of stimulus through a nonspecialized receptor that serve as a nerual code for different modalities.

*perception* An abstraction and elaboration of sensory input.[8]

*plane* A flat surface that is determined by three points in space. In anatomy and biomechanics planes are determined by the perpendicular axes (X, Y, and Z). The sagittal plane is formed by the Y and Z axes. The frontal (coronal) plane is formed by the Y and X axes; and the horizontal (transverse) plane is formed by the X and Z axes. Any motion that occurs in an anatomic joint can be described by the motion around or along a plane. The sagittal plane divides the body into right and left sections. When the body is divided into two equal right and left sections this plane is called the midsagittal plane. The frontal plane divides the body into front and back sections; and, the horizontal plane divides the body into upper and lower sections (Fig. G-9).

*plasticity* The property of a material to permanently deform when it is loaded beyond its elastic range.

*potential energy* Energy that is stored in a structure when it is deformed. When a tensile force is applied to a viscoelastic structure it develops potential energy that will help it return to its original shape once the force is removed. The elastic components of muscle help muscles produce more force when the muscle is stretched because the potential energy in that muscle increases because of the stretching of the elastic components (tendons).

*radicular pain* Pain that is generated by a dorsal nerve root, dorsal root ganglion, or spinal nerve in the vertebral area or in a peripheral nerve. It is controversial if the meninges should be included as part of this list. The patient describes this pain as a sharp-shooting, shocklike distribution of pain that travels to a dermatome. Words such as "the pain travels like an electric wire" is commonly used as a descriptor by the patient.

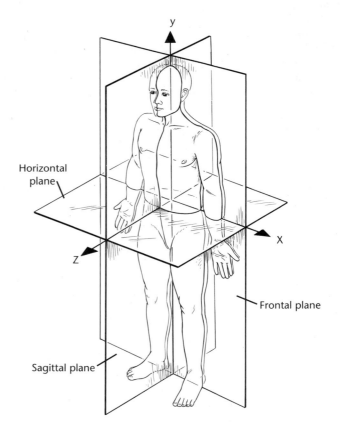

*Fig. G-9* Planes of the human body.

**receptive field** In neuroanatomy a receptive field is a tissue region that is innervated by a receptor terminal and includes the area of surrounding tissue that a stimulus energy is conducted to the receptor terminal.

**receptor adaptation** The mechanism by which the amplitude of the generator potential and thus the firing of action potentials progressively decreases in response to a continuous stimulus.[15] Rapidly adapting receptors (phasic) detect rapidly changing and transient stimuli and inform the nervous system about a change in the environment or position. Slow adapting receptors (tonic) respond to a sustained stimuli and inform the nervous system of the status of the body and its relationship to its environment.

**reflexes*** The shear number and variety of named reflexes is bewildering. There is no standard system for naming reflexes. They may be named according to the location of the motor nuclei, the fundamental tissue types, the diagnostic significance or simply after an individual best known for the reflex (an eponym). Commonly used categories for naming reflexes with representative examples are shown below. This list does not include all categories by which reflexes are named or all possible examples of representative reflexes. In addition, it should be noted that the same reflex can be named according to several categories (for example, the biceps reflex is also a spinal reflex, a deep tendon reflex, and a somatic reflex; the gag reflex is also a cranial reflex, a superficial reflex, and a somatic reflex).

*reflexes named by location of motor nuclei*

Spinal (segmental) reflexes: The motor nucleus of the reflex is located within a spinal cord segment.

Cranial (brainstem) reflexes: The motor nucleus of the reflex is one of the cranial nerve motor nuclei (and therefore located within the brain stem).

*reflexes named by location of sensory receptors*

Superficial reflexes: These reflexes are activated by stimulating receptors located in the skin (and derivatives of skin such as the cornea) or mucous membrane. Superficial reflexes may be named with greater specificity concerning the location of the involved sensory receptors (abdominal reflex, plantar reflex, corneal reflex). Superficial reflexes may also be named for the muscle that contracts in response to skin stimulation (cremasteric reflex) or the functional response (blink reflex, gag reflex, withdrawal reflex).

Deep reflexes: These reflexes are activated by stimulating receptors in tendon, muscle, or joint tissue. An important subdivision of the deep reflexes have their receptors (muscle spindles) located in a muscle belly. Muscle spindle receptors respond to stretch (myotactic) reflexes or deep tendon reflexes (a misnomer). Lastly, muscle stretch reflexes may be named more specifically after the muscle containing the stimulated receptors (Achilles reflex, biceps reflex).

*reflexes named by the basic tissue types involved*

Somatic reflexes: Both the sensory and motor limbs of these reflexes involve somatic tissues. All of the superficial and deep reflexes described above are somatic reflexes.[1] The frequently used term "deep tendon reflexes" is actually a misnomer. These reflexes are really muscle stretch reflexes. Although the reflex is elicited by striking the muscle tendon,

* Written by Charles N. R. Henderson.

the response is due to muscle spindles within the belly of the muscle, not receptors within the tendon. Tendon receptors (Golgi tendon organs) are involved in more complex reflexes, but the mechanism of this involvement is currently a subject of debate within neuroscience.

Visceral reflexes: Both the sensory and motor limbs of these reflexes involve visceral tissues. Mass movement of the contents of the colon following entrance of food into the stomach (gastrocolic reflex) and decreased gastric secretion following entrance of food into the small intestine (enterocoelic reflex) are examples of visceral reflexes.

Somatovisceral reflexes: The sensory limb of these reflexes originates in somatic tissue, whereas the motor limb terminates in visceral tissue. Cardiovascular changes in response to a painful stimulus of muscle, tendon, or joint tissue is an example of a somatovisceral reflex.

Viscerosomatic reflexes: The sensory limb of a viscerosomatic reflex originates in visceral tissue, whereas the motor limb terminates in somatic tissue. Abdominal muscle splinting during appendicitis is an example of a viscerosomatic reflex.

*reflexes named by function*

Pathologic reflexes: These reflexes are abnormal in character or response magnitude for a given sensory stimulus. They are often specific or pathognomonic for a lesion or disease affecting the nervous system. Commonly, they are named after the individual who first discovered the reflex. The Babinski reflex is probably the best known of the pathologic reflexes. This reflex may be observed in an adult after injury to the corticospinal tract. Stroking the sole of the foot produces extension of the great toe. For a long time now it has been said that a newborn infant gives an extensor response to stroking the sole of the foot. This response is said to gradually assume an adult (flexor) form at 6 to 8 months of life. However, more recent studies report that 93% or more of normal newborns have a flexor plantar response. These reports suggest that the presence of a Babinski sign is abnormal, even at birth.

Nonpathologic reflexes are also named according to function. Withdrawal (flexor) reflexes are an example. These reflexes are part of the body's protective mechanism. When the skin over a body part is noxiously stimulated, that part is quickly withdrawn from the stimulus. Because the sensory receptors for this reflex are located in the skin these are also superficial reflexes. These reflexes are often called "flexor reflexes" because withdrawal of the body part usually involves flexion of a limb.[3]

**restriction** A lack of motion in a certain direction. In chiropractic terms a restriction is the inability of a joint to move in a certain direction (for example, the inability of C3 to bend laterally to the right on C4). This definition is defining the motion of a vertebra from its neutral position.[2]

**retrusion** The state of being posterior to the normal position, such as in tooth malposition.

**rolling** In a ball-and-socket joint the contact point on each joint surface changes by an equal amount. Therefore, rotation and translation are occurring simultaneously in a joint.

**rostral** Toward the head. The word is synonymous with cephalid or superior.

**rotation** The clinical term for torque or moment. A rotational moment around the long axis of the spine or the shaft of a bone. In a ball-and-socket joint rotation is defined as the contact point of the socket remains constant while the contact point on the ball moves.

*SAID principle* Specific Adaptation to Imposed Demands. The adaptation of anatomic structures within the human body is very specific. A weight lifter's muscles will hypertrophy and increase in strength but will not significantly increase in endurance. A long-distance runner will have thin muscles that will be able to produce work for a long period of time but may not significantly increase in strength. The body responds to the different stresses applied to it according to the specific demands made by those stressors.

*saltation* Conduction along a myelinated nerve.

*sclerotomal pain* Pain originating from bone or ligament and is usually described by the patient as a deep, dull ache that is more local than a myotomal pain.

*sclerotome* The area of bone innervated from a single spinal segment.[5]

*somatic pain* Pain generated by a skeletal or related structure (muscle, tendon, ligament, facet joint).

*spasm* An involuntary contraction of muscle that may involve the whole muscle or part of a muscle. It can be caused by an injury to a muscle or by a biochemical imbalance (hypercalcemia, hyperkalemia, or other electrolyte imbalances). There is no cerebral cortex involvement.

*spasticity* The involuntary continual contraction of skeletal muscle. This phenomenon usually occurs because of a lesion to the precentral gyrus of the cerebral cortex. Reciprocal inhibition is not lost, and when the muscle is slowly passively stretched it will "give-way," leading to the knife-clasp phenomenon.

*spatial discrimination* The ability of the neurologic system to localize and distinguish two closely spaced stimuli. It is inversely proportional to the size of the receptive field and directly proportional to the receptor density.[15]

*spatial summation (population encoding)* Increasing the number of sensory or motor axonal units to augment the stimulus.[10]

*speed* The instantaneous change of position with respect to time. Speed is simply how fast an object is moving at a given time, and it is a scalar quantity. The unit of speed is distance/time (for example, 35 miles per hour or 32 meters/second).

*spinal stability* The inability of the spine under physiologic loads to limit patterns of displacement so as not to damage or irritate the spinal cord or nerve roots and, in addition, to prevent incapacitating deformity or pain arising from structural changes.[16]

*static muscle activity* A muscle producing force without causing a change in its length (for example, showing off the biceps without changing the joint angle of the elbow).

*stenosis* Narrowing of a canal (for example, narrowing of the intervertebral foramen, spinal canal, or carpal tunnel).

*step* The subphases of the stance phase of gait from ipsilateral heel strike to contralateral heel strike.

*stiffness* A measure of resistance offered to external loads by a material as it deforms. There are three principles of stiffness: (1) a stiffer material needs more stress to deform; (2) stiffness = stress/strain; and (3) the slope of the stress/strain curve exemplifies the stiffness of a material.

*strain* Strain is the change in unit length or angle in a material subjected to a load. Strain is measured as a percentage change in length. Strain is an internal measurement of deformation and its formula (during a tensile load) is as follows: strain = $\text{length}_{final} - \text{length}_{original} / \text{length}_{original} \times 100$.

*stress* (1) A force per unit area of a structure. (2) An internal measurement of force. Stress is to a solid as pressure is to a liquid. The unit of stress is Newton/meter$^2$. There are two types of stress: (1) normal stress, a quantity that is measured perpendicular to the cross-section of a structure (compression and tension stress) and (2) shear stress, a quantity that is measured parallel to the cross section of a structure. The easiest way to understand the effect of stress and strain is to illustrate a stress/strain curve. The slope of the curve describes the stiffness of the material (for example, bone has a higher stiffness than muscle, which in turn, has a higher stiffness than skin).

*stride* The events (subphases of gait) that occur in one lower extremity during the stance and swing phase of gait. From ipsilateral heel contact to ipsilateral heel contact.

*subluxation* (1) Partial or incomplete dislocation. (2) Restriction of motion of a joint in a position exceeding normal physiologic motion, although the anatomic limits have not been exceeded. (3) Aberrant relationship between two adjacent articular structures that may have functional or pathologic sequelae. It can cause an alteration in the biomechanical or neurophysiologic reflexes of these articular structures, their proximal structures, or body systems that are directly or indirectly affected by these articular structures.[6] (4) A motion segment, in which alignment, movement integrity, physiologic function are altered although contact between joint surfaces remains intact.[7]

*subluxation complex* A theoretical model of motion segment dysfunction (subluxation) that incorporates the complex interaction of pathologic changes in nerve, muscle, ligament, and vascular and connective tissues.[7]

*symptom* A subjective finding that is usually present during the history of an examination.

*synapse* The junction between two nerve cells. There are three types of synapses: (1) axodendritic—a synapse between the axon of one nerve cell and the dendrite of another and is the most common type. (2) axosomatic—a synapse between an axon of one cell and the body (soma) of another nerve cell. (3) axoaxonic—the synapse between an axon of one cell and the axon of another cell.

*synarthrosis* A classification of a joint according to its function. A synarthrosis joint is one that has no movement (for example, skull bones).

*synovial joint* A classification of a joint according to its structure. The bones within this joint are freely moveable and a joint cavity separates the bones that make up the joint. The different types of synovial joints are classified according to the shape of the articulating surfaces and the type of motion they allow. There are four different groups of synovial joints:

1. Gliding joint (articulation plane). This joint allows a limited amount of sliding between two flat surfaces (for example, facet, carpal, and tarsal joints).
2. Uniaxial or hinge (ginglymus) joint (movement in only one plane). This joint works like the hinge on a door. The axis of rotation is along the transverse plane and it allows flexion

and extension (for example, radiohumeral joint). A pivot (trochoid) joint is another uniaxial joint in which one bone serves as a pin and the other bone rotates around it. The major motion of this joint is rotation (for example, dens of C2 and C1 and the radioulnar joint of the elbow).

3. Biaxial joint (movement around two axes at right angles to each other). There are two types of biaxial joints: (a) Condyloid (condylar, ellipsoid) joint. this joint has one end in the shape of a shallow ellipsoid socket that articulates with an oval ball and permits all types of motion except rotation (for example, radiocarpal joint, occiput-C1 joint, and the knuckles). (b) Saddle (sellar) joint. This joint has one articulating surface that is convex and the other concave and allows all movement except rotation (for example, carpometacarpal joint of the thumb).

4. Polyaxial joint (movement allowed in all directions, six degrees of freedom). This joint is spheroid (ball and socket). The convex head of one bone fits into a concave socket of another (for example, hip and shoulder joints).

*telencephalon* Head-brain, superior brain

*temporal summation (frequency encoding)* Frequency of action potentials in an afferent or efferent axon.[10]

*tendinitis* Injury to the tendon tissue with capillary damage and acute inflammation.

*tendinosis* Initially an asymptomatic degeneration of tendon caused by aging or cumulative microtrauma without histologic evidence of acute inflammation.[9]

*tenosynovitis (paratendonitis)* Inflammation of the tendon sheath consisting of pain, swelling, and possible local crepitus.

*tenosynovium (paratendon)* The synovial sheath that surrounds long tendons. The long head of the biceps tendon is surrounded by a synovial sheath that bathes the tendon in synovial fluid. The sheath acts similar to a automobile piston that is bathed by surrounding oil.

*threshold potential* The membrane potential at which the action potential begins.

*toe-off* The period of time when the toes are coming off the ground during the stance phase of gait.

*torque* The measurement of a rotational force around an axis that is along the long axis of an object. The difference between moment and torque is that torque occurs around the long axis of an object, whereas moment is a rotational force around any axis of an object. When torque is applied to an object three stresses occur internally: compression, tension, and shear.

*trigger point* (1) A hyperirritable section of muscle that, when compressed, refers pain to other areas and produces a jump sign and, when stroked (transverse), will cause an involuntary muscle twitch. (2) A hyperirritable spot within a taut band of skeletal muscle fibers that is painful upon compression and can give rise to characteristic referred pain, tenderness, and autonomic phenomena.[14]

*twitch duration* The time from beginning to end of a single muscle contraction in each muscle type.

*valgum (valgus)* An increase in an angle; measured from the medial aspect of a joint.

*vara (varum)* A decrease in an angle; usually measured from the medial aspect of a joint.

*vectorial quantity* A quantity characterized by a magnitude, direction, and a point of attachment. When applied to roadmap directions the term encompasses a starting point, a direction of travel, a distance, and an ending point. In chiropractic, the term is applied when an adjustment is performed on a patient. The hands are placed on a certain area (starting point), tissue slack is eliminated (direction), a given amount of force is applied to cause the wanted adjustment (magnitude) in the direction of the zygapophyseal joints (direction).

*velocity* Velocity is the vectorial quantity of speed. It is defined as the instantaneous vector time rate of change of position. Velocity is speed with a particular direction, distance or amount of force, and a starting point (point of attachment). An example of velocity is an automobile starting from Los Angeles heading south toward San Diego and traveling at a speed of 55 mph. In chiropractic, velocity is the thrust of 30 Newtons applied from the contact point of the doctor's hands on the patient (point of attachment) along the direction of the facets of the lumbar spine (direction).

*viscoelasticity* The property of a material to exhibit sensitivity to rate of loading or deformation. All structures in the human body are viscoelastic. Viscoelastic materials contain water (visco) and solid material (elastic).

*Wolff's law* The normal response of bone to stresses (compression, tension, and shear) being applied.

*work (w)* Work is the product of force times the distance an object travels. When work occurs, energy is transferred to or from that object. When the force is in the same direction as the traveling object then energy is gained. If a force is applied in a direction opposite that in which the object is traveling, then energy is lost. There are many examples of work occurring in the human body. When an anatomic joint is moving the muscles are producing work to cause that motion (for example, brachialis muscle produces a concentric action to cause flexion at the elbow). During a throwing motion the shoulder is slowed down at the end of the motion by an eccentric activity of the teres minor and infraspinatus muscles.

*working diagnosis* The diagnosis the clinician will use to treat and manage the patient. As treatment proceeds this diagnosis may change because other information is gained to clarify the patient's condition. The treatment and management of the patient is an integral part of the final diagnosis of the patient's condition.

## REFERENCES

1. Basmajian JV, DeLuca CJ: *Muscles alive: Their functions revealed by electromyography,* ed 5, Baltimore, 1985, Williams & Wilkins.
2. Bergmann TF, Peterson DH, Lawrence DJ: *Chiropractic technique,* New York, 1993, Churchill Livingstone.
3. Biguer B, et al: Neck muscle vibration modifies the representation of visual motion and direction in man, *Brain* 111:1405, 1988.
4. Cotran RS, Kumar V, Robbins SL: *Robbins pathologic basis of disease,* Philadelphia, 1994, Saunders.
5. *Dorland's illustrated medical dictionary,* ed 25, Philadelphia, 1974, Saunders.
6. Gatterman MI: *Chiropractic management of spine related disorders,* Baltimore, 1990, Williams & Wilkins.
7. Gatterman MI, Hansen DT: Development of chiropractic nomenclature through consensus, *J Manip Physio Therap* 17:302, 1994.

8. Jessell TM, Kelly DD: Pain and analgesia. In Kandel ER, Schwartz JH, Jessell TM: *Principles of neural science,* ed 3, New York, 1991, Elsevier.

9. Leadbetter W: Management and treatment of systemic and regional injuries. In Fu F, Stone D, editors: *Sports injuries: mechanisms, prevention, treatment,* Baltimore, 1994, Williams & Wilkins.

10. Martin JH, Jessell TM: Modality coding in the somatic sensory system. In Kandel ER, Schwartz JH, Jessell TM: *Principles of neural science,* ed 3, New York, 1991, Elsevier.

11. Moore KL: *Clinically oriented anatomy,* ed 3, Baltimore, 1992, Williams & Wilkins.

12. Perry J: *Gait analysis: Normal and pathological function,* Thorofare, 1992, Slack Incorporated.

13. Pitner MA: Pathophysiology of overuse injuries in the hand and wrist, *Hand Clin* 6:355, 1990.

14. Travell JG, Simons DG: *Myofascial pain and dysfunction: The trigger point manual,* Baltimore, 1983, Williams & Wilkins.

15. Westmoreland BF, et al: *Medical neurosciences: An approach to anatomy, pathology, and physiology by systems and levels,* ed 3, Boston, 1994, Little, Brown & Co.

16. White AA, Panjabi MM: *Clinical biomechanics of the spine,* ed 2, Philadelphia, 1990, Lippincott.

# Index

## A

Acceleration, defined, 217
Achilles tendinitis, 180
Acromioclavicular joint, 141, 142
  motions, 144-146
Action potential, 33-34
  characteristics, 34, 35
  electric events, 34, 35
Adductor canal, 163
Adductor hiatus, 163
Adjustment, 212
  defined, 204
Alar (sensory) plate, axonal
  development, 28
All-or-nothing phenomenon, defined,
  217
Anesthesia, defined, 217
Angle of lumbar lordosis, 130-131
Ankle, 168-169
  anatomical structures, 165-166, 167
  articulation, 168
  gait, 196, 197, 198
  kinematics, 169
  ligamentous structures, 168
  radiology, 179-181
  retinacula, 168
Antagonist, defined, 217
Anterior antebrachial muscle,
  149-150
Anterior forearm, cutaneous nerve
  supply, 150
Anterior longitudinal ligament, 108
Anterior spinal artery, 65
Arachidonic acid cascade, 206, 207
Arachnoid, 68
Articular capsule, zygapophyseal joint,
  103-104
Articular cartilage, 155, 156
  temporomandibular joint, 79
Articular disc, 78-79
Articular eminence, 78
Articular fossa, 77-78
Articular process
  cervical spine, 93
  lumbar spine, 99-101
Ascending reticular activating system, 57
Ataxia, defined, 217
Atlanto-dens articulation, 94, 96
Atlantodental interspace, 127
Atlas, 94, 95

## B

Autonomic nervous system
  development, 29-30
  head, 86-88
  neck, 86-88
Axis, 94, 95
Axon, myelination, 33
  classification, 33
Axon hillock, defined, 217

## B

Ballism, 50
Basal ganglia, 28, 48-49
  cerebellar interconnections, 46
  disorders, 50
  subcortical loops, 49
Basal (motor) plate, axonal
  development, 28
Bell's palsy, 43
Blood supply
  brain, 64-66
  spinal cord, 64-66
Body righting reflex, 188
Boehler's angle, 181
Bone
  growth, 158-159
  growth in width, 159
  histologic features, 156-159
  remodeling and reconstruction, 159
  shoulder, 173
  types, 158
Bone cell, 157-158
Bone matrix, 157
Brachial plexus, 136, 137
  reflex levels, 140-141
  roots, 136
  sensory and motor innervations, 136,
  137
Bradykinesia, defined, 217
Brain
  anatomic relationships to sensation,
  54
  blood supply, 64-66
  levels, 39
Brain stem, 39-47
  anatomic structures, 41
Brain stem reflex, defined, 223
Broca's area, 50
Brodmann area, 50, 51

## C

Caloric test, 64
Calvaria, bones, 67-68
Cancellous bone, 32-33
Carotid arterial system, 64
Carotid body, 83
Carotid sheath, 83
Carotid sinus, 83
Carpal tunnel, 138, 139
Carpal tunnel syndrome, 138
Cartesian coordinate system, defined,
  217
Cartilage, histological features, 155-156
Cartilaginous joint, defined, 217
Case 1, 1, 35, 192
Case 2, 1-3, 34, 192
Case 3, 3, 41, 43, 71
Case 4, 3-4, 62, 71, 192
Case 5, 4-5, 48
Case 6, 5-6, 42-43, 73, 75, 104, 125, 169
Case 7, 6-7, 73, 76-77, 127
Case 8, 7-8, 73, 93-95, 117
Case 9, 8-9, 93-95, 124, 125
Case 10, 9-10, 125, 136
Case 11, 10-11, 30, 32, 96, 104, 120
Case 12, 11-12, 125, 129-130, 158
Case 13, 12-13, 97-113, 120
Case 14, 13-14, 36, 97-113, 120, 131, 160
Case 15, 14-15, 104, 116, 120, 132, 177
Case 16, 15, 120, 160
Case 17, 15-16, 120, 131
Case 18, 16-17, 104
Case 19, 17-18, 136-141, 150, 171, 173
Case 20, 18-19, 147, 149, 150, 155
Case 21, 19-20, 36, 136, 138, 150, 152, 155
Case 22, 20-21, 150, 151, 152, 155
Case 23, 21-22, 156, 163, 177, 192, 209
Case 24, 22, 178
Case 25, 22-23, 168-171
Case 26, 23-24, 169, 196
Cauda equina, 103, 104
  lumbar region, 111
Center of gravity, defined, 217
Center of mass, defined, 217
Central nervous system
  defined, 36
  development, 27-28
  motor function, 51
  neuroanatomy, 39-47
  physical examination, 63